Telemedicine

Practicing in the Information Age

Telemedicine
Practicing in the Information Age

Edited by
Steven F. Viegas, M.D.
Chairman, Telemedicine Committee
Professor and Chief, Division of Hand Surgery
Department of Orthopaedics and Rehabilitation
Professor, Departments of Anatomy and Neurosciences and Preventive Medicine and Community Health
University of Texas Medical Branch at Galveston
Galveston, Texas

and

Kim Dunn, M.D., Ph.D.
Vice Chair, Department of Internal Medicine
Director, Outcomes Management and Research Program
Texas Department of Criminal Justice
University of Texas Medical Branch at Galveston
Galveston, Texas

With 88 Contributors

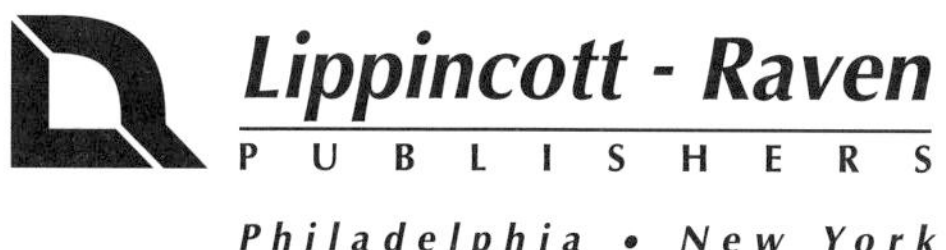
Lippincott - Raven
PUBLISHERS
Philadelphia • New York

8.98

Acquisitions Editor: Danette Knopp
Developmental Editor: Juleann Dob
Manufacturing Manager: Dennis Teston
Supervising Editor: Kimberly Swan
Production Editor: Jane Bangley McQueen, Silverchair Science + Communications
Cover Designer: Jerry Wilky Design
Indexer: Linda Hallinger
Compositor: Tim Hensen, Silverchair Science + Communications
Printer: Maple Press

Printed in the United States of America

9 8 7 6 5 4 3 2 1

Library of Congress Cataloging-in-Publication Data
Telemedicine: practicing in the information age / edited by Steven F. Viegas, Kim Dunn.
p. cm.
Includes bibliographical references and index.
ISBN 0-397-51843-9
1. Telecommunication in medicine. I. Viegas, Steven F. II. Dunn, Kim.
[DNLM: 1. Telemedicine. W 84.1 T268 1998]
R119.9.T452 1998
362.1'028--dc21
DNLM/DLC
for Library of Congress 98-3397
CIP

Care has been taken to confirm the accuracy of the information presented and to describe generally accepted practices. However, the authors, editors, and publisher are not responsible for errors or omissions or for any consequences from application of the information in this book and make no warranty, express or implied, with respect to the contents of the publication.

The authors, editors, and publisher have exerted every effort to ensure that drug selection and dosages set forth in this text are in accordance with current recommendations and practice at the time of publication. However, in view of ongoing research, changes in government regulations, and the constant flow of information relating to drug therapy and drug reactions, the reader is urged to check the package insert for each drug for any change in indications and dosage and for added warnings and precautions. This is particularly important when the recommended agent is a new or infrequently employed drug.

Some drugs and medical devices presented in this publication have Food and Drug Administration (FDA) clearance for limited use in restricted research settings. It is the responsibility of the health care provider to ascertain the FDA status of each drug or device planned for use in their clinical practice.

To my family, the foundation from which,
and on which, the rest of my life is built
—S. F. V.

To our patients, the remote site practitioners,
and the Texas Department of Criminal Justice,
whose commitment to the telemedicine program
has been the secret of its success
—K. D.

Contents

Contributors

Sally Abston, M.D.
Professor
Department of Surgery
University of Texas Medical Branch at Galveston
301 University Boulevard
Galveston, Texas 77555

J. Rick Adams, M.D.
Resident
Internal Medicine Clinic
Michigan State University Kalamazoo Center for Medical Studies
1000 Oakland Drive
Kalamazoo, Michigan 49001

Stanley D. Allen, M.D.
Assistant Professor
Department of Orthopaedics and Rehabilitation
University of Texas Medical Branch at Galveston
301 University Boulevard
Galveston, Texas 77555

Scott K. Alpard, M.D.
Surgical Research Fellow
Division of Cardiothoracic Surgery
Department of Surgery
University of Texas Medical Branch at Galveston
301 University Boulevard
Galveston, Texas 77555

Jack B. Alperin, M.D.
Professor
Departments of Internal Medicine, Human Biological Chemistry and Genetics, and Pathology
University of Texas Medical Branch at Galveston
301 University Boulevard
Galveston, Texas 77555

Karl E. Anderson, M.D.
Professor
Department of Preventive Medicine and Community Health
University of Texas Medical Branch at Galveston
301 University Boulevard
Galveston, Texas 77555

Jake G. Angelo
Manager
Department of Information Services
University of Texas Medical Branch at Galveston
301 University Boulevard
Galveston, Texas 77555

Bruce A. Baethge, M.D.
Associate Professor
Department of Internal Medicine
University of Texas Medical Branch at Galveston
301 University Boulevard
Galveston, Texas 77555

Alexandra Bambas, M.P.H.
Research Associate
Program on Legal and Ethical Issues in Correctional Health
University of Texas Medical Branch at Galveston
301 University Boulevard
Galveston, Texas 77555

Jim E. Barrett, Ed.D.
Director
Health Sciences Center for Educational Resources
Affiliate Associate Professor
Department of Medical Education
Division of Biomedical Informatics
University of Washington School of Medicine
Room T-252, Box 357161
Seattle, Washington 98195
Director of Education and Senior Fellow
International Telemedicine Center, Inc.
Seattle, Washington 98195

Nancy B. Bell, Ph.D.
Assistant Professor and Director
Office for Research
University of Texas Medical Branch at Galveston
301 University Boulevard
Galveston, Texas 77555

Oliver M. Black
Engineering Technician
Department of Information Services
University of Texas Medical Branch at Galveston
301 University Boulevard
Galveston, Texas 77555

Patricia Davis Blair, J.D., M.S.N., R.N.
Associate Professor of Nursing and Director
Center for Nursing Ethics, Law, and Policy
School of Nursing
Department of Maternal-Child
Program on Legal and Ethical Issues in Correctional Health
University of Texas Medical Branch at Galveston
301 University Boulevard
Galveston, Texas 77555

Betsey S. Blakeslee, Ph.D.
Telemedicine Liaison
Center for Total Access
Fort Gordon, Georgia 30905

Jon C. Bowersox, M.D., Ph.D.
Clinical Assistant Professor of Surgery
Department of Surgery
Stanford University School of Medicine/Santa Clara Valley Medical Center
751 South Bascom Avenue
San Jose, California 95128

Michael Charles Boyars, M.D.
Associate Professor
Division of Pulmonary and Critical Care Medicine
Department of Internal Medicine
University of Texas Medical Branch at Galveston
301 University Boulevard
Galveston, Texas 77555

Anne Brasier, M.L.S.
Senior Reference Librarian
Office for Research
University of Texas Medical Branch at Galveston
301 University Boulevard
Galveston, Texas 77555

Robert M. Brecht, Ph.D.
Chief Executive Officer and Senior Fellow
International Telemedicine Center, Inc.
7580 Fannin Street
Houston, Texas 77054

Thomas A. Broughan, M.D.
Professor and Chairman
Department of Surgery
University of Oklahoma Health Science Center
2808 South Sheridan Road
Tulsa, Oklahoma 74129

Jason H. Calhoun, M.D., F.A.C.S.
Professor and Chairman
Department of Orthopaedics and Rehabilitation
University of Texas Medical Branch at Galveston
301 University Boulevard
Galveston, Texas 77555

Beverly C. Campbell, B.S., M.T. (A.S.C.P.)
Manager
Laboratory Information Services
Department of Pathology
University of Texas Medical Branch at Galveston
301 University Boulevard
Galveston, Texas 77555

Kleanthe C. Caruso, R.N., M.S.N., C.N.A.A., C.C.H.P.
Administrator
University of Texas Medical Branch at Galveston/Texas Department of Criminal Justice System Nursing Services
301 University Boulevard
Galveston, Texas 77555

Jeff W. Chen, M.D., Ph.D.
Assistant Professor of Neurosurgery
Department of Surgery
University of Texas Medical Branch at Galveston
301 University Boulevard
Galveston, Texas 77555

David A. Chiriboga, Ph.D.
Professor and Chair
Department of Health Promotion and Gerontology
School of Allied Health Sciences
University of Texas Medical Branch at Galveston
301 University Boulevard
Galveston, Texas 77555

Beth L. Cory, B.S.N., M.N.
Director of Nursing
Department of Nursing Services
Texas Department of Criminal Justice Hospital, University of Texas Medical Branch at Galveston
301 University Boulevard
Galveston, Texas 77555

Daniel F. Cowan, M.D., C.M.
Director
Laboratory Information Services
Professor
Department of Pathology
University of Texas Medical Branch at Galveston
301 University Boulevard
Galveston, Texas 77555

William S. Crump, M.D.
Professor
Department of Family Medicine
University of Texas Medical Branch at Galveston
301 University Boulevard
Galveston, Texas 77555

Jeffrey R. Davis, M.D., M.S.
Associate Professor of Family Medicine
Departments of Preventive, Occupational, and Environmental Medicine
University of Texas Medical Branch at Galveston
301 University Boulevard
Galveston, Texas 77555

Casi T. Doughty, M.A
Program Manager
Department of Education and Professional Development
University of Texas Medical Branch at Galveston
Correctional Managed Care
301 University Boulevard
Galveston, Texas 77555

Jennifer C. Dudley, B.A.
Research Coordinator
Office for Research
University of Texas Medical Branch at Galveston
301 University Boulevard
Galveston, Texas 77555

Kim Dunn, M.D., Ph.D.
Vice Chair
Department of Internal Medicine
Director
Outcomes Management and Research Program
Texas Department of Criminal Justice
University of Texas Medical Branch at Galveston
301 University Boulevard
Galveston, Texas 77555

Fernando Elijovich, M.D.
Associate Professor of Medicine
Department of Internal Medicine
University of Texas Medical Branch at Galveston
301 University Boulevard
Galveston, Texas 77555

Tom K. Epley, III, B.S.
Information Services Leader
Department of Information Services
University of Texas Medical Branch at Galveston
301 University Boulevard
Galveston, Texas 77555

Oliver Esch, M.D.
Assistant Professor
Department of Radiology
University of Texas Medical Branch at Galveston
301 University Boulevard
Galveston, Texas 77555

Alan R. Felthous, M.D.
Marie B. Gale Centennial Professor of Psychiatry
Director, Adult Division and Chief, Forensic Service
Department of Psychiatry and Behavioral Sciences
University of Texas Medical Branch at Galveston
301 University Boulevard
Galveston, Texas 77555

Daniel H. Freeman, Jr., Ph.D.
Professor
Departments of Preventive Medicine and Community Health and Psychiatry and Behavioral Medicine
University of Texas Medical Branch at Galveston
301 University Boulevard
Galveston, Texas 77555

Jean L. Freeman, Ph.D.
Associate Professor
Departments of Internal Medicine and Preventive Medicine and Community Health
University of Texas Medical Branch at Galveston
301 University Boulevard
Galveston, Texas 77555

Michelle Gailiun, M.A., M.S.W.
Director of Telemedicine
Department of Medical Administration
Ohio State University Medical Center
320 West 10th Avenue
Columbus, Ohio 43210

Bernard F. Godley, M.D., Ph.D.
Associate Professor
Department of Ophthalmology and Visual Sciences
University of Texas Medical Branch at Galveston
301 University Boulevard
Galveston, Texas 77555

Keith Gran, B.S., M.B.A., C.P.A.
Director of Financial Affairs
Department of Internal Medicine
University of Texas Medical Branch at Galveston
301 University Boulevard
Galveston, Texas 77555

J. Andrew Grant, M.D.
Professor of Medicine, Microbiology, and Immunology
Department of Internal Medicine
University of Texas Medical Branch at Galveston
301 University Boulevard
Galveston, Texas 77555

Jeanette C. Hartshorn, R.N., Ph.D.
Professor and Associate Dean for Academic Administration
School of Nursing
University of Texas Medical Branch at Galveston
301 University Boulevard
Galveston, Texas 77555

Nancy Hughes, M.D.
Department of Internal Medicine
University of Texas Medical Branch at Galveston
301 University Boulevard
Galveston, Texas 77555

Meena Husein, B.S., M.S.
Director of Technical Solutions
Texas Department of Criminal Justice Outcomes Management and Research
University of Texas Medical Branch at Galveston
301 University Boulevard
Galveston, Texas 77555

Matthew R. Keith, B.S.Ph., B.C.P.S.
Associate Clinical Professor of Pharmacy Practice
Managed Health Care Division
College of Pharmacy
University of Houston
Estelle Pharmacy
Huntsville, Texas 77340

Emmie H. Ko, M.D.
Chief Resident
Department of Orthopaedic Surgery
University of Texas Medical Branch at Galveston
301 University Boulevard
Galveston, Texas 77555

David Krasnow, O.D., M.P.H.
Director
Clinical Telemedicine
Massie Research Laboratories
9033 Wilshire Boulevard
Beverly Hills, California 90211

Cheryl L. Laffer, M.D., Ph.D.
Assistant Professor of Medicine
Associate Director of Clinical Hypertension
Department of Internal Medicine
University of Texas Medical Branch at Galveston
301 University Boulevard
Galveston, Texas 77555

Russell A. LaForte, M.D.
Assistant Professor
Department of Internal Medicine
University of Texas Medical Branch at Galveston
301 University Boulevard
Galveston, Texas 77555

Helen K. Li, M.D.
Assistant Professor and Director of Vitreoretinal Diseases and Surgery
Department of Ophthalmology and Visual Sciences
University of Texas Medical Branch at Galveston
301 University Boulevard
Galveston, Texas 77555

Jeffrey R. Lisse, M.D.
Director
Division of Rheumatology
Professor
Department of Internal Medicine
University of Texas Medical Branch at Galveston
301 University Boulevard
Galveston, Texas 77555

Mark H. Lowitt, M.D.
Assistant Professor
Department of Dermatology
University of Maryland School of Medicine
405 West Redwood Street
Baltimore, Maryland 21201

John S. Mancoll, M.D.
Assistant Professor of Surgery
Division of Plastic Surgery
Department of General Surgery
University of Texas Medical Branch at Galveston
301 University Boulevard
Galveston, Texas 77555

Emil P. Miskovsky, M.D.
Director of Hepatology
Assistant Professor
Department of Medicine
University of Texas Medical Branch at Galveston
301 University Boulevard
Galveston, Texas 77555

Mary Moore, Ph.D.
Associate Dean for Library and Information Resources
Associate Professor
College of Communications
Arkansas State University
108 Cooley Drive
State University, Arkansas 72467

Michael B. Moore, B.S., P.A.-C.
Physician Assistant
Department of Cardiovascular and Thoracic Surgery
Abilene Regional Medical Center
1630 Antilley Road
Abilene, Texas 79606

Owen J. Murray, D.O.
Associate Medical Director
Department of Correctional Managed Health Care
University of Texas Medical Branch at Galveston
301 University Boulevard
Galveston, Texas 77555

Sterling A. North, B.A.
Director
Office of Continuing Education
University of Texas Medical Branch at Galveston
301 University Boulevard
Galveston, Texas 77555

Kenneth J. Ottenbacher, Ph.D.
Professor
School of Allied Health Sciences
University of Texas Medical Branch at Galveston
301 University Boulevard
Galveston, Texas 77555

David P. Paar, M.D.
Assistant Professor
Department of Internal Medicine
University of Texas Medical Branch at Galveston
301 University Boulevard
Galveston, Texas 77555

Alice L. Parker, M.S.
Vice President
Teletraining Systems, Inc.
1524 West Admiral Avenue
Stillwater, Oklahoma 74074

Lorne A. Parker, Ph.D.
Chairman
Teletraining Institute
1524 West Admiral Avenue
Stillwater, Oklahoma 74074

Casey D. Peterson, M.B.A.
Administrative Director
Department of Clinical Affairs
Texas Department of Criminal Justice Hospital
301 University Boulevard
Galveston, Texas 77555

Linda G. Phillips, M.D.
Chairman
Truman G. Blocker, Jr., M.D., Distinguished Professor
Chief
Division of Plastic Surgery
Department of General Surgery
University of Texas Medical Branch at Galveston
301 University Boulevard
Galveston, Texas 77555

Sue Prill, M.D.
Department of Oncology
University of Texas Medical Branch at Galveston
301 University Boulevard
Galveston, Texas 77555

Carolyn T. Purcell, B.A., M.B.A.
Executive Director
Texas Department of Information Resources
300 West 15th Street
Austin, Texas 78701

Richard Roland Rahr, Ed.D.
Professor and Chairman
School of Allied Health Sciences
University of Texas Medical Branch at Galveston
301 University Boulevard
Galveston, Texas 77555

Karen A. Rasmusson, M.D.
Associate Professor
Department of Neurology
University of Texas Medical Branch at Galveston
301 University Boulevard
Galveston, Texas 77555

Vonda G. Reeves-Darby, M.D.
Assistant Professor
Department of Internal Medicine
University of Texas Medical Branch at Galveston
301 University Boulevard
Galveston, Texas 77555

Norbert J. Roberts, Jr., M.D.
Professor
Departments of Internal Medicine, Microbiology, and Immunology
Director
Division of Infectious Diseases
University of Texas Medical Branch at Galveston
301 University Boulevard
Galveston, Texas 77555

Sally Sue Robinson, M.D.
Professor
Department of Pediatrics
University of Texas Medical Branch at Galveston
301 University Boulevard
Galveston, Texas 77555

Roberto J. Rodrigues, M.D.
Coordinator
Health Services Information Systems Program
Pan American Health Organization/World Health Organization
525 23rd Street, Northwest
Washington, D.C. 20037

Richard M. Satava, M.D.
Professor
Department of Surgery
Yale University School of Medicine
40 Temple Street
New Haven, Connecticut 06510

Jade S. Schiffman, M.D.
Clinical Associate Professor
Department of Ophthalmology and Visual Sciences
University of Texas Medical Branch at Galveston
301 University Boulevard
Galveston, Texas 77555

Sue Schneider, B.S.
Senior Database Consultant
Department of Pathology
University of Texas Medical Branch at Galveston
301 University Boulevard
Galveston, Texas 77555

Deborah E. Seale, M.A.
Assistant Professor of Clinical Laboratory Science
East Texas Area Health Education Center
University of Texas Medical Branch at Galveston
301 University Boulevard
Galveston, Texas 77555

Stephen J.B. Sibbitt, M.D.
Assistant Professor
Department of Internal Medicine
University of Texas Medical Branch at Galveston
301 University Boulevard
Galveston, Texas 77555

Laura K. Slaughter, M.D.
Resident
Department of Psychiatry and Behavioral Sciences
University of Texas Medical Branch at Galveston
301 University Boulevard
Galveston, Texas 77555

David J. Solomon, Ph.D.
Associate Professor
Department of Internal Medicine and Office of Educational Development
University of Texas Medical Branch at Galveston
301 University Boulevard
Galveston, Texas 77555

T. Howard Stone, J.D., L.L.M.
Research Director and Assistant Professor
Program on Legal and Ethical Issues in Correctional Health
Institute for the Medical Humanities
Department of Preventive Medicine and Community Health
University of Texas Medical Branch at Galveston
301 University Boulevard
Galveston, Texas 77555

Rosa A. Tang, M.D., M.P.H.
Clinical Professor
Department of Ophthalmology and Visual Sciences
University of Texas Medical Branch at Galveston
Clinical Sciences Building G-87
Galveston, Texas 77555

C. Sloan Teeple, B.A.
Second-year Medical Student
University of Texas Medical Branch at Galveston
610 Texas Avenue
Galveston, Texas 77555

Paula D. Townley, B.S.N., R.N.C.
Education Specialist
Department of Education and Professional Development
University of Texas Medical Branch at Galveston
Correctional Managed Care
301 University Boulevard
Galveston, Texas 77555

Jeanine Warisse Turner, Ph.D., M.A.
Assistant Professor of Management
School of Business
Georgetown University
Adjunct Research Assistant Professor
Department of Radiology
Georgetown University School of Medicine
G-04 Old North
Washington, D.C. 20057

Steven F. Viegas, M.D.
Chairman
Telemedicine Committee
Professor and Chief
Division of Hand Surgery
Department of Orthopaedics and Rehabilitation
Professor
Departments of Anatomy and Neurosciences and Preventive Medicine and Community Health
University of Texas Medical Branch at Galveston
301 University Boulevard
Galveston, Texas 77555

Michael M. Warren, M.D.
Professor and Chief of Urology
Departments of Surgery and Urology
University of Texas Medical Branch at Galveston
301 University Boulevard
Galveston, Texas 77555

Maurice Willis, B.S., M.D.
Third-year Resident
Department of Internal Medicine
University of Texas Medical Branch at Galveston
301 University Boulevard
Galveston, Texas 77555

Joseph B. Zwischenberger, M.D.
Professor
Division of Cardiothoracic Surgery
Department of Surgery
University of Texas Medical Branch at Galveston
301 University Boulevard
Galveston, Texas 77555

Preface

We are at the beginning of a journey to a new age of communication, involving information sharing and real-time video connection. This book is intended to help readers begin this journey and to serve as a guidebook as new communication technology becomes increasingly integrated into our lives.

As they try to decide whether to start this journey, many have asked if telemedicine is cost-effective. The same was asked when the telephone was being considered as a new communication tool soon after it was invented. It was not cost-effective at first. There was no telegraph in the home or drugstore, so why would anyone ever think that a telephone would have a place in every household and business? Costs were high, access was limited, and technical problems were routine. Despite these obstacles, the need and desire to communicate drove the technology forward, and telephones, including cellular technology and fax machines, are now an integral part of almost every component of our lives.

As with the telephone, telemedicine encompasses many different pieces of technology. In that respect, telemedicine can, and often does, mean different things to different people. This book contains varied perspectives and interpretations of what telemedicine is and what it can do. The chapters highlight various ways that telemedicine is being used. The chapter authors, like blind men feeling different parts of an elephant, have different perspectives and experiences. The different uses of telemedicine outlined in this volume provide the reader with a global perspective of telemedicine.

It is important to remember that we are not discussing new medicine or new types of healthcare, but rather new technology that is being incorporated into medicine. Incorporation of technology is not unique—in fact, the development and use of new technology and equipment in medicine is common. What is different, however, is that the communication technology that enables telemedicine has the potential to impact all general and subspecialty areas in medicine, and eventually all people.

The specific technology will change, and the networks used will evolve and expand. The process by which people communicate and interact and the extent to which communication takes place are also changing quickly and continually. Unlike the characters in the television show *Star Trek*, who go where no one has gone before, physicians go where their healthcare delivery system, education, research, and managed care contracts take them. It is telemedicine technology that will enable physicians to do what they have always done, only better.

Steven F. Viegas

Introduction

As the telemedicine program and the recognition of the telemedicine activities at the University of Texas Medical Branch at Galveston grew, the number and frequency of visitors inquiring about telemedicine and how to start a successful telemedicine program also grew. As a result, the decision was made to develop a book on telemedicine that would address these kinds of questions and cover all the different aspects and applications of telemedicine.

The organization of this book also resulted in a conference held at the University of Texas Medical Branch at Galveston in the spring of 1997. One goal of the conference was to bring practitioners at the remote sites in the Texas Department of Criminal Justice prison system together with subspecialists to explore how telemedicine could be more useful in providing care for inmates. The principles explored in the conference and the subsequent information, which are shared in this book, are germane to any institution interested in implementing telemedicine as part of practice.

Conference support was obtained from the Department of Internal Medicine and the Correctional Managed Care Program at the University of Texas Medical Branch at Galveston; Pfizer, Inc.; Boehringer Ingelheim Pharmaceuticals, Inc.; Berlex Laboratories; MedVision; and American Medical Development.

Kim Dunn

Telemedicine: Practicing in the Information Age,
edited by Steven F. Viegas and Kim Dunn.
Lippincott–Raven Publishers, Philadelphia © 1998.

1

Past as Prologue

Steven F. Viegas

Departments of Orthopaedics and Rehabilitation, Anatomy and Neurosciences, and Preventive Medicine and Community Health, University of Texas Medical Branch at Galveston, Galveston, Texas 77555

The future does not just happen. It is the result of a long journey from the past with a brief stop for the marriage between the reality of the present and dreams of what might be. The past is full of examples demonstrating humans' need to communicate. One example of pioneering ways to communicate with one another is the pony express, which was dedicated to fulfilling people's need to communicate by written word as fast as possible. The telegraph's speed put a quick end to the exciting story of the pony express. The dream to communicate by speech over great distances became a reality with the telephone.

The current dream, which is starting to become reality, is not only to communicate by voice but also visually in real time. Real-time video transmission will have a tremendous impact on education, business, and healthcare. Videoconferencing technology will likely follow a similar journey as that of the telephone.

THE TELEPHONE: A HISTORICAL REVIEW

Invention

The telephone was invented on March 10, 1876, by Alexander Graham Bell and Tom Watson (Fig. 1-1). When Alexander Graham Bell showcased his invention at the Grand Centennial Exposition in Philadelphia, it caused great excitement and enthusiasm. Dom Pedro II, the Emperor of Brazil, was reportedly the first at the exposition to listen to Bell speaking on his new invention from 500 ft away (Fig. 1-2). Another individual who used Bell's new invention at the exposition was Colonel Alfred Belo, who was the senior proprietor of the *Galveston Daily News* (Fig. 1-3). Colonel Belo subsequently obtained two of Bell's new telephones, placing one in his home and one in the editor's room at the newspaper. These were the first telephones in Texas.

The Early Years

At first, there was a general belief that the telephone was a toy, and there was uncertainty as to its practical application. In the early years, only the wealthy and

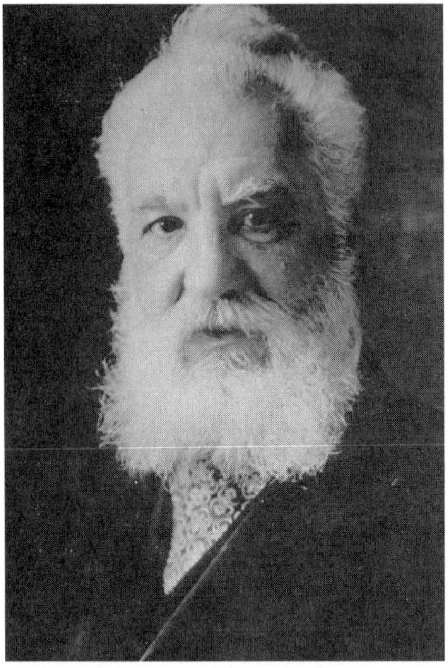

FIG. 1-1. Alexander Graham Bell many years after he invented the telephone with Tom Watson. (From ref. 1, with permission.)

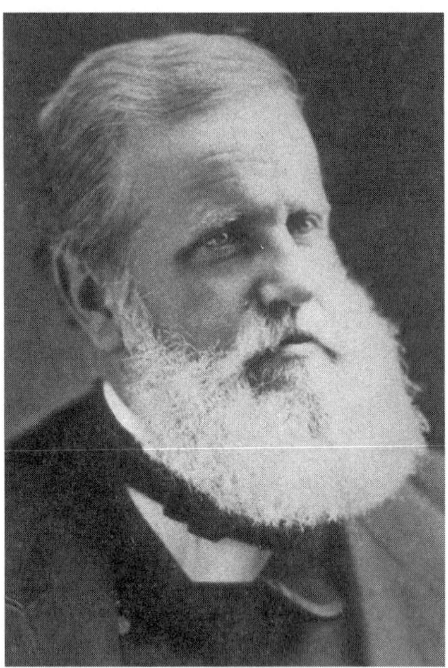

FIG. 1-2. Dom Pedro II, the Emperor of Brazil. (From ref. 1, with permission.)

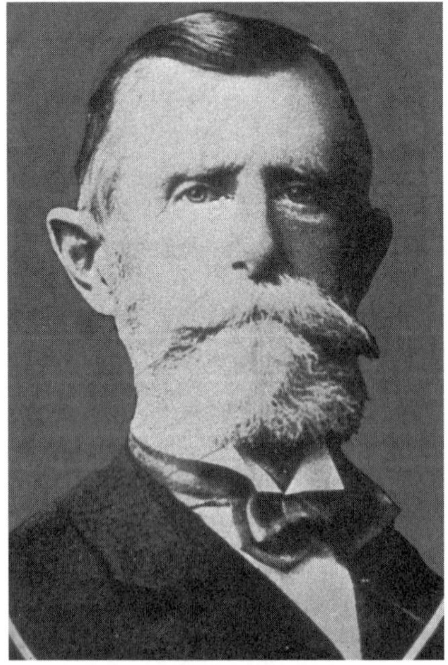

FIG. 1-3. Alfred Horatio Belo, former Confederate Army Colonel and senior proprietor of the *Galveston Daily News*. (From ref. 1, with permission.)

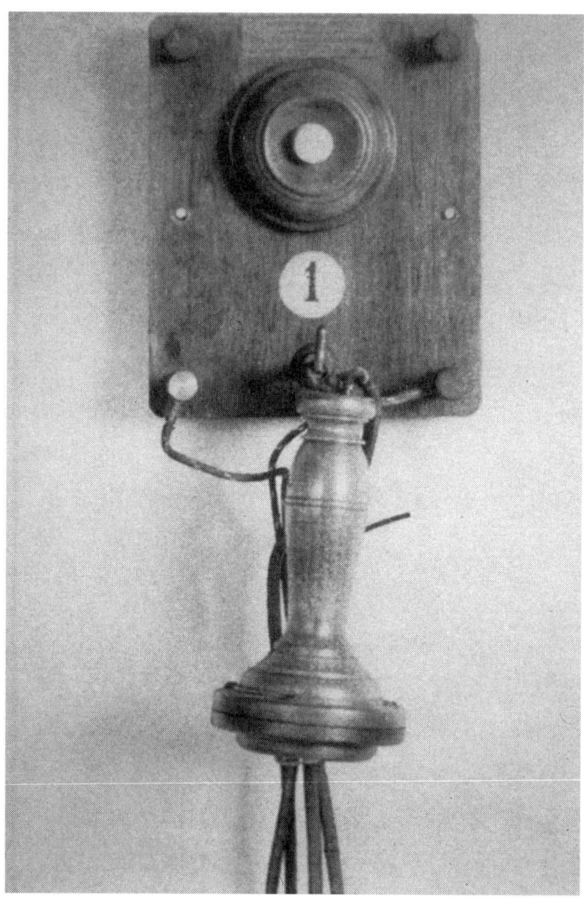

FIG. 1-4. One of the first types of telephones. The 1878 Butterstamp model had a "handle" that looked like a butter mold, which was used for both listening and talking. (From ref. 1, with permission.)

influential installed telephones in their homes. Even then it was usually a novelty, as the home had not been a place for the electronic communication of the time, the telegraph. Mark Twain, frustrated by the poor sound quality, which often was indistinguishable even when shouting into the telephone, called the telephone a device used to practice cursing (Fig. 1-4). Doctors and pharmacists were often the first to sign up for a telephone, because they saw the potential for the technology to assist them in their professions. There was a flat monthly fee for telephone service at the time, and people often congregated at the corner drugstore to make and receive calls. Although the telephone was beginning to find a place, in 1878 after the first year of Bell Telephone Company's operation, there were only 230 telephones in service in the United States.

Bell offered to sell his patents to the Western Union Company for $100,000. The company declined, thinking that the telephone was just a novelty. That deci-

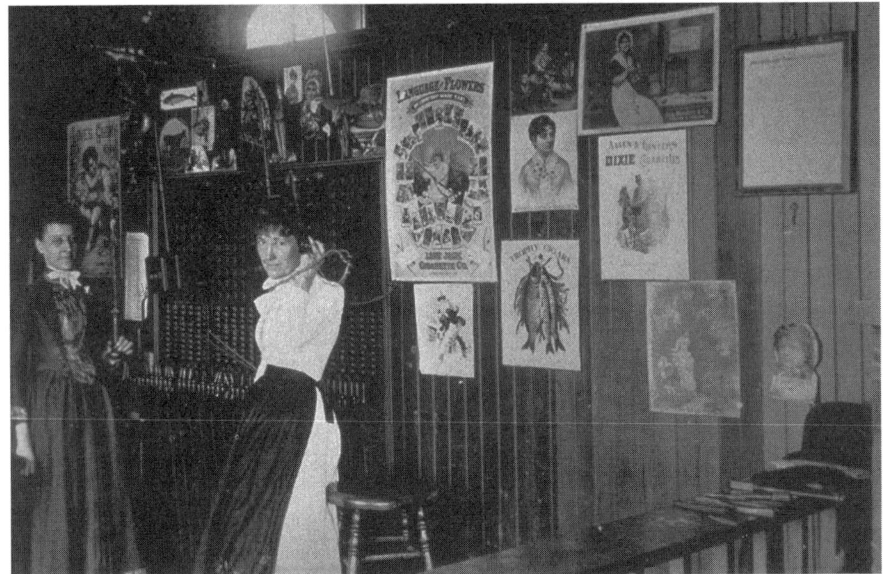

A

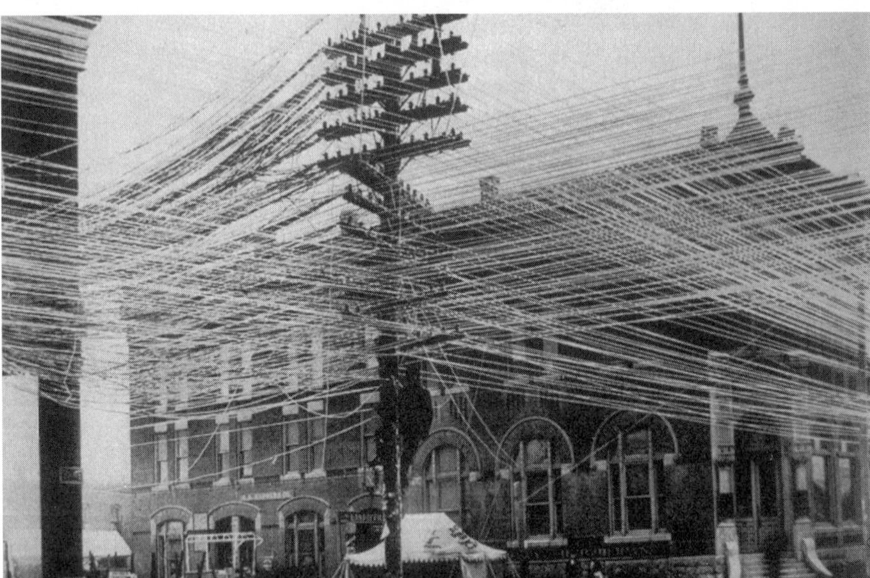

B

FIG. 1-5. A: A photograph of operators working at an early telephone switchboard in Springfield, Missouri, in 1880. **B:** A photograph of a street in Pratt, Kansas, taken in 1911, shows the maze of telephone lines that covered the town to support the telephone system. (From ref. 2, with permission.)

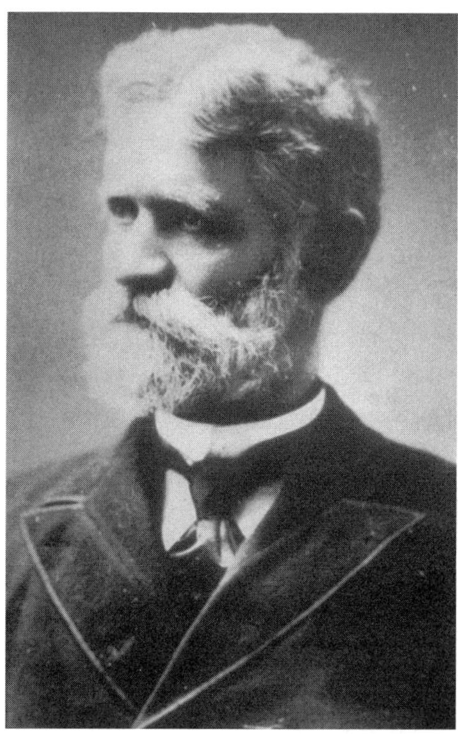

FIG. 1-6. Almon Brown Strowger, an undertaker in Kansas City, Missouri, who invented the "automatic telephone exchange" in 1889. (From ref. 1, with permission.)

sion is generally regarded as one of the worst business decisions ever made. Thomas Edison and Elijah Gray were later asked to develop a telephone system for Western Union.

Expansion

The telephone network expanded using the infrastructure of the telegraph lines. Building on its telegraph lines, Western Union tried to establish its own telephone system and had 30,000 telephones in place in less than 1 year. Western Union would later lose a legal battle over patent infringement of Bell's invention. The value of one share of Bell Telephone Company's stock increased from $300 to $1,000 the day after that decision.

The technical concerns and support needed for the early telephone systems were significant because of the need for large, manual switchboards, operator assistance, and individual line dedication (Fig. 1-5). Almon B. Strowger, an undertaker in Kansas City, Missouri, invented the first direct-dial telephone. He was convinced that he was losing business because the switchboard operators were failing to complete calls to him (Fig. 1-6). These phones were first advertised as "girl-less, cuss-less, cut-out-of-order-less, wait-less telephones" (Fig. 1-7). Dr. Moses Greeley Parker in Lowell,

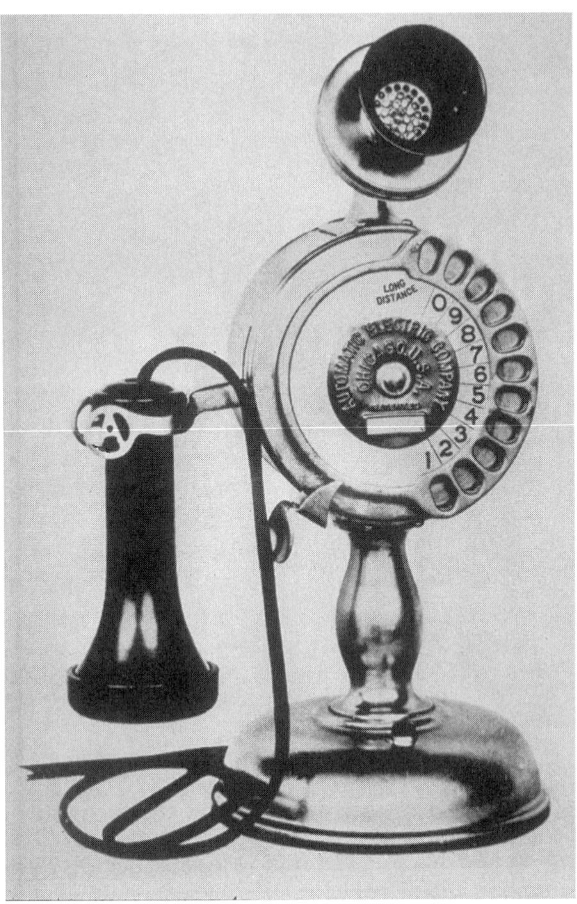

FIG. 1-7. A photograph of a 1905 model of the Strowger automatic telephone. (From ref. 1, with permission.)

Massachusetts, suggested changing telephone listings from names to numbers because a measles outbreak risked losing all four switchboard operators. In the same year that train fare from New York to Philadelphia was $4.50, the telephone long-distance charge for a New York to Philadelphia call was $0.80. In 1880, there were 60,000 telephones in the United States, including at least one in every town with a population of more than 10,000.

During the period that the Bell patents were in effect, through 1894, a total of 230,000 telephones were installed in the United States. Bell successfully defended his patents in more than 600 cases. Many different systems and companies developed, resulting in the existence of separate, incompatible telephone systems. This meant that businesses sometimes needed many different telephone companies to reach the people they wanted to talk to (Fig. 1-8).

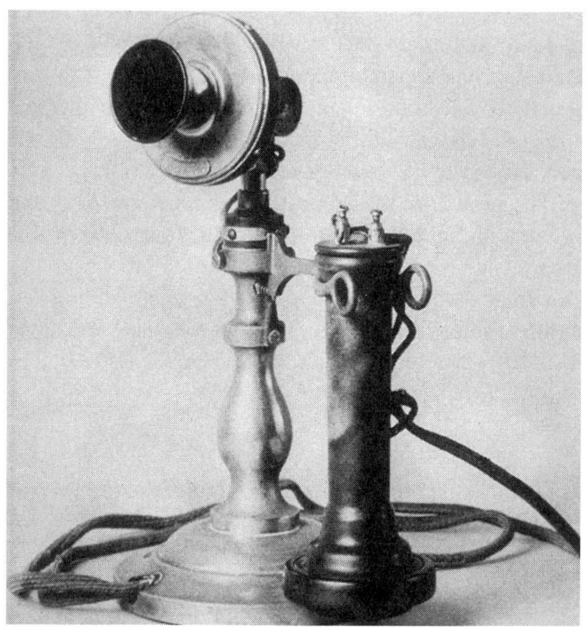

FIG. 1-8. A photograph of an 1897 model deskset telephone. (From ref. 1, with permission.)

Technological Advances

The first transcontinental telephone call in 1915 from New York to San Francisco lasted 23 minutes and had 50,000 men assigned for technical support. There were five men stationed over every mile who were assigned to watch the 14,000 miles of copper wire across the 130,000 telephone poles from the East Coast to the West Coast. Despite these technical demands, the telephone continued to gain increasing acceptance, having moved from a toy to a necessity. Thirty-nine years after its introduction, there were 11 million telephones in operation.

Those who were among the first to own a telephone were rather isolated from the early dreams of being able to talk to anyone they wanted to talk to, because few people had telephones and the networks were limited. The telephone system has come a long way. Mobile telephones have also traveled far since the 1970s, when mobile telephone equipment was large, expensive, and technically limited and the ranks of mobile telephones were in the thousands, to the current trend toward smaller and smaller phones, increasingly global coverage, and tens of millions of subscribers in the United States alone.

VIDEOCONFERENCING

As was the case with the telephone, the healthcare profession has been one of the first to identify the potentially beneficial impact of real-time videoconferencng on its mission. The problems are similar to those in the early days of the telephone, with limited numbers of telemedicine sites and separate, incompatible systems. The limitations and inconvenience of having only one telephone in a hospital or medical center would be quickly realized, especially with the increasing trend to rely on the convenience of cellular phones. However, most telemedicine programs have only one telemedicine unit per site. The growth in the number of telemedicine sites and networks will both be complicated and aided by the different infrastructures that already exist. These infrastructures can be beneficial; as the telegraph infrastructures were beneficial to the early growth of the telephone network. The telemedicine networks can be built on the satellite, radio, fiberoptic, cable, Internet, and telephone systems of today.

CONCLUSION

As exciting and dynamic as I believe the impact of telemedicine technologies will be on healthcare and medical education, one should remember there is not a separate department of telephone medicine. The telephone has become an integral part of healthcare and medical education and has been integrated and incorporated into almost every aspect of life. I also believe that telemedicine will not exist as a distinct department or division of healthcare but will be assimilated into and ultimately improve every aspect of healthcare and education.

REFERENCES

1. Hall JF. *Hello, Texas: a history of telephony in the lone star state.* Austin, TX: Texas Telephone Association, 1990.
2. Park DG Jr. *Good connections. A century of service by the men and women of Southwestern Bell.* St. Louis: Southwestern Bell Telephone Company, 1984.

Telemedicine: Practicing in the Information Age,
edited by Steven F. Viegas and Kim Dunn.
Lippincott–Raven Publishers, Philadelphia © 1998.

2

Historical Context of Telemedicine

Jim E. Barrett and Robert M. Brecht

Health Sciences Center for Educational Resources and Department of Medical Education, University of Washington School of Medicine, Seattle, Washington 98195, and International Telemedicine Center, Inc., Seattle, Washington 98195; and International Telemedicine Center, Inc., Houston, Texas 77054

Tele is the Greek root word meaning "far off" or as *Webster's* defines it, "distant, remote, whence, from, or to a distance" (1). Just as *telephone* means sound (phone) across distance, *telemedicine* is medicine across distance. As far back as 1844, when the telegraph service was established, those involved in healthcare used innovations in communications when they provided an improved solution. The telephone was a logical extension and is still a major communication tool used in telemedicine.

Radiologic images were likely the first documented medical visual communication across distance. In 1948, x-rays were transmitted over telephone lines between West Chester and Philadelphia, Pennsylvania (2). In 1959 at the University of Nebraska, the use of two-way, closed-circuit television began with the transmission of motion visuals across campus, showing neurologic examinations for medical education (3). In 1962 at the University of Nebraska, a two-way microwave connection to the Nebraska Psychiatric Institute and the Norfolk State Hospital, more than 100 miles away, was established. For 6 years, the system was used for consultation and demonstrated the long-distance capability of interactive video (4,5).

FIRST-GENERATION TELEMEDICINE

Clinical Care

After the early examples of medical communication across distance were a number of historic clinical-care projects. An extensive program began in 1968 between Massachusetts General Hospital and Boston's Logan International Airport's clinical station, which was staffed by nurse clinicians. More than 1,600 patients were seen under this early interactive video system (6,7). Massachusetts General expanded its services to include dermatology, radiology, cardiology, and telepsychiatry. These were all regularly used to provide care to a variety of local sites until the mid-1980s (7).

Feasibility

During the 1970s and into the early 1980s, there were 15 telemedicine sites receiving federal funding (5), and several of the projects demonstrated the feasibility of even longer distance telemedicine. Satellites were used to carry signals to and from remote areas of Canada and Alaska and on board ships at sea. The National Aeronautics and Space Administration, Lockheed, and the U.S. Public Health Service began a project called STARPAHC between the Papago Indian Reservation in Arizona and Massachusetts General Hospital's clinic at Logan Airport. The project was to research telemedicine and provide medical service to astronauts, as well as to the reservation. Portions of the project continued for nearly 20 years (5). Much of these early experiments were concerned with the technology's feasibility. Could audio and video be transmitted in a multipoint fashion? Could diagnostic and educational objectives be accomplished across distances using interactive video technology?

Even though the majority of the first generation projects were based on standard analog television, the projects involved operationally complex and relatively expensive studios, engineering staff, and equipment. In addition, the projects were almost all federally funded as demonstration projects, with little done to validate the quality of medical care as compared to alternative methods. The availability of adequate bandwidth necessary for long-distance interactive video was scarce and, when available, very expensive. When the funding ran out for these projects, none of them was converted to self-supporting services (7). The start-up funding may have been withdrawn prematurely in a reaction to political pressures to curtail funding for programs based on extending access to healthcare (8). In spite of the rapid reduction in funding, the important milestone for telemedicine became clear—the feasibility of extending a scarce medical resource across distance had been demonstrated.

SECOND-GENERATION TELEMEDICINE

Digital Communication

During the late 1980s and into the early 1990s, the number of telemedicine projects reported in the literature diminished considerably. A major change in distance communication was occurring, however, one which would have a significant impact on the future of telemedicine.

Digital communication methods were on the rise, with computers becoming commonplace as information and communication devices. Advancements in compression technology occurred to the point at which interactive video could be carried over wide-area surface networks. The pleasant surprise was that this new advanced technology was becoming available at a fraction of the cost of the analog interactive video used in the first-generation telemedicine projects. In all other areas of healthcare, advanced technology is a major culprit in what has been referred to as the runaway costs of U.S. healthcare (9). As a result of these technology advances, the vast majority of all second-generation projects used computer-based, digital, teleconferencing systems. The advantages included not only lower transmission costs but also reduced equipment size, simplicity of operations, and an easy-to-use computer interface rapidly becoming common to healthcare providers (6).

Two significant telemedicine projects in Texas using digital land-based systems and researching success factors, as well as healthcare access issues, were started in 1989. They were the Texas Tech University Health Sciences Center's Med-Net and the Texas Telemedicine Project between Austin and Giddings, 65 miles away (5). Similarly, in 1991, the Medical College of Georgia started a link from Augusta to Dodge County Hospital in Eastman, Georgia. This system has grown to more than 60 sites and has become a statewide telemedicine network (10). These and other projects helped focus attention away from the feasibility of technology issues and onto a growing list of other barriers that must be addressed if telemedicine is going to have a widespread impact on healthcare. These barriers have often been grouped as (a) technology and standards; (b) liability, licensure, and confidentiality; and (c) reimbursement. Each presents formidable challenges as the field advances (11).

Rural Telemedicine

Of the projects begun during the second generation phase, rural telemedicine programs became the largest reported application. The most obvious focus has been the extension of the specialist out to the rural domain of the general practitioner. As desired, the benefit and savings from these projects included those of increased access to specialists and savings in treatment time and associated travel costs. Potential savings are considerable, not only in the form of direct travel costs but also lost employment from time away from work, extended costs to family members, and the loss of productivity to employers.

TELERADIOLOGY

Teleradiology and, to a slightly lesser extent, telepathology play a special role in the history of telemedicine; during the first generation as a consultative service and more recently as a diagnostic service.

Early Use

The early use of teleradiology, using video transmissions of a film by focusing a camera on a light box, was inadequate for primary diagnoses. When these transmissions were used in consultation with a general practitioner, the practice was judged valuable. The U.S. Department of Defense supported several pilot projects to bring the input of radiologists to distant sites, including ships at sea. Much of this use led to advances in specialized digital scanning hardware, which brought second-generation diagnostic applications into use (12).

Development of Standards

Although debate still exists regarding quality issues in primary teleradiology and telepathology (7), the high use of images and data in these disciplines has led to the development of the first standards by the American College of Radiology–National Electrical Manufacturers Association. The adoption of such standards is a major contribution to the uniform application and expansion of telemedicine.

Another factor special to teleradiology and telepathology is that they were the first applications that allowed Health Care Financing Administration (HCFA) reimbursement. Receiving governmental Medicare support has allowed considerable refinement in the applications and the important addition of standards to be developed. In addition, because reimbursement is possible, teleradiology has been suggested as a financial outgrowth of many medical centers' use of excess capacity to leverage themselves into a larger market under the new era of competition in a cost-containment environment (13). Overall, teleradiology has been identified as approximately 50% of all telemedicine occurring and has grown from 50,000 cases per year in 1994 to more than 115,000 in 1996 (14).

TELEMEDICINE EXPANSION

Societal Factors

Approaching the mid-1990s, changes were occurring in society that set the stage for the further expansion of telemedicine. Namely, the use of the Internet was growing at an exponential rate. During this time, the use of the Internet was literally doubling every 4 to 5 months. Physicians and patients alike were learning to use multimedia browsers to access information and pictures and to communicate with each other via electronic mail. The computer and its digitized imagery was becoming common as a professional tool.

Another societal element focusing federal funding was the rise of managed healthcare. From the White House throughout the nation, it was becoming clear that a check in rising healthcare costs must occur. Telemedicine, being seen as a possible partial solution, continued to receive federal support (15). During a 1995 survey project funded by the U.S. Office of Rural Health Policy, 2,472 nonfederal rural hospitals were surveyed as to whether they had telemedicine projects. With a 95% response rate, it was found that 17.6% (or 416 respondents) were using telemedicine (16). Another study by Abt Associates, Inc. of western rural hospitals found that more than 25% of the hospitals had ongoing telemedicine projects (17).

Sustainable Environments

Several successful telemedicine projects have found a sustainable environment. The University of Texas Medical Branch at Galveston working with the Texas Department of Criminal Justice, the Ohio State University Medical Center's correctional project, and the East Carolina University Central Prison Program, are three such examples. The editors of the publication *Telemedicine Today* completed three surveys of interactive, video-mediated telemedicine programs in 3 years. They found ten programs performing 1,750 interactions in 1993, 25 programs performing 2,110 consultations in 1994, and 50 performing 6,267 consultations in 1995.

The home-care segment of telemedicine is also demonstrating considerable growth. Active projects in Kansas and Georgia have demonstrated success and have spun off into commercial services. In Kansas alone, Linda Roman, chief executive officer of HELP Innovations, estimated that if just 10% of all traditional home-care visits were substituted with electronic home care, a savings of $1.5 billion would occur annually.

Overall, the home-care market has demonstrated tremendous opportunity for telemedicine growth, and significant advances in low-cost telephone and cable two-way interactive technology have occurred to meet this market.

Blue Cross Blue Shield of Minnesota provides an example of payers that have turned to telephone-based service to reduce clinic visits. Blue Shield reports more than 86% patient acceptance, as well as a reduction in cost from $65 to $12 down to $15 per contact. By handling 800 contacts a day, with a reduction of 45% in visits by those using the system, major cost savings are being estimated. Because of this type of cost savings, the number of telemedicine programs within managed-care organizations continues to grow.

American Telemedicine Association

One of the signs of telemedicine growth was the creation of the American Telemedicine Association in 1993. The production of a scholarly journal and the first successful professional meeting in early 1996 were also strong indicators that telemedicine is here to stay. In early 1997, the announcement of the creation of the Association of Telemedicine Service Providers was another indicator that telemedicine is becoming its own industry within healthcare.

DEVELOPMENTS IN TELEMEDICINE

Many events and changes in the mid-1990s set the stage for the next generation of telemedicine. Compression technology continues to make major advancements in faster, more capable multimedia computers and in wide-area networks sharing data and images across faster and faster communication channels. The deregulation of the telephone industry opened competition between both the telephone providers themselves and the cable providers seeking a growth market in two-way data. These factors brought costs down and brought new cost savings to the telemedicine field. Federally, the Telecommunications Act of 1996 ensured broad dissemination of service and lower costs relating to telemedicine applications.

Popular opinion has moved from viewing telemedicine as a future novelty to a practical application. For example, the November 1995 issue of *Fortune* magazine included an article entitled "Telemedicine begins to make its case." The article described the practicality of electronic home healthcare, of medical telemetry at reasonable costs, and of providing access for patients to self-care information. In light of such growing public and professional interest in telemedicine, the HCFA has authorized a long awaited national telemedicine demonstration project. The data collected on cost, confidentiality of information, efficiencies, and quality are expected to lead to Medicare reimbursement and further Medicaid reimbursement.

On the legal front, California set the stage for other states to follow by passing the Telemedicine Development Act of 1996. The previous requirement was for face-to-face interaction to practice medicine within any state. The California law requires registration in California and a current license in the home state (as well as some minor conditions), thereby allowing out-of-state physicians to practice telemedicine in California.

THIRD-GENERATION TELEMEDICINE

Another round of funding from the U.S. Department of Health and Human Services totaling $42 million for 19 new telemedicine projects was announced in late 1996. The focus of these multiyear projects is on evaluation; specifically, the impact of telemedicine on costs, quality of care, and access to health care. Assessment of methods of confidentiality and combining consulting with medical information systems are both part of the contracts. Attention is being given to sustainability, comparable outcomes, and the development of standards that can be accepted by traditional medicine. In short, the maturing of telemedicine into modern healthcare is being seen.

Acceptance and use of telemedicine involves more than just lower cost technology and information access: It requires acceptance by healthcare providers. Wells and Lemak include "provider availability, consumer support, the nature of contractual arrangements, physician-physician relationships, rural physician familiarity with hub sites, and overall ease of use" as factors that will lead to the sustained use of telemedicine by remote users.

Most important, in this new generation of telemedicine, informatics, the electronic patient record, and distance education have all become natural partners with traditional clinical consultation. An increasing number of authors are embracing telemedicine as part of the systems view of networked electronic healthcare. In addition, the use of secure Internet and intranets using common browser software to deliver patient data, images, and basic teleconferencing to distant partners in healthcare have been shown to be practical.

CONCLUSION

Many in the healthcare field recognize telemedicine by a broader definition than was common in the first two generations of projects. *Telemedicine* is being replaced by *telehealth*, the systematic application of telecommunication technology to the field of healthcare. In short, telemedicine is moving to the desktop as a new systems approach to healthcare—one in which information, expertise, and patient data are all being brought to the location and time of care. Electronic alerts, practice guidelines, and access to centralized informational databases are all within the new realm of telehealth.

REFERENCES

1. Guralnik DB, ed. *Webster's New World Dictionary*, 2nd ed. Cleveland: World Publishing Co., 1967.
2. Gershon-Cohen J, Cooley AG. Telediagnosis. *Radiology* 1950;55:582–587.
3. Wittson CL, Benschoter R. Two-way television: helping the medical center reach out. *Am J Psychiatry* 1972;129:624–627.
4. Perednia PA, Allen A. Telemedicine technology and clinical applications. *JAMA* 1995;273:483–487.
5. Preston J, Brown FW, Hartley B. Using telemedicine to improve health care in distant areas. *Hosp Commun Psychiatry* 1992;2:25–32.
6. Bird KY. Cardiopulmonary frontiers: quality health care via interactive television. *Chest* 1972;61: 204–205.
7. Crump WJ, Pfeil TA. Telemedicine primer: an introduction to the technology and an overview of the literature. *Arch Fam Med* 1995;9:796–803.
8. Grigsby J. Current status of domestic telemedicine. *J Med Systems* 1995;1:19–26.
9. Bashshur RL. Telemedicine and the health care system. In: Bashshur RL, Sanders JH, Shannon GW, eds. *Telemedicine theory and practice*. Springfield, IL: Charles C. Thomas Publisher, 1997:5–35.
10. Bashshur RL, Sanders JH, Shannon GW, eds. *Telemedicine theory and practice*. Springfield, IL: Charles C. Thomas Publisher, 1997.
11. Whitehead R. The evolution of telemedicine. *Teleconference Magazine* 1995;14:9–11, 26.
12. Gitlin JN. Teleradiology. In: Bashshur RL, Sanders JH, Shannon GW, eds. *Telemedicine theory and practice*. Springfield, IL: Charles C. Thomas Publisher, 1997;111–177.
13. Field MJ, ed. *Telemedicine a guide to assessing telecommunications in health care.* Washington, DC: National Academy Press, 1996.
14. Wachter G. Teleradiology service provider. *Telemed Today* 1996;4:14–15.
15. Weissert WG, Silberman S. Healthcare on the information highway: the politics of telemedicine. *Telemed J* 1996;1:1–15.
16. Hassol A, Gaumer G, Grigsby J, Mintzer CL, Puskin DS, Brunswick M. Rural telemedicine: a national snapshot. *Telemed J* 1996:1:43–48.
17. Abt Associates, Inc. *Exploratory evaluation of rural applications of telemedicine*. Prepared for the Office of Rural Health Policy, 1996.

Telemedicine: Practicing in the Information Age,
edited by Steven F. Viegas and Kim Dunn.
Lippincott–Raven Publishers, Philadelphia © 1998.

3

International Perspective

David Krasnow and Roberto J. Rodrigues

Massie Research Laboratories, Beverly Hills, California 90211; and Health Services Information Systems Program, Pan American Health Organization/World Health Organization, Washington, D.C. 20037

The mission of telemedicine from an international viewpoint replicates many of the issues facing telehealth in the United States but further includes various challenges unique to foreign countries. The technology needs to be appropriate in situations for which physical barriers or distance prevent transfer of information between providers and patients and in which the availability of information is essential to proper care. Telehealth applications necessarily must add value to what is presently being done by health professionals. Any system should address the problems of access and equity to explore novel ways to deliver healthcare, to promote healthy provider behaviors, and to facilitate dissemination of knowledge between providers and consumers.

Inherent to the implementation of new systems are the structural issues of healthcare reform in the resident country. Changing the paradigm of healthcare delivery involves the reengineering of existing processes and forms of care. New models integrate a mixture of governmental, managed care, and private providers. Any program must address the issue of increased access to basic healthcare services clearly defined in terms of cost-benefit analyses. New models require usage of standardized sets of public interventions, disease management programs, and focus on decentralized operations.

International telemedicine programs require emphasis on managerial and professional decision making, accountability and feedback mechanisms, cost containment and recovery (financial sustainability), orientation toward support of health promotion, and increased client participation. It is wise to engender patient participation in the understanding and maintenance of his or her health status. The applied information systems should integrate health information, patient management, telecommunications, and extrasectoral components.

CULTURAL DIFFERENCES

Knowledge of the local sociopolitical environment is essential to market development. Successful companies operating in the international arena understand the importance of the sociopolitical environment and address it at every level of decision making. The cultural awareness capacity of nonlocal firms determine their success or failure. Telemedicine outside the United States represents a brand new market potential. It may not be a trivial task to locate international expertise in the United States or hire appropriately skilled counterparts in the country in which one chooses to work. The health system in a given country can vary significantly from region to region. The local personnel must exhibit an appropriate level of expertise and knowledge of the possibilities to interact with local healthcare systems. Local infrastructures and politics also vary greatly. The local realities of one city or province may not apply to another locale.

Social values, perceptions of illness, and patterns of client-provider interactions differ among different countries, inside the same country, and between social classes. Language remains a major hindrance to overseas telemedicine applications. Besides the "official" language, there exist native and ethnic languages or dialects that can create serious difficulties when establishing a program. For example, there are 23 Mayan languages spoken in Guatemala by the Indian residents who comprise 50% of the population. Literacy levels create another limiting factor in the broader use of telemedicine by the population at large.

Validation of knowledge content to local problems and practices is important. The allocation and evaluation of costs, time, and responsibilities, as well as potential litigation issues, require consideration when transplanting applications developed for other environments.

INFRASTRUCTURE

Human and organizational resources and capabilities vary widely internationally. On a country-to-country basis, the stage of technological development of providers and consumers changes. Available indigenous telecommunication technology issues are important. In Latin America, between $250 billion and $350 billion have been earmarked for investment from 1998 to 2003 to upgrade infrastructure. Computer literacy and the capability to purchase and maintain relatively expensive capital equipment is a concern.

The importance of an appropriate behavioral and institutional infrastructure dictates that a framework be provided to allow information to be used in a way that encourages individuals to work toward the overall objectives of the organization. Unless such an appropriate framework is in place, information cannot be translated into action. The telehealth framework mandates clear responsibility and accountability structures, setting of objectives and targets for individuals and departments, and mechanisms for motivating people and for providing feedback about their achievements. An environment must be created in which managers are able to take action to influence events in their areas of responsibility.

A broad spectrum of potential applications exists across the globe, even in developing countries. Different health problems can demand different levels of information and transmission requirements. There is need for varied options regarding

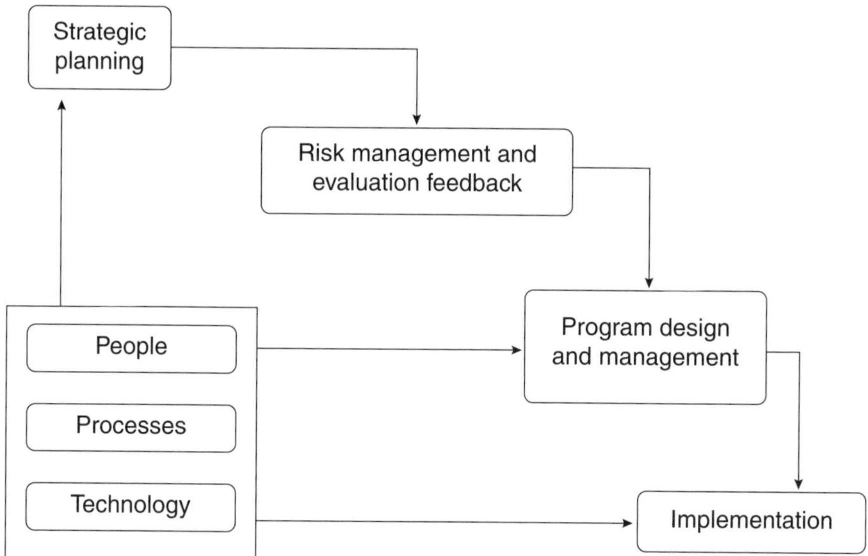

FIG. 3-1. Project planning and evaluation.

bandwidth from simple twisted pair and off-the-shelf solutions to videoconferencing using analog television to compressed video and data transmissions across broad band resources. In most instances, deployment depends on making use of existing local communication channels.

Internationally, the need for Internet access is high. This is a rapidly expanding source of health information with increasing variety, depth, and quality of information in many languages. Currently, however, Internet connectivity is limited outside the United States. Maintenance of knowledge contents and the disparities of alternate sources of health information present major problems for end users. The Internet often contains more misinformation than appropriate information regarding contemporary medical practices. Furthermore, the available search engines are woefully inadequate to conduct specific searches. Often, specific medical databases are not accessible. Linkage to the medical databases of neighboring countries and allied medical schools can provide current, same-language information.

Standardized technologies, open architecture interoperability, modular design with expandability, and scaleability are required to ensure widespread compatibility and market expansion.

PROGRAM PLANNING

In Fig. 3-1, a model is used that includes three elements: people, processes, and technology. People form the most crucial element. The processes involve both person-to-person interaction on all levels (government to local village) and the interface

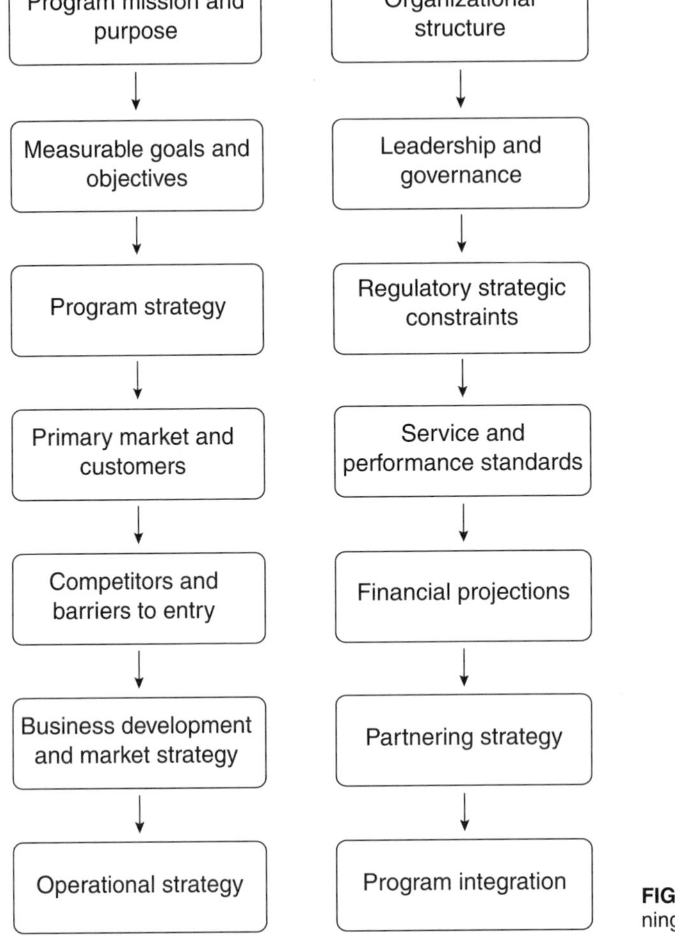

FIG. 3-2. Strategic planning module.

issues of people with technology. It is imperative to remember that the technology exists only to facilitate healthcare delivery. The planning and evaluation model flows from strategic planning to implementation, including risk management, evaluation feedback, program design, and management and feedback loops during every phase. This loop permits rapid prototyping and almost immediate feedback. This program design allows for ongoing changes to meet individual program requirements. It creates an evolving and flexible model as opposed to an inflexible structure.

The second flowchart (Fig. 3-2) carefully segregates the issues of measurable goals, primary markets, barriers to entry, organizational structure, leadership, regulatory constraints, standards-based practices, finance, and partnering strategies. All of these modules require careful consideration and planning for any international telemedicine implementation to survive. Deliberately, they are not country specific. Each region and locale necessitates individual crafting of policy and planning.

Many projects have shown low rates of use. There appears to be increasing evidence that managerial and acceptance issues play vital roles in both program effectiveness and use of services. Leadership, official "buy-in," and organizational and training factors directly relate to the ultimate failure or success of many programs. To ensure long-term viability, early adopters should be encouraged to be champions of the program. The local providers and their assistants must accept and actively support the deployment of any telemedicine application. Systems must easily integrate into routine clinical practice. Interfaces should not be burdensome to the user.

TELECOMMUNICATIONS

Strategic Planning Issues

Identification of primary markets and consumers, barriers to market entry, business development, and marketing strategy are highly region specific. Even in the same country there can be marked differences regarding needs, infrastructure, language, and culture. Technology service companies, consultants, integrators, and providers must understand the specific nature of healthcare markets. Many proposed solutions involve unrealistic scenarios. Some vendors describe their products in terms of applications not relevant to the health sector or fail to perceive that the fundamental basis of healthcare is the relationship between the patient and the healthcare professional. Technology must enhance this relationship, not encroach on it. The key to entering the health market is to understand the need to adapt or modify technology to serve the real and important needs of providers and patients. As indicated in Fig. 3-2, participant buy-in (i.e., government, academic, and private sector providers, telecommunication companies, industry partnerships) is fundamental for success.

Financing requires cooperation between government, development agencies, and the private sector. Retrospective experience shows that nearly all externally funded projects collapse when funding is terminated. This fact demonstrates that all projects need justification in terms of cost benefit and long-term financial sustainability. This further indicates that spreading the financial risk across several stakeholders may be appropriate. Cost sharing increases overall awareness, use, and the long-term potential for success.

Telehealth managers should be sensitive to the cultural and professional perceptions related to the introduction of technology. Two of the most important driving forces in most projects have been related to market pressure to sell services and the politics and economics of managed care. In some instances, the pitch for technology can be seen only as a commercial venture. Competitive entities fighting for market share among different providers and between national and international companies tend to accentuate this notion. Among health professionals, issues, such as competition for clients and contracts, payment for services, professional licensing, and "turf," can effectively block telemedicine development.

Considering the requirements for technical expertise and specialized professional management, an assessment must be made of the number, experience level, and balance of skill mixes required. Particularly in less developed countries, the identification and recruitment of competent individuals along with difficulties in staff retention can be significant hindrances to systems development.

Project Formulation

International project planning hopefully avoids the common approach of searching for a problem that fits the existing technology in favor of determining the appropriate health problems that could be solved by technology. Currently, clinical problems most amenable to effective telemedicine solutions are cognitive in nature. They relate primarily to transmission of data, image, or audio to a distant site staffed by a consultant. They potentially include database searches, medical management through call center triage, and a more basic exchange of messages or reports.

Needs assessments duly consider all implementation environment factors and constraints, as well as the requirements and expectations of the providers and patients. Technology ideally exists as an almost invisible overlay to clinical activity. Education and training lay the foundation for future applications and program expansions. A starting point for implementation planning is to determine what services are currently absent or insufficient and determine if those services could be enhanced by technology to facilitate transfer of data, images, or voice.

Technological specifications are key to the scope, function, and operation of telemedicine applications. These requirements represent the major thrust of both public and private sector telecommunication endeavors. Perhaps more crucial to effective implementation on the local level is the appropriateness of content and information usability.

Financial projections, risk management, and continuous evaluation feedback represent key elements that must be inherent to any program from the initial stages onward. Evaluation criteria should be constructed considering fulfillment of defined needs; long-term sustainability; demonstration of organizational support; acceptance and use of health professionals; and ability to track data on costs, quality, efficiency, and outcomes. These elements are graphically illustrated in Figs. 3-1 and 3-2.

Implementation Issues

The technical system selected to support telehealth can be as simple as a telephone or as sophisticated as computers linked to satellite. The management needed to assure optimization of the proposed system is critical. Management may be simple or sophisticated, depending on the technical system chosen for implementation. However, the process required in any case is a common one. Gaining achievable results depends on clinical and management structures to support the technology.

Key elements necessary for consideration include (a) deciding who is going to define, describe, and write the program; (b) defining the program mission and purpose; (c) determining measurable goals and objectives; (d) describing the strategy for achieving these goals, including a plan to overcome barriers to implementation; (e) establishing administrative support (i.e., identifying and selecting candidates); (f) writing an operational plan with time lines for all phases of implementation; (g) writing a plan to monitor and evaluate each stage of implementation; (h) establishing feedback mechanisms for each stage; (i) establishing small-scale implementation before expanded roll-out of the program; and (j) providing for change or modification in each phase based on the feedback mechanism.

Implementation goals should address a variety of issues that include, but are not limited to, (a) reducing the cost of delivery of care; (b) reducing the number of visits to more costly health centers; (c) reducing societal costs (e.g., dislocation and loss of income); (d) expanding the scope of services and expertise in more remote areas; (e) facilitating prevention programs; (f) providing distance learning for health professionals and staff; and (g) reducing the interval between presentation of a clinical problem and its effective treatment.

INTERNATIONAL LINKAGE

There is a desire in the international community to have access to a wide range of colleagues and ideas across the globe. Lessons learned in one geographic locale can apply to situations in a disparate location. Free transfer of technological, medical, legal, and regulatory information can prove beneficial to professionals across the globe. Many regions underserved by medical specialists can potentially benefit from tertiary consults in North America, Europe, or Asia. The adage to think globally but act locally applies to telehealth on an international scale.

One prime area in which global linkage has greatest potential lies in distance learning. Many universities already provide vast arrays of subject matter for distribution anywhere. This global education permits access to basic, intermediate, and advanced course work. Continuing medical education transcends geographic or geopolitical isolation. Physicians, technicians, nurses, and allied health workers can substantially enhance their skills using this teaching modality. Courseware is now being developed in hundreds of subject areas, in several languages, that is directly applicable to international telemedicine.

The sharing of information regarding legal, regulatory, liability, and professional standards could assist in addressing transborder practice of medicine, local standards of care, and malpractice. Standards-based practices would facilitate cross-border interactions.

CONCLUSION

International telemedicine program development integrates technological considerations with various combinations of culture, geography, geopolitics, language, and healthcare systems. No single model functions with effectiveness across all national boundaries. A North American paradigm is not transferable to the myriad of cultural complexities encountered in the international arena. Acute sensitivity and flexibility function as fundamental elements for implementation overseas. Most senior international governmental and academic leaders prefer carefully crafted strategic partnerships to a vendor-client relationship. Programs and alliances reflect long-term relationships and commitments. Adaptability, flexibility, sensitivity, and patience remain the hallmarks of successful program planning and development in foreign markets.

Telemedicine: Practicing in the Information Age,
edited by Steven F. Viegas and Kim Dunn.
Lippincott–Raven Publishers, Philadelphia © 1998.

4

Telemedicine in the United States

Robert M. Brecht and Jim E. Barrett

International Telemedicine Center, Inc., Houston, Texas 77054; and Health Sciences Center for Educational Resources and Department of Medical Education, University of Washington School of Medicine, Seattle, Washington 98195, and International Telemedicine Center, Inc., Seattle, Washington 98195

Telemedicine has been practiced and talked about since the late 1950s and a substantial amount of money has been spent on research and demonstrations, but telemedicine still has no universally accepted, all-inclusive definition. One of the most comprehensive definitions was proposed by Bashur (1). A more common definition, however, used with minor deviations by a number of statewide planning groups, is the following: Telemedicine is the use of telecommunications technology to send data, graphics, audio, and video images between participants who are physically separated (i.e., at a distance from one another) for the purpose of clinical care (2–4). The term *telehealth* is often used for an even broader perspective of the application of telecommunications to the healthcare environment.

The lack of availability of qualified health professionals continues to be a major barrier to accessing healthcare for many areas. Although there may appear to be enough health professionals in the United States, these professionals are poorly distributed. Many urban and especially suburban areas of the United States enjoy an oversupply of professionals, particularly specialty physicians, whereas rural areas continue to experience an inadequate number of health professionals. The rural environment is not a low-density reflection of its urban counterpart. A 1990 study by the U.S. Office of Technology Assessment (5) cited three problems that are specific to residents of rural areas:

1. Although the rural population has relatively low mortality rates, a disproportionate number of rural people experience chronic illnesses. Furthermore, infant mortality is higher than in urban areas, and the number of deaths from injury is dramatically higher.
2. The lack of a public transportation system and the existence of few local providers make it difficult for rural individuals to reach facilities where they can obtain care. Individuals living in areas with six or fewer residents per square mile (i.e., frontier rural areas) have geographic access problems of immense propor-

tions. Moreover, in such counties there is often an insufficient population base to adequately support local health services.

3. The physical barriers to access, difficult as they are, may be outweighed by financial barriers. In 1987, one out of every six rural families lived in poverty, compared to one out of every eight in urban areas. Also, rural residents below the federal poverty level were less likely to be covered by Medicaid than urban residents (35.5% versus 44.4%).

Other problems facing rural healthcare systems include professional isolation, lack of access to specialists, declining hospital use, discontinuity of care when patients are transferred to tertiary centers, financial difficulties, and trouble recruiting and training physicians. Although the severity may differ among communities, virtually all rural communities share similar problems. Although much of the discussion has focused on the needs of rural Americans, there are access problems for many population groups in urban areas as well (6). As a result of such needs, a large number of telemedicine initiatives are under way. In the United States, telemedicine programs exist in at least 40 states. Vast amounts of federal, state, foundation, and private money has been spent on developing these programs.

FACTORS DRIVING EXPANSION

Given the policy and economic barriers, the expansion of telemedicine programs is impressive. There is widespread public enthusiasm for telemedicine. Since 1994, many bills have been introduced in Congress with ties to telemedicine. The federal government has spent hundreds of millions of dollars in grants and defense spending for telemedicine projects. Telemedicine in the 1990s became one piece of a much wider movement aimed at building a national telecommunications infrastructure. The development of image enhancement and data-compression technologies, along with great improvement in price and performance of computer and videoconferencing technology, also played a large part in the expansion. The introduction of international standards for telecommunications and teleconferencing also played a significant role. These factors have been driving the expansion of telemedicine. Although these factors will continue to play a major role in further expansion, others will play a larger role as we move into the twenty-first century. These other factors include (a) telecommunications deregulation and the resulting competition and imposed advanced services and infrastructure to rural areas; (b) the move to managed care in both privately and publicly funded programs; and (c) the individual state initiatives to remove the barriers to telemedicine, especially in the area of reimbursement.

CURRENT ENVIRONMENT

Despite the many economic and policy barriers to telemedicine, the number of telemedicine programs continues to grow rapidly. In January 1997, the U.S. Office of Rural Health Policy released the first major national survey of rural telemedicine. The

Exploratory Evaluation of Rural Applications of Telemedicine conducted by Abt Associates, Inc. includes information about the extent of telemedicine penetration, use, and cost data (7). Nearly 30% of the 2,472 rural hospitals surveyed were predicted to be using some sort of telemedicine technology for delivering patient care; approximately two-thirds of them used only teleradiology. The number of reported programs doubled from 40 to 82 from 1995 to 1996 in *Telemedicine Today's* annual survey (8). The actual number of telemedicine programs is underreported due to the perspective that telemedicine provides a market advantage. Of the 53 telemedicine programs with which he was involved in late 1996, Chuck Jones, Southwestern Bell's Director of Telemedicine for Oklahoma, indicated that 45 were under nondisclosure agreements (9).

Surveys (7,10) also confirmed that the most common clinical applications of telemedicine are radiology, cardiology, orthopedics, dermatology, and psychiatry. The most significant contributions to filling the specialty-care "gaps" in rural communities are in radiology, dermatology, cardiology, neurology, orthopedics, oncology, and pediatrics. Seventy-six percent of telemedicine programs perform fewer than 16 consults per month (8). Continuing medical education and administrative uses constitute the bulk of the uses for telemedicine systems. The most cited reason for underuse of telemedicine programs was that many programs studied did not complete adequate strategic and operational planning. Instead, programs concentrated on technology issues rather than need and human factor issues. The resulting budgets did not provide for the level of planning, training, and process reengineering necessary to build sustainable programs. On the other hand, the programs studied provided experience and demonstrated that telemedicine could be an effective tool to provide better access to healthcare for many populations. These programs have the potential to reduce overall patient case costs by providing the support necessary to allow patients to spend more time at home during their illness.

These surveys (7,8) also confirm that telemedicine services are being delivered using a number of different technologies. Although the specific technologies may vary somewhat with different features or by combining several technologies, they basically include two fundamental approaches; store and forward and interactive video. These are discussed in more detail in later chapters of this book.

The types of clinical care that are being typically supported through store and forward technology include radiology, cardiology, dermatology, pathology, and ophthalmology.

An example of a successful store and forward radiology program is INPHACT of Nashville, Tennessee. At last reporting, they were performing approximately 7,200 diagnostic study reads per month (10).

Much of the nonradiology focus of telemedicine has been on using interactive, compressed, digital video systems to deliver clinical services in almost every clinical specialty area. Correctional health is particularly amenable to this approach (11). A successful interactive video project with which I was involved was the University of Texas Medical Branch's correctional telemedicine project with the Texas Department of Criminal Justice (12). This program has resulted in high inmate satisfaction, saved numerous trips, and achieved provider acceptance.

OBSTACLES TO TELEMEDICINE EXPANSION

There continue to be obstacles to telemedicine expansion. Some are currently being addressed at the federal and state levels. The policy barriers to telemedicine include the lack of reimbursement for telemedicine services, malpractice liability and jurisdiction, licensure and credentialing, confidentiality and telecommunications costs, and availability. Other inhibiting factors include the lack of clinical standards, objective evaluation of data, and provider resistance. A number of these issues are discussed in other chapters of this book. Some of the more significant ones are discussed in the following sections.

Reimbursement

One of the most significant barriers to telemedicine expansion is that many telemedicine applications are not reimbursed. The U.S. Health Care Financing Administration (HCFA), the federal agency responsible for Medicare and Medicaid, requires a face-to-face consultation for reimbursement, except for image applications such as radiology. HCFA influences major commercial carriers and other third-party insurers about reimbursement policy. At the time of this writing, HCFA is conducting a 3-year demonstration project to assess reimbursement issues, but individual states had already begun to foster reimbursement for telemedicine. In the Federal Balanced Budget Act of 1997, Congress mandated that HCFA begin paying for telemedicine services to Health Professional Shortage Areas beginning in 1999. Louisiana legislated telemedicine reimbursement. California, Oklahoma, and Texas have legislated the elimination of face-to-face requirements for reimbursement when telemedicine is an appropriate alternative. Third-party payors are reimbursing telemedicine in a number of states, and as many as 12 states have some Medicaid reimbursement (13). Most telemedicine payment schemes only reimburse the specialist consultant fee with no provision for infrastructure, communications, and remote provider costs.

Communication Costs

Fundamental to the development of telemedicine is the availability of telecommunications infrastructure and the costs involved for use of that infrastructure. Many rural areas lack basic services, such as Internet access, let alone the digital and broadband services used in many applications of telemedicine. The services used by telemedicine programs to these rural areas have historically been very expensive. Under the Universal Access Fund provision of the 1996 Telecommunications Deregulation Bill, funds have been allocated to subsidize certain telecommunications services to rural, nonprofit, healthcare providers, including telemedicine services, beginning in 1998.

Licensure

States retain the authority to license medical professionals. A number of states have passed laws restricting the practice of telemedicine by persons who are not fully licensed in that state. Given the expected low volume of telemedicine consultations, practitioners are reluctant to incur the costs and administrative requirements associated with multiple state medical licenses.

Liability and Legal Jurisdiction

Most malpractice rates and coverage extent vary by state or region within a state. There is significant uncertainty regarding whether malpractice policies cover services provided by telemedicine, especially across multiple state lines. A malpractice lawsuit could be filed in the jurisdiction where either the physician or patient resides. A plaintiff may be able to select the venue most advantageous to the plaintiff's suit.

Provider Resistance

Little information is available about rural physicians' attitudes concerning the use of telemedicine. Studies have been limited in scope. In a Minnesota assessment of the attitudes and opinions of rural Minnesota family physicians toward telemedicine, surveyed physicians overwhelmingly agreed that they do not have sufficient information about telemedicine (15). Their awareness of telemedicine's applications, capabilities, benefits, and policy issues were minimal.

The Abt Associates study conducted for the U.S. Office of Rural Health Policy (7) found that, of rural physicians who had conducted a handful of telemedicine consults, many appeared to be willing to participate in a teleconsult visit, even without reimbursement, because they learn through the process. The lack of time to devote to teleconsults may be a more important barrier than the lack of reimbursement.

FUTURE TRENDS

The telemedicine industry is maturing. Greater emphasis is placed on planning and developing a business model for the program, which should result in sustainable telemedicine undertakings. Telemedicine is rapidly shifting from the high-end room teleconferencing systems to desktop computer systems, resulting in a significant reduction in technology costs. Coupled with deregulation and other provisions (e.g., universal access) of the federal Telecommunication Act of 1996, costs continue to decline significantly. Even less expensive is the use of the Internet for telemedicine applications. Such Internet applications continue to evolve and expand. While the 3-year HCFA telemedicine demonstration project runs its course to 1999, more states will take the lead in providing Medicaid reimbursement and legislating telemedicine reimbursement. California and Texas are two states to monitor for progress in the arena—California because of its Telemedicine Development legislation, and Texas because of the Telecommunications Infrastructure Fund, which provides $900 million to $1.5 billion to invest in distance learning and telemedicine infrastructure. As more of the obstacles continue to be addressed, a rapid expansion of telemedicine will be seen, with telemedicine ultimately moving into the home.

With the integration of telemedicine into an overall health information environment, the *tele* will disappear, and telemedicine will be looked on as an essential tool in the delivery of healthcare services.

REFERENCES

1. Bashur RL. On the definition and evaluation of telemedicine. *Telemed J* 1995;1:19–30.
2. Brecht RM, ed. *Texas telemedicine strategy planning project: preliminary report.* Lubbock, TX: Texas Telehealth/Education Consortium, 1997.
3. California Telehealth/Telemedicine Coordination Project. *Telehealth & telemedicine: taking distance out of caring.* Fresno, CA: California Health Collaborative, 1997.
4. Iowa Telemedicine Advisory Council. *Iowa Telemedicine Advisory Council report.* Association of Iowa Hospitals and Health Systems, Des Moines, IA: Association of Iowa Hospitals and Health Systems, November 1994.
5. Office of Technology Assessment. *Rural America at the crossroads: networking for the future.* US Government Printing Office, 1990.
6. Ginzberg E. Improving health care for the poor. *JAMA* 1994;271:464–467.
7. Abt Associates, Inc. *Exploratory evaluation of rural applications of telemedicine.* Washington, DC: Office of Rural Health Policy, 1996.
8. Grigsby B, Allen A. Fourth annual program review. *Telemed Today* 1997;5:30–38.
9. Jones CP. Discussion of common telemedicine problems. TeleMed II Conference. Anaheim, CA, 1996.
10. Allen A, Patterson J. Annual survey of teleradiology service providers. *Telemed Today* 1997;5:24–25.
11. Brecht RM. Correctional telemedicine: an overview. In: Neuherger N, Scott UJ, eds. *Telemedicine sourcebook.* New York: Faulkner & Gray, 1998.
12. Brecht RM, Gray CL, Peterson C, Youngblood B. The UTMB-Texas Department of Criminal Justice Telemedicine Project: findings from the first year of operation. *Telemed Today* 1996;2:25–35.
13. Kane J, Marken J, Boulger J, et al. Rural Minnesota family physicians' attitudes toward telemedicine. *Minn Med* 1995;78:19–22.

Telemedicine: Practicing in the Information Age,
edited by Steven F. Viegas and Kim Dunn.
Lippincott–Raven Publishers, Philadelphia © 1998.

5

Telemedicine: The Perspective of One State

Carolyn T. Purcell

Texas Department of Information Resources, Austin, Texas 78701

In his state strategic plan, *Vision Texas*, Governor George Bush wrote, "[t]he mission of Texas state government is to support and promote individual and community efforts to achieve and sustain social and economic prosperity" (1). The deployment of a telecommunications infrastructure is important for the enfranchisement of communities in rural Texas, particularly with respect to accessible medical services. According to a report by Texas Comptroller of Public Accounts John Sharp, "[a]s of January 1995, 58 Texas counties did not have a hospital, 227 counties did not have a psychiatric bed, 22 counties did not have a doctor, and 167 counties did not have an Ob-Gyn specialist" (2). The report acknowledged that developments in telecommunications offer a technological remedy for the dearth of medical resources in rural Texas.

The efficiencies provided by telecommunications that could make scarce resources virtually ubiquitous make telemedicine a compelling strategy for a fiscally conservative legislature. As a testament to its support, when the 74th Legislature deregulated telecommunications in Texas, the bill included a provision for funding "distance learning programs and telemedicine services projects [to] improve the effectiveness and efficiency of health care delivery" (3). One and a half billion dollars will be made available over 10 years to fund this initiative.

CURRENT STATUS OF TELECOMMUNICATIONS IN TEXAS

Texas government relies heavily on telecommunications to conduct official business with Texans. For example, in a survey of agencies and universities, the Texas Department of Information Resources found that 81% of respondents consider electronic mail (e-mail) a mission-critical aspect of conducting business (4). In addition to using e-mail for internal communications, 92% of the agencies reported that their employees had access to Internet e-mail. Eighty-eight percent of the agencies and universities surveyed used the Internet to disseminate important public information. A Harte Hanks' Texas poll survey indicated that 55% of Texans (or approximately 9 million Texans) use a computer, and 46% of those (or approximately 4 million Texans) have access to the Internet (5). Most Internet watchers agree that the number of subscribers doubles every year.

The state strategic plan for information resources management promises "access to the coordinated, interoperable communications infrastructure necessary to support state computer and videoconferencing needs" (6). Building the infrastructure requires planning and leveraging enterprise volume to gain advantages for buying products and services. The Texas General Services Commission negotiates with local and long distance service providers to obtain volume discounts for bandwidth. The Texas Department of Information Resources negotiates with manufacturers of hardware and publishers of software for volume purchase discounts. In both cases, these rates are made available to state agencies and universities and to local political subdivisions. The Texas health and human services agencies share a common network management operation to lower costs and raise the quality of service across the agencies. In some rural areas, state government assumes the role of anchor tenant for deployment of advanced telecommunications services.

The promise of interoperability is realized through the adoption of standards, and Texas has adopted open standards for telecommunications. A report commissioned by the Texas Senate Committee on International Relations, Trade and Technology provides a statewide inventory of interactive video telecommunications resources and services provided by Texas state agencies and universities (7). According to the survey, state facilities exist in 43 Texas cities and towns. In addition to identifying the major networks, the report concluded that the existing videoconferencing facilities are interoperable and that, through connectivity to public networks (such as Southwestern Bell Telephone Co. or GTE), the facilities can conduct interstate and even international conferences. This ability to interconnect sites is of paramount importance to the legislature, whose view of the enterprise acknowledges no boundaries between agencies and universities.

CONTENT

Telemedicine includes more than interactive video: It includes all occasions by which pertinent healthcare data are shared among authorized parties electronically through networks. For example, access to medical libraries and their contents can be an important link for a physician otherwise isolated in a remote Texas community. The ability of the physician to communicate with colleagues via e-mail may provide him or her an opportunity to stay current with leading-edge studies in medicine. Continuing education opportunities may be made available via telecommunications in his or her office, permitting the physician to tend patients while advancing his or her skills and knowledge. Most dramatically, the ability to consult with a physician remote from the patient through two-way teleconferencing can improve the quality of decisions made by healthcare providers and hopefully lead to better outcomes.

The implications of data collection facilitated through telemedicine are significant. The combination of patient data with demographic information offers many opportunities to "slice and dice" data to render statistical observations, not only about the patients, but also their diagnoses, treatment modalities, service providers, and insurers. Correlating this information with government program participation characteristics could tell policy makers how effective a program is in achieving the expected outcome.

The Texas legislature and the governor's office write budgets that are outcome oriented. The material from longitudinal studies could inform policy makers in their evaluation of a program's effectiveness and guide funding decisions.

The 74th Legislature created the Texas Health Care Information Council, whose purpose is to define a universe of data that would be useful to consumers in determining the quality of care they expect in a variety of settings (8). The availability of on-line information resources for healthcare can mean that healthcare providers in remote, medically underserved areas have access to the most current and complete sources of information on which to base diagnoses and treatments. The availability of comprehensive data about a patient regardless of where he or she seeks medical care means administering treatment that takes into account the patient's complete medical history.

OBSTACLES

Public policy issues exist that can slow the deployment of telemedicine until adequate solutions or positions are found. Most of these issues have to do with accepting electronic transactions with the same confidence as face-to-face encounters. This is especially critical when dealing with an issue as important as an individual's health.

Transactions that occur on-line, whether an interactive exchange of data or merely an inquiry into an existing data repository, travel via a network. Most secure transactions use Value Added Networks, or VANs. A VAN restricts traffic to a known population of participants at an identified number of sites. Automated teller machines use VANs to limit the possibility of invasion by unauthorized users. The Internet, on the other hand, provides the attractive feature of easy access at low cost, although its very openness suggests that it is less secure. Securing the Internet will be an eternal struggle for those who wish to take advantage of its characteristic accessibility. Not only are nodes on the Internet subject to unauthorized intrusions, but "spoofing" undermines the assumption that the parties on either end of a transaction are who they say they are.

Paramount in the discussion of any automated system designed to transfer information about a person's health is a concern about maintaining confidentiality. Although public policy makers want to develop efficient, enterprisewide public assistance systems, the rules and statutes governing relationships between various government healthcare programs have resulted in a complex maze of prohibitions and requirements for explicit authority to share data. In Texas, the legislature is frustrated by the lack of information shared between agencies but, at the same time, is conscientious about maintaining a citizen's right to privacy.

In the 1996 version of Comptroller John Sharp's Texas Performance Review (9), one problem cited is the failure of the federal Health Care Financing Administration to authorize Medicare reimbursement for telemedicine services unless provided through a managed care organization. Furthermore, the document cited Texas for its failure to reimburse telemedicine services delivered to Medicaid recipients. The 75th Texas Legislature passed legislation to remedy this situation in 1997 (10).

Finally, healthcare consumers and practitioners alike must have confidence in the system that is used. Solutions to the problems of security, confidentiality, and authentication will increase confidence in the Internet as a vehicle for a health information system that is widely available. The efficiency of on-line transactions will speed acceptance; much like electronic funds transfer was quickly adopted by employees who fought end-of-pay-period bank teller lines to deposit their paychecks.

ACCELERATORS

In 1995, the 74th Texas Legislature deregulated telecommunications and established an industry-supplied fund to be used to advance telecommunications infrastructures in public schools, libraries, and in public healthcare facilities throughout Texas (11). Industry will contribute approximately $150 million a year for 10 years. Grant proposals that "improve the effectiveness and efficiency of health care delivery" are among projects given priority. *Telemedicine* is defined as "consultive, diagnostic, or other medical services delivered via telecommunications technologies to rural or underserved public, not-for-profit hospitals, and primary health care facilities in collaboration with an academic health center and associated teaching hospitals or tertiary center" (11). By this definition, telemedicine includes, at least, "interactive video consultation, teleradiology, telepathology, and distance education for working health care professionals" (11). In addition to grant money, the legislation provided for deep discounts on recurring line charges for the targeted facilities.

Rapid expansion of electronic commerce will accelerate responses to security and authentication barriers to widespread use of the Internet. For example, digital signature legislation has been proposed or enacted in 29 states. These laws would consider a communication signed if accompanied by a digital signature that warrants the identity of the sender and the integrity of the contents. Encryption standards are building public confidence that content can be secured and remain confidential.

Governments around the world are grappling with public-policy issues to advance electronic commerce. Creating an infrastructure that will allow users to be confident of the identity of the parties, the contents of the transaction, and the secrecy of the contents in an open environment will result in more and better uses of electronic transactions.

Finally, the Internet has taught the world the value of ubiquitous access and dynamic composition. Instead of building new databases, old databases are being linked together in new and dynamic ways, thus eliminating redundant data collection and retention. By eliminating data redundancy, data integrity will improve. Designating a primary custodian for each data element assumes a hierarchy of integrity of each element and assigns accountability to the custodian.

TRENDS

Government is in the midst of a sea change. Virtually every assumption that has guided government operations in the past is under scrutiny. The technology that enables telemedicine is both a cause and an effect of this vast change.

Bureaucracies are built to intermediate between the haves and the have nots, between the government and its citizens. Traditionally, this intermediation occurs through personal contact. The trend is to downsize government by eliminating the middle man. Disintermediation occurs through many devices, but in most cases depends on some sort of electronic exchange of information or products. In administrative operations, it is mostly achieved through electronic commerce. In program areas, information is made available electronically on the Internet, through kiosks, on bulletin boards, and through automated voice-response telephone systems. As technology becomes more sophisticated, functions performed by people, such as detection of fraud in the Medicaid system, will be performed more reliably and cheaper by computers.

A prerequisite of this trend to replace human functions with electronic ones is the elimination of considerations of time and place. In cyberspace, governments have learned that they can conduct business any way and any time without adding bricks and mortar or employees. Telemedicine is giving Texans an opportunity to receive quality medical care regardless of their geography.

Budget crises in state government have forced agencies to look for partners to share expenses. The incentive to collaborate to reduce budget demand led the Texas Department of Criminal Justice to contract with the health science centers of various Texas universities for the delivery of medical services to inmates. This program resulted in a huge application of telemedicine that advanced its use throughout the state. In addition to improved medical care for inmates and a reduced cost for physician travel, the public safety of Texans is enhanced as there are fewer opportunities for escape during inmate transport.

Deregulation of telecommunications in Texas and at the national level has resulted in the accelerated deployment of advanced infrastructure while telephone, media, and cable companies jockey for position in this wide-open market. The opening of this highly competitive market benefits the public in significant ways. Public access to faster communication links capable of transmitting large amounts of data will result in many new products and services. As competition increases, costs for local telephones and other services are expected to drop. As telecommunications and videoconferencing product lines mature, the public will see a remarkable improvement in the quality of products, as well as lower pricing.

CONCLUSION

Telemedicine is a technology that lies at the intersection of universal quality services and efficient government. Policy makers in Texas enthusiastically embrace this new technology, and the legislature has endorsed it with a sizable commitment of funds. As the barriers to full implementation capitulate to the assault of capitalism, Texas will emerge in the vanguard of virtual government.

REFERENCES

1. Texas Office of the Governor. *Vision Texas: the statewide strategic planning elements for Texas state government.* Austin, TX: Texas Office of the Governor, 1996.
2. Texas Comptroller of Public Accounts. *Health care atlas of Texas.* Austin, TX: Texas Comptroller of Public Accounts, 1997.
3. Tex. Rev. Civ. Stat. Ann. art. 1446c-O, sec. 3.606 (Vernon Supp. 1997).
4. Texas Department of Information Resources. *Going forward: achieving the state's vision for information and technologies.* Austin, TX: Texas Department of Information Resources, 1996:12, 13.
5. Hawkins L. Wealth, race play roles in who uses computer. *Austin American-Statesman.* 1996 Nov 3.
6. Texas Department of Information Resources. *Facing the future: a vision for information and technologies to serve tomorrow's Texans.* Austin, TX: Texas Department of Information Resources, 1995:13.
7. Texas Department of Information Resources. *Statewide inventory of interactive video telecommunications resources and services: final report to the Texas Senate Committee on International Relations, Trade and Technology.* Austin, TX: Texas Department of Information Resources, January 27, 1997.
8. Tex. Health and Safety Code Ann. sec. 108.001 (Vernon Supp. 1996).
9. Texas Comptroller of Public Accounts. *Disturbing the peace: the challenge of change in Texas government,* Vol. 2. Austin, TX: Texas Comptroller of Public Accounts, 1997:154.
10. Texas H.B. 2017, 75th Leg., R.S. (1997).
11. Tex. Rev. Civ. Stat. Ann. art. 1446c-O, sec. 3.606 (Vernon Supp.1997).

Telemedicine: Practicing in the Information Age,
edited by Steven F. Viegas and Kim Dunn.
Lippincott–Raven Publishers, Philadelphia © 1998.

6

Telemedicine Program Implementation at University of Texas Medical Branch

Steven F. Viegas, Kim Dunn, Jason H. Calhoun, and Jake G. Angelo

Departments of Orthopaedics and Rehabilitation, Anatomy and Neurosciences, and Preventive Medicine and Community Health, University of Texas Medical Branch at Galveston, Galveston, Texas 77555; Department of Internal Medicine, Texas Department of Criminal Justice, University of Texas Medical Branch at Galveston, Galveston, Texas 77555; Department of Orthopaedics and Rehabilitation, University of Texas Medical Branch at Galveston, Galveston, Texas 77555; and Department of Information Services, University of Texas Medical Branch at Galveston, Galveston, Texas 77555

The University of Texas Medical Branch (UTMB) at Galveston has implemented a telemedicine program in the Texas prison system that has quickly grown and become recognized as a leader in the telemedicine field. UTMB has been involved in addressing the healthcare needs of inmates in the Texas Department of Criminal Justice (TDCJ) for more than 50 years. Since 1983, UTMB has had a prison hospital on its campus that provides subspecialty care to inmates, as well as outpatient clinic facilities, minor operating room suites, and inpatient beds for patients treated in Galveston.

HISTORY

Until 1994, healthcare costs across the state were rising at a rate of 16% per year per inmate. In 1994, the Texas Legislature established a capitated contract with the University of Texas Medical Branch and Texas Tech University.

As of 1997, the inmate population in the TDCJ was approximately 136,000. This inmate population is distributed across approximately 100 units, primarily in rural settings. UTMB is responsible for healthcare delivery for 80% of patients in prison units.

From 1992 to 1993, experimentation was done with videoconferencing for education and patient care by means of teletechnology at UTMB. Starting in October 1994, a telemedicine program was implemented with one local telemedicine unit at the prison hospital at UTMB and four remote telemedicine units at four different prison unit facilities. The initial implementation of the telemedicine program was primarily technology driven, stimulated by the TDCJ healthcare contract to provide subspecialty care.

In 1996, there was a reorganization to a more physician-driven program. Four additional remote prison-unit telemedicine sites were added in late 1996, with the local telemedicine unit number increasing to four. This brought the total telemedicine site count to 12 by February 1997, comprising eight remote and four local telemedicine room units. The remote units range in distance from 50 to 280 miles, with an average distance of 177 miles from Galveston. The local units are located in the outpatient clinic facility (two units), a separate telemedicine room, and in the trauma ward of UTMB in Galveston.

As of February 1998, 90 to 100 telemedicine visits were seen on the network per week, and more than 7,700 telemedicine consults had been completed. Eighty-eight percent of the UTMB/TDCJ telemedicine network is used for telemedicine clinics, 11% for teleconferences (use, quality review, and continuing education), and 1% for training. A total of 23 general and subspecialty services have been involved with the telemedicine program: cardiology, dermatology, otolaryngology, general medicine, general orthopedics, general surgery, gastroenterology, hematology/oncology, infectious diseases, neurology, neurosurgery, ophthalmology, an orthopedic foot and hand clinic, pulmonary, rheumatology, thoracic surgery, urology, vascular surgery, endocrinology, oral surgery, plastic surgery, obstetrics/gynecology, and psychiatry.

INITIAL REACTIONS

Surveys were completed using questionnaires early in the telemedicine program for the first 647 patient encounters. The findings determined that the satisfaction level was high among patients, presenters, and consultants. Ninety-three percent of the patients thought that they were adequately informed about what to expect from a telemedicine clinic visit. Seventy-one percent of patients thought that telemedicine was the same or better than face-to-face, live clinic encounters, and 22% thought it was only slightly less optimal. Eighty-six percent of the patients were very comfortable with the presenter, and ninety-three percent of the patients were very comfortable with the consultant. A total of 74% of these patients preferred telemedicine to traveling to Galveston.

The healthcare presenters at the remote site thought the consults were completed without any technical difficulty 99% of the time. Eighty-five percent of the presenters thought that the patient was comfortable with the encounter, and 92% of the presenters thought problems that were addressed in the telemedicine clinic visit were appropriate for telemedicine technology.

The consultants thought 71% of the problems were completely appropriate for telemedicine. Seventy-two percent of the consultants thought that the telemedicine clinic visit was equal to a face-to-face, live diagnosis, while 27% thought it was slightly less adequate. Seventy-two percent of the consultants thought that the consult was useful for generating an adequate treatment plan, while 27% thought it slightly less adequate. The consultants found telemedicine completely sufficient

72% of the time, while an additional 26% of the consultants thought that it met most of their needs.

Early in the telemedicine program, the same kinds of problems and inefficiencies of any small, new clinic or office were evident. If there were only one remote telemedicine site (just as if a clinic had only one examination room), the physician's time was not optimally used and it became inefficient and frustrating for the physician. In fact, in the telemedicine setting, the one clinic is often used by *all* the general and subspecialty services using telemedicine. By adding telemedicine sites, placing a telemedicine unit actually in a live clinic setting, or both, the capability could switch from one remote unit to another, between live, local patient clinic visits and remote telemedicine clinic encounters, or a combination of the two.

Advancements

Desktop technology was tested and integrated into the telemedicine network. Medical peripherals are continually being evaluated and upgraded to address the needs of individual services and physicians. Medical peripherals that have been used in the telemedicine networks include stethoscopes, ophthalmoscopes, otoscopes, slit-lamps for ophthalmologic examinations, scopes, and dermatologic scopes.

All managed-care guidelines have been revised to incorporate telemedicine assessment on both an elective and an emergent basis. Follow-up clinic appointments are also screened for appropriateness of follow-up appointments at either the prison unit healthcare facility, UTMB, or a telemedicine site consult.

Cost Savings

Cost savings in the areas of inmate transportation and security have been identified for the state. Calculation of the cost savings regarding transportation and security costs for transporting inmates to Galveston is difficult due to many factors, including that transportation and security are scheduled and funded by TDCJ. The estimates, however, which include transportation of security officers, special meals for inmates during transport, transient cell costs for housing en route to and from Galveston, transportation scheduling, and vehicle costs, have been calculated over the telemedicine program's first 2 full years of operation with four remote telemedicine prison sites. The estimation is that more than $500,000 was saved in transportation and security costs during the first 2 full years of operation of the telemedicine program. There is, of course, the additional benefit of avoiding the loss of medical compliance during transportation to and from Galveston. Avoidance of transportation of inmates is also viewed as a benefit to public safety.

The ability to deliver subspecialty care to rural settings, where often there is no subspecialty consultation capability for great distances, is accomplished through telemedicine. Although actual healthcare costs saved by the program have not been calculated, the alternative costs that would be involved in actually staffing medical clinics in rural towns with the general and subspecialty physicians that staff the 19 clinics now covered by the telemedicine network are estimated to be more than $310,000 per year per remote location. In addition, actual individual 24-hour a day emergency room physician coverage is estimated at more than $650,000 per remote location, for a total of more than $960,000 per year per remote site for physician staffing costs.

In addition to man hours, an increase in the use of the primary facilities can also result in cost savings. This has been shown to be the case in telemedicine networks. Approximately 80% of the patients that would have been sent to a tertiary facility can, with telemedicine support, stay in the local community facility. Additionally, increasing the safety of the general population by addressing the healthcare needs of prisoners via telemedicine has also been acknowledged.

CONCLUSION

The telemedicine program at UTMB for TDCJ is continuing to grow and be increasingly integrated into the healthcare delivery plans of the managed-care system. Telemedicine technology, telecommunication lines and networks, medical peripherals, and telemedicine protocols are continuing to be evaluated and updated. The telemedicine program is expected to be a strategic component for reengineering the healthcare delivery system at UTMB at Galveston.

Telemedicine: Practicing in the Information Age,
edited by Steven F. Viegas and Kim Dunn.
Lippincott–Raven Publishers, Philadelphia © 1998.

7

Organizational Telecompetence: Creating the Virtual Organization

Jeanine Warisse Turner and Casey D. Peterson

School of Business, Georgetown University and Department of Radiology, Georgetown University School of Medicine, Washington, D.C. 20057; and Department of Clinical Affairs, Texas Department of Criminal Justice Hospital, Galveston, Texas 77555

Many expectations have been formed regarding the impact of new communication technologies on the healthcare industry. Telemedicine promises to alleviate travel concerns associated with the delivery of healthcare, to bring specialty care to areas where none currently exists, and to improve opportunities for physician recruitment in rural areas. However, the introduction of a communication technology to an organization does not bring about these widespread changes in the environment without the organization acknowledging and addressing the changing processes and work practices required. These organizational changes take time. Although communication technologies are evolving and changing rapidly, the parallel organizational understanding of the human communication processes that must evolve to adopt and implement a communication technology is not keeping pace. Organizational change is necessary for the expectations of new communication technologies to be fully realized.

Little attention is given to organizational aspects of telemedicine implementation (1). In discussions of telemedicine, the focus is often on technology products. Attention is paid to the characteristics of the technological innovation (i.e., image clarity, transmission speed) rather than how easily the technology can be integrated within the processes of the organizational environment. The introduction of any technology into an organization involves the implementation of both product and process (2,3). The *product* refers to the technology and the changes to the technological infrastructure. The *processes* are the organizational goals and strategies and individual work practices that must change to adopt a new way of accomplishing tasks.

It is possible that the intense scrutiny given to the specifics of the technology, rather than the ways that the organization will be influenced by the technology's adoption, is due to the challenge of predicting the use of a tool that few, if any, within the organization have experience with. For example, how could someone anticipate how having a car that flies would influence his or her everyday life? Guesses could be made based on familiarity with aircraft and nonflying cars, but it is not until an individual actually uses the car to travel from place to place that he or she can understand how his or her life will be affected. Similarly, telemedicine introduces a familiar but totally new way of practicing medicine. In clinical teleconsultations, the physician may be denied physical touch as a means of gathering information or conveying intimacy. The physician may need to improve his or her verbal skills in instructing a healthcare practitioner or patient at the remote location to accomplish tasks. Distinct organizations and unfamiliar individuals must work together in familiar yet totally new ways.

This chapter explores how new communication technologies can influence and change organizations and the individuals working with them. This chapter also provides suggestions for planning for organizational changes so that new communications technologies can encourage familiarity and effective communication between organizations. Although *telemedicine* can refer to many different types of communication technologies, many of the examples in this chapter draw from electronic clinical consultations using videoconferencing technology.

DIFFUSION OF TELEMEDICINE

The initial decision to pursue telemedicine is often made by a small group of people within an organization. These individuals can be thought of as *innovators*. Rogers (4) described innovators as risk takers who have the ability to cope with a high degree of uncertainty about an innovation at the time of adoption. Innovators are responsible for launching an idea by bringing a new idea inside the organization. Innovators are often able to apply complex technical knowledge to an organizational problem. Keen (5) argued in describing teleconferencing technology that innovators are often focused on a specific technology with little reference to the current communication context in which it is being introduced. When the innovator is someone high in the organizational hierarchy, the innovation has a better chance of legitimate consideration by the organizational "agenda" than when it is introduced by a vendor or lower-level member of the organization.

However, innovators make up a small percentage of an organization (4,6). Rogers (4) described a second category of innovation users as *early adopters*. Early adopters comprise a more integrated part of the organization and can be opinion leaders for the rest of the organization. Organizational members often look to these early adopters for advice when considering whether to try an innovation. The *early majority* and *late majority* are the third and fourth category of adopters and often take their cue from the early adopters. The early and late majority members adopt an innovation as a result of increased pressure from the organization and from their peers. Finally, Rogers (4) described *laggards*, who are the last to adopt an innovation and who may never adopt. Laggards wait to adopt until the innovation is a proved concept.

Rogers' diffusion theory is helpful for organizations that are adopting telemedicine (4). This theory describes the audience of users that must accept telemedicine before it can be integrated within the organization. Often, the individuals who are instrumental in bringing telemedicine into the healthcare environment have a hard time understanding why other organizational members are slow to accept the idea. Although innovators are excited by the possibility of watching to see whether telemedicine will work, other members of the organization may need more proof before adopting. Still others may wait until someone whom they respect as a leader suggests that telemedicine is an effective method of delivering care. Rogers' theory emphasizes the importance of developing opinion leaders and champions in each of the organizations involved in the network (4). Rogers' theory helps organizations understand how individuals adopt innovations. Two additional areas that are important involve the organization's culture and elements that contribute to communication technology integration.

RECOGNIZING CULTURE

A culture is defined as the integrated pattern of human behavior that creates a goal-oriented environment in which individuals work (7). Every organization develops its own culture. In a telemedicine environment, a new culture is created made up of the distinct organizations involved in the network that share the common goal of integrating their own work practices to deliver healthcare. Telemedicine technologies, as other communication technologies, require cooperation between at least two different parties for communication to occur (8). A communication technology links individuals and organizations together, but use depends on collaboration and coordinated strategies by each of the organizations involved in the network. These organizations combine to form a virtual organization that is made up of the combined goals and practices of each of the organizations in the network.

Although each organization works within its own culture, these distinct organizations must find ways to work together for the good of the virtual organization. In strong cultures, the majority of organizational members understand the goals of the organization; whereas in weak cultures, the organization's beliefs and values are not clear and employees do not appear to work toward a common goal. One of the challenges in the management of a virtual organization is in the lack of clear goals and common structure. This challenge comes from the absence of personnel and organizational power, which is often reinforced by the conflicting cultures of each distinct organization. As people that work within the virtual organization have a first allegiance to the organization in which they are employed, the new virtual organization often has little power with which to make demands regarding telemedicine implementation. The virtual organization often takes a cultural back seat to the original organizations. Therefore, successful implementation requires that the leadership within each individual institution recognize the importance of cultural acceptance of telemedicine within organizational missions and strategies.

In some telemedicine networks, previously competitive organizations must work together. In these situations, it is important that the rationale to collaborate and cooperate be greater than the incentives to remain competitive. In spite of the best intentions, it can be difficult for organizations that have fostered cultures built on competition to work together toward common goals.

SUGGESTIONS FOR IMPLEMENTATION: BECOMING TELECOMPETENT

Warisse (2) described effective integration of a new communication technology by an organization as *telecompetence*. The construct of telecompetence explores the ability of the organization or the individual within the organization to be a competent communicator within a telecommunications environment. Warisse (2) recognized telecompetence in three dimensions: the technological, the organizational, and the interpersonal. Because the organizational dimension is most helpful in this chapter, discussion is limited to that dimension.

In examining telecompetence within the organizational dimension, Warisse (2) suggested that six elements must be considered: (a) rationale, (b) access, (c) expertise, (d) communication environment, (e) norms and rules, and (f) protocols. Each is important to implementation, and they can overlap.

Rationale

Rationale describes the importance of establishing a need for telemedicine implementation. This need should reflect the organizational strategy and mission. It can be helpful if this rationale is recognized by the highest members of the organization so that support and resources for implementation can be created. With telemedicine, a rationale must be established by each organization involved. Therefore, a needs assessment includes exploring telemedicine's potentials in each organization involved. In this way, the key individuals who are integral to the successful functioning of the virtual organization can be identified and involved in the early stages of the implementation process (9).

Tichenor and colleagues (10) underlined the importance of gaining input from key individuals throughout the organization in their emphasis on teamwork. Teams are comprised of members of each of the sites involved and can include technology coordinators, healthcare practitioners, and program coordinators. Each organization may not have the same reasons for participating. For example, a prison system may want to avoid inmate transports, while an academic medical center is interested in more efficient care mechanisms. A rural hospital may need access to a certain specialty, while an urban hospital may hope to gain patient referrals. Although different incentives may bring organizations together to implement telemedicine, it is important that a common strategy for implementation be developed.

Access

Access is usually understood as a purely technological issue. However, organizational access is also important. Organizational access suggests that each organization involved in the network is adaptable and flexible in coordinating with one another. In this way, a new organizational structure can be created to support the values and goals of the virtual organization. In addition, individuals within each organization need to believe that telemedicine is supported by their organization and be encouraged to extend the effort to spend time learning a new method of delivering healthcare. This effort may require the identification and development of opinion leaders within the various groups (e.g., nurses, specialists, technicians, administrators) who are associated with the success of the systems, so that telemedicine can be diffused and adopted as quickly as possible.

Expertise

Expertise describes the importance of developing evaluation tools and training curricula that measure the success of telemedicine within each organization and for the virtual organization as a whole. Early in the implementation process, each organization should identify key success factors that quantify an effective telemedicine program. These should be concrete objectives that can be easily measured. Instead of having a goal of a "successful telemedicine program," programs should describe specifically what success means (11). Success factors should also be identified by the key groups involved in implementation. This may mean developing physician, presenter, and patient evaluations. It could also mean tracking the number of consultations or saved transportation costs. The data gathered from these evaluation tools will contribute to the organizational expertise regarding telemedicine implementation. As the organization develops an understanding of what works and what does not, training programs can be created and distributed. This expertise can also be used to persuade groups and individuals within the organization who have not yet adopted telemedicine.

Often, training is limited to the specifics of operating the equipment. However, many telemedicine organizations have realized that training must also include preparing presenters for their role. For example, some of the healthcare practitioner presenters may have been trained in school to perform a neurologic examination but may not have used that skill for some time. In such a case, the development of training programs for the relearning of that skill may be necessary. Similarly, as a videoconferencing environment is different from the traditional doctor-patient encounter, consultants need to be trained in the new work practices, communication strategies, and protocols that accompany their new role.

An extensive telemedicine training program has been developed by the Georgia Statewide Telemedicine Program (12). This training program takes a three-pronged approach addressing the technology, operational protocols, and clinical needs of the new environment.

Communication Environment

The *communication environment* created by the networked organizations must support collaboration. The communication environment element describes the creation of the virtual organization. Members of each of the organizations involved in the network must have opportunities to share ideas and solutions regarding telemedicine implementation. These opportunities can be created through weekly or monthly meetings of the coordinators and key individuals from each organization. These individuals should represent the technological issues, as well as healthcare and overall management and coordination concerns.

A mission and strategy for telemedicine deployment for the virtual organization should be created so that priorities and protocols can be developed. To assist in this effort, each organization within the network should create a coordinator or point person to manage the telemedicine implementation within that organization. This person can conduct a needs assessment within the organization and develop an understanding of the benefits that telemedicine can provide. He or she can also serve as a point person to coordinate scheduling and operations. The coordinator plays a critical role in the diffusion of telemedicine within the organization by identifying opinion leaders who can help stimulate interest. Hiring personnel can be problematic during the early stages of telemedicine deployment, because smaller organizations may not be able to afford new personnel. In these cases, it may be important to designate a coordinator within the organization and then remove other responsibilities if his or her duties become overwhelming. Ideally, one overall coordinator should be designated for the virtual organization to serve as a point person and coordinator for each individual organization.

Norms and Rules

Norms and rules of how telemedicine should be accomplished by the organizations in the network must be created among the network members as they decide which procedures work best. Norms that may be acceptable in one organization may need to be reassessed. For example, in some organizations, the norm that physicians are not always on time for consultations may have developed. However, timely arrival of a specialty physician during a teleconsultation is critical. Not only is the patient kept waiting, but many other members of the virtual network can be inconvenienced. As telemedicine constitutes a new method of accomplishing healthcare delivery, understandings of scheduling, clinical evaluations, evaluative feedback, consultant recommendations, and so on must be developed. Some programs advise that network development start small. For example, it may be helpful to begin telemedicine with two or three sites so that norms and rules can be worked out before expanding into a larger network.

Often, norms and rules regarding telemedicine use are created by the innovators who propelled the program. These rules are not written down but are kept in the heads of those involved in the program. As new specialties and groups adopt telemedicine, however, the lack of written procedures and rules may make implementation difficult. Therefore, it is important to make these norms and rules explicit through the development of protocols.

Protocols

Protocols represent the explicit understandings of the practices that make telemedicine work among a networked organization. Some of these may be similar to protocols developed from other telemedicine programs, while others are unique to a specific context. Some specialties may need to develop their own protocols for specific clinical areas, including

1. Which patients should be referred for telemedicine?
2. What data should be available to the specialist before the patient is seen?
3. How should feedback be coordinated?
4. In what form should recommendations be made?

Other protocols may involve uses of the system, including

1. Which uses of the system will take priority in the face of a scheduling conflict?
2. How will staff be trained?

Telecompetent implementation of telemedicine within organizations requires attention to each of the six elements described: rationale, access, expertise, communication environment, norms and rules, and protocols. In this way, the goals and strategies of each organization, as well as the virtual organization, can be recognized.

CONCLUSION

Promises surrounding the implementation of telemedicine technology can only be realized through the efforts and collaboration of the organizations comprising the network. The creation and development of a strong culture supportive of telemedicine within the virtual organization requires a recognition of the values and goals of the new organization by all of the networked members. It also requires that a culture that is supportive of telemedicine be created within each of the organizations involved.

The six elements discussed promote the creation of a telecompetent organization whose culture is supportive of collaboration and use among network members. Attention to the processes and practices surrounding healthcare delivery among institutions can help to facilitate the creation of new practices that can support successful implementation of telemedicine.

Obviously, emphasis on the technological infrastructure is critical to creating efficient telecommunications connections. When the videoconferencing system cannot be turned on or the network is down, use is problematic. However, technical feasibility is just one step toward optimal use. Understanding and addressing many of the organizational elements that can influence use can create a culture of telecompetence supporting telemedicine.

REFERENCES

1. Whitten P, Allen A. Organizational structure in telemedicine programs. *Telemed Today* 1996;4: 28–29.

2. Warisse J. *Communicative implications of implementing telemedicine technology: a framework of telecompetence*. Ph.D. diss., Ohio State University. Dissertation Abstracts International, 57-10A. Columbus, OH: University Microfilms no. 9710679, 1996:4180.
3. Roberts K, Grabowski M. Organizations, technology, and structuring. In: Clegg S, Hardy C, Nord W, eds. *Handbook of organization studies*. London: Sage Publications Inc., 1996:409–423.
4. Rogers E. *Diffusion of innovations*, 5th ed. New York: Free Press, 1995.
5. Keen P. *Competing in time: using telecommunications for competitive advantage*. Cambridge, MA: Ballinger Publishing Company, 1986.
6. Bashshur R. Telemedicine in medical care. In: Bashshur R, Armstrong P, Youssef Z, eds. *Telemedicine: explorations in the use of telecommunications in healthcare*. Springfield, IL: Charles C. Thomas Publisher, 1974:15–40.
7. Deal T, Kennedy A. *Corporate cultures: the rites and rituals of corporate life*. Reading, MA: Addison Wesley, 1982.
8. Markus L. Toward a critical mass theory of interactive media. In: Fulk J, Steinfeld C, eds. *Organizations and communication technology*. Newbury Park, CA: Sage Publications Inc., 1990:194–218.
9. Dakins D. Innovative solutions propel program operations. *Telemed Telehealth Networks* 1996;2: 14–17.
10. Tichenor J, Balch D, Gutske S, Schecter A. Operational issues at the East Carolina University School of Medicine. *Telemed Today* 1996;4:28–29.
11. Leslie K. Searching for telemedicine's bottom line. *Telemed Telehealth Networks* 1996;2:30–33.
12. Adams L, Grigsby RK. The Georgia state telemedicine program: initiation, design, and plans. *Telemed J* 1995;1:227–235.

Telemedicine: Practicing in the Information Age,
edited by Steven F. Viegas and Kim Dunn.
Lippincott–Raven Publishers, Philadelphia © 1998.

8

Legal and Ethical Issues

Patricia Davis Blair, Alexandra Bambas, and T. Howard Stone

Center for Nursing Ethics, Law, and Policy, School of Nursing, Department of Maternal-Child, Program on Legal and Ethical Issues in Correctional Health, University of Texas Medical Branch at Galveston, Galveston, Texas 77555; Program on Legal and Ethical Issues in Correctional Health, University of Texas Medical Branch at Galveston, Galveston, Texas 77555; and Program on Legal and Ethical Issues in Correctional Health, Institute for the Medical Humanities, Department of Preventive Medicine and Community Health, University of Texas Medical Branch at Galveston, Galveston, Texas 77555

The development and use of new technology or new applications of existing technology have legal and ethical implications that arise subsequent to the use of such technology. Often, these legal and ethical implications themselves are not new but rendered so because their context may be new or changed. Such may be the case in telemedicine, in which the use of "electronic information and communications technology to provide and support healthcare when distance separates the participants" (1) alters the context in which healthcare services are provided. For example, is the standard of care for treatment transformed by telemedicine's affect on quality of care? Do health professionals who consult with distant patients through telemedicine assume obligations consistent with therapist-patient relationships? How is confidentiality, privacy, or informed consent assured through this medium of healthcare?

These are just a few of the questions colored by legal and ethical considerations. Rather than await the inevitable legal or ethical conundrum that may be posed by a particular case or controversy, this chapter reflects on considerations that most likely will perplex or should give pause to those persons who are involved in the uses of telemedicine. Some of the more significant legal issues are reviewed, including how laws are likely to be applied in analogous contexts. Ethical issues are also explored, with some thought to how adverse consequences that arise from the use of telemedicine can be anticipated and resolved.

LEGAL ISSUES

Telemedicine raises a number of legal issues, of which only the most perplexing are noted here. These issues are licensing, medical malpractice, and standards of care. Other issues that may not be as legally perplexing but are nonetheless important to consider are antitrust, confidentiality and privacy, and reimbursement. Although these topics by themselves are not new, the telemedicine context gives each topic an added dimension and therefore deserves examination.

Licensing

Licensing is possibly one of the most confounding legal issues raised by telemedicine practice. This is due in large part to the sovereign police power held by every state under the U.S. Constitution, Amendment X, to secure and regulate public health. It is pursuant to these police powers that individual states control the practice of medicine and delivery of health services through, for example, licensing regulations (2). Licensing is intended in part to protect a state's citizens from the unlawful or unauthorized practice of medicine. As each state is essentially free to choose how and under what conditions the state will license practitioners, no two states' licensing provisions in law or practice are the same.

Telemedicine, with its potential for greatly facilitating cross-state medical practice, confounds the ability of any single state to regulate such practice. National licensing that supersedes state licensing has been suggested, but commentators suggest that national telemedicine licensing would create constitutional conflicts between the states' rights and federal powers. Opponents of national licensing also contend that national licensing will hamper state efforts to protect its citizens and undermine local medical practice. Preserving state prerogatives to protect citizens and therefore regulate, as well as protect, medical practice appears to have significant support among medical and healthcare professionals.

Some states have already enacted laws regarding telemedicine licensing, ranging from laws that delegate to state medical boards the authority to determine the criteria for cross-state telemedicine practice to laws by which such criteria are set forth by the state legislature. For example, Chapter 5 of California's Business and Professional Code permits the state's medical board to develop a registration program through which physicians and surgeons licensed in other states can practice medicine in California, while the Texas Administrative Code requires a special purpose license, and similar legislation has been proposed in other states.*

National licensing is not, however, inherently unworkable. Practicing across state lines is already permitted for many medical and health professionals employed with federal agencies (e.g., the U.S. Veterans Administration, the Indian Health Service, the military), so long as the professional is licensed in any state (3,4). For these employees, however, constitutional law protects the federal prerogative with respect to federal

*See California Business and Professional Code, sec. 2052.5(a)(1), (2), and (b); Texas Administrative Code, sec. 174.3; Montana H.B. 513, 55 lh Reg. Sess. (Mont. 1997) (prohibiting telemedicine practice without a telemedicine certificate); Oregon S.B. 467, 69th Leg. Reg. Sess. (Or. 1997) (requiring separate license to practice medicine across state lines; provisions in S.B. 467 are based on the Federation of State Medical Board's Ad Hoc Committee on Telemedicine's Model Act to Regulate the Practice of Medicine Across State Lines); and North Carolina H.B. 814, Sess. 1997 (N.C. 1997) (requiring nonresident physicians practicing telemedicine to be licensed in North Carolina).

employees who might otherwise be restricted from using their state license to practice in another state. However, it is far from clear that national licensing for nonfederal professionals would ever be implemented. A more limited approach, such as the Federation of State Medical Board's Model Telemedicine Act, which includes a special limited license for telemedicine purposes only, may work in place of national licensing (5). The model act itself establishes no new regulatory or licensing agency and provides for a state's existing licensing agency to issue a special telemedicine license. The special license subjects the licensee to the medical practice act of each issuing state and to the regulatory authority of those states' medical boards. The special purpose license would be required of only those physicians who "regularly engage" in the practice of medicine across state lines.

As with any model act, a state's enactment and implementation of the model telemedicine act is entirely voluntary and subject to revisions. Whether any "national" telemedicine licensing scheme will ever be realized, much less made uniform, among different states is therefore quite uncertain. Incongruous as it may seem, the federal government may be the final arbiter over national telemedicine licensing. Constitutional law permits the federal government to regulate commerce that occurs *between* states, which in essence precludes state governments from doing so. Cross-state telemedicine practice clearly implicates interstate commerce, which in turn invites federal regulation. Additionally, federal regulation will inevitably result in the event telemedicine practice is reimbursed under Medicare and Medicaid. Although this does not imply that the federal government will impose a national telemedicine licensing scheme, federal reimbursement does suggest the federal government's ability, should it feel so compelled, to influence both practitioners and state legislatures with respect to cross-state licensing.

Medical Malpractice

Medical malpractice refers to professional misconduct that includes an unreasonable lack of skill or failure to execute professional or fiduciary duties that are owed to a patient (6). Such misconduct could include, for example, negligence in providing or failing to provide treatment, failure to obtain a patient's informed consent to treatment, or improper disclosure of confidential or private medical information.

Two of the most vexing questions concerning malpractice in the telemedicine context are exposure to malpractice liability when telemedicine practice transcends jurisdictional lines and whether a telemedicine encounter suffices to establish the requisite "professional-patient" relationship on which any finding of liability must rest. The short answer to both questions is "it depends." As it now stands, exposure to malpractice liability rests on the threshold issues of whether the telemedicine encounter involves a patient in one state and a clinician in another and how attenuated the telemedicine encounter is.

To compel a health professional to answer in court for alleged malpractice, a court must have personal jurisdiction over the health professional. Such jurisdiction may be difficult to establish based on a telemedicine encounter in which the consulting or treating health professional was physically located in one state and the patient in another at the time of the encounter. Courts are reluctant to impose personal jurisdiction absent, in part, the health professional's systematic or continuing contact or presence in the state (7). In the case *Prince v. Urban*, for example, numerous telephone consultations between a California patient and her Illinois physician, together with ensuing prescription refill arrangements made by the Illinois physician over the telephone, were deemed an insufficient basis to establish the California court's jurisdiction over the physician for purposes of making the physician answerable in that court to the patient's malpractice claims (8). Had the Illinois physician marketed his or her services in California, provided treatment to other California patients, or otherwise directed more purposeful acts in California, the result would probably have been different. Clearly, those physicians who have frequent telemedicine contacts in other states should expect to be subject to those states' jurisdictions in malpractice cases.

Exposure to liability also depends on whether a telemedicine encounter is sufficient to establish a professional relationship between the professional being sued for negligence and the patient claiming damages. The existence of a professional-patient relationship establishes the professional's duty to exercise reasonable care in treating his or her patients. Lack of a professional-patient relationship precludes such a duty and also liability for negligence. A professional-patient relationship "arises out of a consensual contract of employment . . . under which the patient seeks medical assistance and the physician agrees to render treatment" (9). Such a relationship may be established by the referral of a patient to a consulting physician, a formal consultation between two or more physicians regarding a patient, or a contractual relationship between a physician and, for example, a hospital under which the physician is on-call to provide consultative or supervisory services to other physicians regarding their patients. In fact, a professional-patient relationship may be established in the absence of any direct contact between a patient and the consulting or on-call physician. As the court in the case of *McKinney v. Schlatter* (9) found, so long as the physician participates in the diagnosis of the patient's condition, participates in or prescribes a course of treatment for the patient, and has an obligation to a hospital, its staff, or its patients for whose benefit the physician is on-call, a professional-patient relationship is established.

Although intuitively no different, malpractice claims brought by patients who are incarcerated in prison where telemedicine use is quickly expanding may in fact be quite dissimilar from "free world" malpractice claims. Logistically, prisoners may have difficulty proving compensable loss as a result of a health professional's negligence because such loss will usually be based on the prisoner's lost wages (almost certainly minimal) and future earnings (doubtful for prisoners without a well-established history or promise of gainful employment). Moreover, prisoners may have difficulty hiring expert, and expensive, witnesses—generally other health professionals—that are required in negligence lawsuits to testify as to the appropriate standard of care against which the defendant health professional's conduct will be measured.

Prisoners may also be foreclosed from bringing or prevailing on negligence claims against health professionals where such professionals are provided with immunity from suit or in jurisdictions that do not recognize that a health professional-patient relationship exists between a prison inmate and, for example, the inmate's treating physician.*

Case law, such as *McKinney v. Schlatter*, suggests that telemedicine encounters provide a sufficient basis to establish professional-patient relationships, including encounters that are a direct result of a referral or consultation regarding patient care, encounters that are at least as interactive as telephone conversations, and encounters that involve professionals who have contractual or other obligations to provide such services in these settings. All professionals who engage in telemedicine practice should assume that their telemedicine encounters impose on them at least the same obligations arising from a professional relationship as do their nontelemedicine encounters.

Standards of Care

Standards of care are essentially criteria against which a clinician's conduct pertaining to patient care is measured. Standards of care are used in medical malpractice negligence lawsuits to gauge whether a clinician charged with negligence conformed his or her conduct to the legal fiction of how a reasonable and prudent physician would act under the same or similar sets of circumstances.† Any applicable standard of care in a medical malpractice suit generally depends on the in-court testimony of clinicians whose training, skills, and experience establish their expertise to express opinions on such matters."‡ Establishing a standard of care particular to a patient's malpractice claim, such as the finding of a professional-patient relationship, is a prerequisite to holding a clinician liable for negligence.

There is no clarity with respect to the standards of care in telemedicine practice. This is not surprising because the widespread use of communications technology to provide or support healthcare over distances is relatively new, and there has been little opportunity for the development of standards of care. Additionally, no legal case has yet been put forth as sufficiently precedent-setting or influential to establish standards of care for telemedicine practice, a situation that may persist for some time. Changes in practice brought on by technological developments serve to render any future stan-

---

*See, for example, *Schmidt v. Adams*, 438 S.E.2d 659 (Ga. Ct. App. 1993), in which the Georgia Court of Appeals found that a physician assistant does not act within the scope of a traditional health professional-patient relationship when the physician assistant's primary concern and duty is the governmental function of caring for persons confined in jail. Id. at 660. The court stated that in making patient care decisions, the physician assistant acts in an official capacity, and is also therefore protected by immunity from suit under the doctrine of sovereign immunity. Id. at 660-61. See also *Ross v. Schackel*, 920 PI.2d 1159 (Utah 1996), in which the Utah Supreme Court found that prison physicians cannot be held liable for malpractice injuries in the absence of fraud or malice because prison physicians acting in a discretionary, official capacity as government employees generally have immunity from negligence suits. Id. at 1164; but see *Kagan v. State of New York*, 221 A.D.2d 7 (N.Y. App. Div. 1996), in which the court indicated that prison health professionals are subject to malpractice liability for failure to exercise professional judgment when, for example, the treatment decision was not based on intelligent reasoning or adequate examination.

†See *Helling v. Carey*, 519 P.2d 981, 983–984 (1974); see generally Zitter JM. *Standard of care owed to patient by medical specialist as determined by local, "like community," state, national or other standards* [annotation]. 18 A.L.R.4h 603 (1996).

‡See generally *Necessity of expert evidence to support an action for malpractice against a physician or surgeon* [annotation]. 81 A.L.R. 2d 597 (1995).

dards of care somewhat transient. Moreover, even when standards of care are established, health professionals may not always be cognizant of what those standards are or may simply choose—reasonably or unreasonably—to disregard those standards. To complicate matters, courts of law across jurisdictions are free to adopt different standards of care, which has often resulted in different verdicts for similar malpractice claims. Nonetheless, telemedicine practice over distances and across jurisdictions suggests that the conduct of clinicians who are charged with telemedicine malpractice will be measured against national, rather than local, standards of care.

In fact, a national standard of care for telemedicine has been suggested (10), one against which all clinicians working in telemedicine would be measured. Quite simply, the national standard of care would require that a professional who uses telemedicine in a particular care area possess the skill expected of a reasonably competent professional who uses telemedicine under the same or similar circumstances nationwide. It remains to be seen whether courts will adopt such a standard. But because courts will look to those who work in telemedicine to provide in-court testimony as to the applicable standard of care, it is essentially left to telemedicine practitioners to discern the level of knowledge and skill required of persons who practice telemedicine, to conform their own practice accordingly, and to expect that their telemedicine practice will be measured against a national standard.

ETHICAL ISSUES

Telemedicine represents a novel medical technique or practice environment and raises ethical issues centered around maintaining traditional aspects of medical practice. Among the humanistic ethical concerns raised by telemedicine, three are addressed here: (a) health professional-patient relationships, (b) confidentiality and privacy, and (c) consent to treatment. As with the legal issues discussed in the previous sections, these ethical issues in themselves are not new but pose fresh questions when applied to telemedicine. By recognizing, delineating, and exploring these issues, healthcare administrators, providers, and policy makers have an opportunity to create constructive responses to them through systems design, policy implementation, and training.

Health Professional–Patient Relationships

Concerns about professional-patient relationships in telemedicine arise primarily for two reasons. First, telemedicine practice generally enlarges the clinical encounter to include not only patient interaction with but also a strong degree of patient dependence on professionals outside the traditional physician-patient relationship, including persons at the patient's location and at a remote site. Many of these professionals, despite functioning in a therapeutic capacity, may be nonphysicians heretofore obliged under different ethical codes (or no codes at all) than those governing physician conduct. These professionals must therefore reinterpret their roles and obligations in light of expanded responsibilities.

Second, one of the most striking aspects of telemedicine is the removal of patients and caregivers from each other's physical presence—often over great distances. Although this feature provides the primary advantage of greater access to care, the distance itself can interfere with the therapeutic relationship as the laying on of hands traditionally has been an integral part of the physician-patient relationship and has played an important role in establishing trust between the two. Also, the introduction of vastly different cultures to each other can hinder the development of a therapeutic relationship in an environment in which little time is available to establish familiarity and meaningful contact.

The relationship between physicians and patients has always played an important role in therapy, especially in relation to the development of trust between patients and their physicians. If physical separation and distance between patients and caregivers retards the development of the patient's trust in the caregiver, the traditional relationship may suffer noticeably. It is therefore important to examine ways in which patient trust can be preserved in a telemedicine encounter. Changes in the professional-patient relationship because of telemedicine practice depend in part on how encounters are designed at particular institutions. For instance, consider a case in which a primary physician and patient in one location consult with another distant physician, a situation familiar to nontelemedicine encounters. Although two physician-patient relationships then exist between the patient and the presenting physician and between the patient and the consulting physician, *the primary* relationship typically resides between the presenting physician and patient. As the patient's primary physician, the presenting physician may have the long-term relationship with the patient, and therefore the patient would justifiably expect greater obligation within that relationship.

The more complex and novel situation involves the case in which a nonphysician caregiver presents the patient to a physician at a remote location. As mentioned in the previous paragraph, physical separation can prohibit some of the traditional methods of establishing and sustaining the physician-patient relationship. Besides the physician's inability to touch the patient, the disjunctive environments, as well as the technology itself (such as clutter or equipment failure), can adversely affect the ability of the patient and physician to establish a strong personal rapport and understanding. In this situation, the role of the presenting caregiver is the key. Hopefully, the presenter will develop either an independent therapeutic relationship with the patient, function as a physical surrogate for the consulting physician, or both.

As telemedicine becomes routine, nurses and allied health professionals will become more common as patients' primary caregivers. In those situations when a nonphysician caregiver is in the best position to establish a strong therapeutic relationship with the patient, that caregiver will need to be able to take on some of the responsibilities that have previously been reserved for physicians but have been increasingly represented in healthcare professionals' codes of ethics. Principles, such as patient-advocacy, beneficence, veracity, and confidentiality common in nursing codes of ethics, would be particularly useful in this context (11,12).

Medical and health professionals at both the patient's location and at a remote site can enhance the relationship by focusing on empathic medical practice, improving their listening skills, interpreting and using body language effectively, becoming attuned to other nonverbal communication, and creating an office environment that visually enhances communication and intimacy between the patient and consultant.* Visual cues, for instance, not only help a patient understand the mechanics of the encounter, such as knowing what the consultant is doing or who is present at the remote location, but also reveal interpersonal information, such as how the professional responds to the patient's comments or questions. The professional should present a comfortable, attentive image to the patient and should not be preoccupied or interrupted if possible.

Professionals should also be aware of certain communication patterns and techniques to enhance rapport during a telemedicine encounter. Because the presenting professional plays a central role in the encounter and may have a well-developed rapport with a consultant, the encounter may tend to focus on communication between the presenter and the consultant rather than between the patient and the consultant. This pattern of excluding the patient should be avoided. Questions that in a traditional setting might have been directed to the patient should also be addressed to the patient in a telemedicine setting. At a minimum, the consultant should always greet the patient and conduct a brief history to establish some contact.

Privacy and Confidentiality

Respect for patient privacy and confidentiality is essential to the long-term health of the professional-patient relationship. These are also important issues in the telemedicine setting, because they can potentially be breached in any of several ways: during the telemedicine encounter (including through taping the encounter); during transmission of information regarding the encounter over communications lines to the remote station; or when patient records and information regarding the encounter are stored, either electronically or on paper.

Because medical examinations often reveal highly sensitive information that can be communicated verbally, visually, or in other ways, it is important that the presenter indicate to the consultant the presence of all persons who are on- or off-camera and vice-versa, including other patients (especially when the examination room doubles as a patient waiting room), nonclinical technical staff, persons who have no therapeutic relationship with the patient (such as students), or persons who would not be present in a nontelemedicine encounter. This information appropriately limits or influences the circumstances under which medical information is disclosed by both patient and consultant to maintain confidentiality. Ideally, the presence of such external parties would be kept to a minimum as the disclosure of such information can be vital to proper treatment. But because it may not be possible or even desirable to permanently exclude these parties from the telemedicine encounter, other

*The literature offers excellent methods for improving interpersonal contact. One particularly useful approach is explored in Cassell EJ. *Talking with patients, vol. 1: the theory of doctor-patient communication*. Cambridge, MA: MIT Press, 1985; and Cassell EJ. *Talking with patients, vol. 2: clinical technique*. Cambridge, MA: MIT Press, 1985.

safeguards should be explored and implemented, such as asking nonessential personnel to leave the consulting or presenting sites for a period if the patient desires it or if the consultant believes it to be prudent. Additionally, monitor screens should be placed carefully so as not to allow passersby visual or aural information. Another method of preventing abuses and reducing errors is to develop meaningful confidentiality policies that apply to all staff and protect the rights of patients.

For the same reasons, a patient's consent to a taped examination should also be obtained; taped examinations should not occur without, at the least, prior disclosure to the patient. The taping of an examination for nontherapeutic purposes, such as for education or research, may be as easily obtained in cooperation with another consenting patient or through a simulated examination, and for these reasons should never be imposed on a nonconsenting patient. The subsequent use of such taped encounters must be restricted to their originally intended use and the audience for which the patient's consent was obtained.

Breaches of patient privacy and confidentiality can also occur during data transmission of patient medical information, such as radiology images, laboratory results, and so on. Although external interception of patient information from video or data transmission lines is considered unlikely at the time of this writing (13), it is nevertheless possible and therefore justifies that precautions be taken. Certain technical safeguards, such as encryption, can be used to help ensure that data obtained without authorization are neither translatable nor linked to identifiable patients. Using passwords and key cards to access patient records may also reduce threats to confidentiality. Transmitting patient medical information by facsimile presents another challenge, because human error can easily occur by either misdialing telephone numbers or receiving, storing, or both, faxes in unsecured areas. Many of these risks can be reduced by using automated dialing or built-in security features on the fax and by developing and teaching standardized security procedures, such as confirming receipt or nonreceipt of information (14). The main risks to patient privacy and confidentiality are posed by human errors, not technological ones, and the most serious threats to patient confidentiality result from intentional but inappropriate use of or access to confidential patient information by personnel with authorized access to such information. Stored information and records can also be accidentally or incidentally accessed, although again intentional access to stored information appears to pose more potential for serious damage (15).

As these risks cannot be completely avoided without sacrificing telemedicine altogether, the risks to patient privacy and confidentiality must be addressed in part through administrative devices such as training and policies. Training should apply to all staff and professionals and should be ongoing to reflect changes or new developments, and policies should be consistently enforced. To be effective, a policy regarding patient confidentiality should be addressed to the entire care team, including the traditional healthcare team physicians, nurses, and allied health practitioners, as well as technologists or other persons who may be involved in telemedicine encounters. Confidentiality agreements and education programs should similarly be geared toward both care and support staff to be effective, and these newest members of the expanded healthcare team may require specific education and training regarding the proper respect for and treatment of sensitive information.

Informed Consent

Informed consent is one of the cornerstones of responsible medical practice and applies equally to telemedicine practice. Patients always should be informed of and understand the risks and benefits of all treatments and agree to those treatments before those treatments are applied. The importance of informed consent for a particular treatment can vary somewhat according to the level of risks involved with the proposed treatment, the availability of alternatives, the expected benefits of the proposed treatment, and the consequences of not proceeding with the proposed treatment or its alternatives.

Insofar as telemedicine is one of an array of options involved in the medical encounter, informed consent to use telemedicine during the medical encounter may be necessary. Regardless of the general popularity of telemedicine among patients and providers, some patients may not feel comfortable with the technology. Patients obviously retain the right to refuse telemedicine without refusing treatment altogether, just as patients can refuse a particular treatment without refusing general care altogether. Separate consent for telemedicine may be appropriate for the near future, however, given the potentially increased risks to confidentiality of information, the lack of data regarding the effectiveness of telemedicine encounters, and the technology's unusual nature. Over time, if protective measures are further developed and telemedicine becomes routine, special consent may become less important.

To establish a high level of informed consent for telemedicine, the document should include certain information relevant to the patient's decision to use this type of encounter, including how telemedicine works; who will be present during the examination; known or potential risks to privacy or confidentiality of patient information, including institutional policies regarding instruction or the recording of the telemedicine encounter; and the consequences of refusal, including delays in treatment due to the complications of scheduling a hospital visit.* Regardless of whether an institution decides to incorporate telemedicine consent into a general consent document for care or to address telemedicine in a separate document, the issue should be approached consistently by referral to an institutional policy.

CONCLUSION

This discussion of the legal and ethical issues raised by telemedicine should by no means be considered exhaustive. Other legal and ethical implications are posed

*For articles on confidentiality in the telemedicine context, see Meux E. Encrypting personal identifiers. *Health Serv Res* 1994;29:247–256; Wemert JJ. Maintaining confidentiality of computerized medical records. *Indiana Med* 1995;88:440–444; Gilbert F. How to minimize the risk of disclosure of patient information used in telemedicine. *Telemed J* 1995;1:91–94; and Lawrence LM. Safeguarding the confidentiality of automated medical information. *J Qual Improve* 1994;20:639–646.

by the use of electronic information and communications technology to deliver healthcare over distances for which time and space constraints do not permit examination. This chapter provides an overview of some of the more perplexing, as well as confounding, issues. Some of these issues, such as those involving licensing, confidentiality, and the professional-patient relationship, may very well be settled by the promulgation of laws or the adoption of ethical standards. Issues pertaining to malpractice may become clearer over time as cases are developed and settled. Practitioners should come away with the understanding that although law and ethics may tend to follow developments in new technology or applications of existing technology to new fields, consideration of potential legal and ethical issues can help prepare practitioners for the inevitable conundrums that will arise.

REFERENCES

1. Committee on Evaluating Clinical Applications of Telemedicine. Institute of Medicine. *Telemedicine: a guide to assessing telecommunications in health care.* Field MJ, ed. Washington, DC: National Academy of Sciences, 1996:16.
2. Grad FP. *The public health law manual*, 2nd ed. Washington, DC: American Public Health Association, 1990.
3. Vibbert S. *Telemedicine sourcebook 1996–1997: a progress report and resource guide on telemedicine's growing marketplace impact: projects, players, policies and strategies.* 1996:25.
4. Notice of matching program verification of Veterans Administration professional licensure and registration records. *Federal Register* 1985;50:30, 327.
5. Ad Hoc Committee on Telemedicine. Federation of State Medical Boards. A model Act to Regulate the Practice of Medicine Across State Lines: An Introduction and Rationale. Federation of State Medical Boards, 1996.
6. American College of Legal Medicine Textbook Committee. *Legal medicine II*, 3rd ed. St. Louis: Mosby, 1995:8.
7. Bonelli DR. *In personam jurisdiction, under long-arm statute, over nonresident physician, dentist, or hospital in medical malpractice action* [annotation]. 25 A.L.R. 4th 706 (1983).
8. Prince v. Urban, 49 Cal. App. 4th:1056,1066; 57 Cal. Rptr 2d 181 (Ct App, 4th App Dist, Div 3 (1996).
9. *McKinney v. Schlatter*, No. CA96-05-100, 1997 Ohio App. LEXIS 544, at *6–7 (Ohio Ct. App. Feb. 18, 1997) (citations omitted).
10. Herscha L. Is there a doctor in the house? Licensing and malpractice issues involved in telemedicine. *Boston Univ J Sci Technology Law* 1996;2:8.
11. American Nurses' Association. *Code for nurses with interpretive statements.* Kansas City, MO: American Nurses' Publishing, 1985.
12. Fowler MDM. The nurse's role: responsibilities and rights. In: Mappes TA, Zembaty JS, eds. *Biomedical ethics.* New York: McGraw-Hill, 1991:157–162.
13. Oliver DW. Operational medicine: telemedicine—a paramedical and specialist tool. *J R Nav Med Serv* 1994;80:124–125.
14. Capen K. Facts about the fax: MDs advised to be cautious. *Can Med Assoc J* 1995;153:1152–1153.
15. O'Reilly M. Use of medical information by computer networks raises major concerns about privacy. *Can Med Assoc J* 1995;153:212–214.

Telemedicine: Practicing in the Information Age,
edited by Steven F. Viegas and Kim Dunn.
Lippincott–Raven Publishers, Philadelphia © 1998.

9

The Corrections Environment

Jeanine Warisse Turner, Michelle Gailiun, Kleanthe C. Caruso, Owen J. Murray, and Michael M. Warren

School of Business, Georgetown University and Department of Radiology, Georgetown University School of Medicine, Washington, D.C. 20057; Department of Medical Administration, Ohio State University Medical Center, Columbus, Ohio 43210; University of Texas Medical Branch at Galveston/Texas Department of Criminal Justice System Nursing Services, Galveston, Texas 77555; Department of Correctional Managed Health Care, University of Texas Medical Branch at Galveston, Galveston, Texas 77555; and Departments of Surgery and Urology, University of Texas Medical Branch at Galveston, Galveston, Texas 77555

Telemedicine technology has the potential to alleviate many of the problems faced by the delivery of healthcare to hard-to-reach populations. Growing at a rate of between 8% and 9% per year, the U.S. prison population constitutes one hard-to-reach group confronting complicated obstacles to receiving healthcare (1). Security concerns are compounded by the fact that corrections institutions are often located in remote, rural areas. Although complicated to deliver, healthcare is a constitutional right for prison inmates, making efficient and quality care an important concern (1). The use of telecommunications technologies can provide effective alternatives to augment the delivery of primary and specialty care by overcoming the constraints imposed on this medically underserved population. Although *telemedicine* is an umbrella term used to refer to any use of telecommunications technology in the delivery of healthcare, much of this chapter draws from experience gained from programs using interactive videoconferencing technology.

In addition to confronting some of the health concerns in the prison setting, the prison setting itself presents a unique environment for the exploration of the possibilities for telemedicine as a form of healthcare delivery. Without many of the barriers facing telemedicine within nonprison programs (i.e., credentialing and licensure issues), the prison environment offers a rich opportunity for studying telemedicine implementation and use, including a defined population, guaranteed clinic visits, provision of general as well as specialty medical services, and independence from the problems of third-party reimbursement.

The University of Texas Medical Branch (UTMB) at Galveston telemedicine program has consistently generated more inmate consultations using interactive video than any other telemedicine program in the United States, reporting a total of more than 7,700 consultations across 24 specialties as of February 1998. Ohio State University Medical Center (OSUMC) in cooperation with the Ohio Department of Rehabilitation and Corrections (ODRC) conducted 2,434 consultations across 15 specialties as of May 1997. As these two telemedicine programs illustrate, telemedicine within the corrections environment creates the opportunity for studying larger samples of patient and physician perceptions of telemedicine across a variety of specialties. This chapter explores the use of telemedicine by correctional organizations and discusses challenges to and suggestions for successful implementation in a corrections environment.

NATIONAL SURVEY OF STATES PURSUING TELEMEDICINE TECHNOLOGY

A 1997 survey of telemedicine activity in corrections programs in every state conducted by Gailiun (2) revealed more formally what many proponents already know: that there seems to be a natural "fit" between what telemedical technologies offer and what correctional healthcare systems appear to need (2). The survey revealed that 36% of state correctional systems have active programs under way, whereas another 22% are considering telemedicine. Just because the fit may be clear, however, does not mean that implementation of corrections telemedicine does not face many obstacles and challenges. Most programs have reported substantial problems in building familiarity and usage with the system, mirroring many of the findings in the private sector (2).

TELEMEDICINE SOLUTIONS WITHIN THE INMATE ENVIRONMENT

Decreased Costs Associated with Inmate Travel

Healthcare delivery within the inmate environment faces many complicated obstacles. One of the primary obstacles cited by prison programs is the issue of inmate transportation. A major contribution that telemedicine can potentially make within the corrections environment is to alleviate the cost of inmate transportation. These costs include the expense of inmate travel and the potential danger to society if an inmate escapes during a transport. The transportation process itself offers arguably the greatest opportunity for an inmate to escape as the ride to the medical facility is much less secure than the institution itself (3).

Transportation of inmates includes both direct and indirect costs. Direct costs consist of the cost of security officers and gasoline for vehicles, whereas indirect costs cover the vehicle maintenance and the processing and preparation of inmates for travel. Some healthcare delivery systems that treat inmates, such as the UTMB system, require overnight accommodations, as the inmates can be required to travel from as far as 850 miles away (1). Depending on the distance and resources, transportation costs can average from $100 to $300 per prisoner. Exact cost figures are difficult to estimate, as the total costs of healthcare per inmate depends on a variety of factors, including distance traveled, security of the treatment facility, mode of transportation, number of individuals involved in the processing of inmates, and the number of escort officers required.

In some situations, the healthcare practitioner travels to the institution or to a prison hospital to provide specialty care. In these cases, the costs of travel for the healthcare practitioner must also be included. Adding complication to the process, the scheduling of the patient with a specialty physician for further diagnosis or testing at an outside facility must not only accommodate the schedule of the physician but also the transportation schedule and the scheduling of security officers. Inclement weather conditions can force the cancellation of trips. These complications can create delays in inmate appointments, thus disrupting continuity of care.

Telemedicine can alleviate many of the costs of inmate transportation and processing by keeping the inmate within a secured environment, thereby eliminating travel expenses for the prison system and the healthcare practitioner. Some programs have found that interactive video teleconsultations provide a helpful means of screening patients so that they are routed to the appropriate specialty, and wasted trips can be avoided. Obviously, the telemedicine system itself brings with it a number of costs, including equipment, transmission, processing, and scheduling, along with initial costs accompanying the implementation of any new technology. However, many prison programs are finding telemedicine to be effective as a means to augment the inmate population's medical care.

Increased Access to Care

Access to appropriate care in a timely manner can also be problematic in an inmate population. Removing the challenges of transportation can create quicker appointments for inmate patients. Several studies of the use of interactive video as an appropriate means of improving access to quality care within inmate settings have had positive results (1,4–6). The OSUMC, in partnership with the ODRC, reported 88% appropriateness of telemedicine in an assessment of 131 consultations across 11 specialties over 1 year (6). Similarly, an evaluation of telemedicine appropriateness with 130 patients conducted by the UTMB program indicated telemedicine was found to be effective in providing care while reducing inmate travel (1). In many situations, inmates have been able to see a healthcare practitioner sooner with telemedicine than they would have if they had to wait to be scheduled through the normal transportation process.

Positive Patient Assessment

Surprising to many, the response from inmate patients has been positive. Two large-scale studies of patient satisfaction have been conducted. In a study conducted with 221 Ohio inmate patients within the OSUMC/ODRC telemedicine program, researchers found that patients were generally satisfied with telemedicine as a means of information exchange (7). The UTMB program also conducted a study of inmate satisfaction. The UTMB study of 647 inmate patients suggested that patients were satisfied with telemedicine as a replacement for traditional, face-to-face encounters (1). Although few other formal studies have been conducted, anecdotal evidence corroborates these findings.

In examining inmate satisfaction, it is important to remember the entire context of a medical trip that an inmate faces. A medical trip is not just a "get-out-of-jail-for-a-day-free card." The inmate may be gone for the whole day or several days, shackled and chained during the entire time he or she is away from the institution. Some inmates have said that being escorted in chains by security officers through academic medical centers is embarrassing and uncomfortable. Other inmates have suggested that they prefer telemedicine because they are afraid of many of the people that they have to ride with on the prison vans on the way to medical appointments (8).

Improved Communication Among Healthcare Practitioners

Telemedicine has improved communication between healthcare practitioners by potentially placing more members of an inmates' healthcare team in the "same room." For example, within the OSUMC/ODRC program, inmates left their home institution for specialty care and traveled to the academic medical center or the prison hospital. In doing so, the correctional physician responsible for primary care was limited in his or her contact with the specialist's recommendation to notes provided by the specialist on a consultation form and the memory of the inmate him- or herself. With telemedicine, however, the correctional physician can be present for the specialty consultation. In one example of telemedicine, the specialist is at the academic medical center while the inmate and the correctional physician are at the inmate's home institution. This configuration has several important implications for improving communication. Said one hospital administrator, "[telemedicine] hinders the inmate's ability to manipulate certain issues, by putting everyone involved with the patient's care in the same room. With a population that tends to manipulate and deceive, this is important" (9).

Telemedicine can also allow the correctional physician to observe the specialist's examination. In doing so, the healthcare practitioner at the institution can consult with and learn from the specialist. For example, observing and participating in several of the consults between remote dermatologists and prison inmates may provide the prison physician with the ability to conduct initial screening and diagnosis of patients with skin disorder complaints. Fred Schilling (10), director of health services for the Virginia Department of Corrections, underlined the important role that telemedicine played in educating healthcare practitioners located at the remote sites through a human immunodeficiency virus (HIV) clinic. Schilling (10) noted that he had seen the level of care improve for HIV-infected prisoners because of telemedicine. Although there have not been formal studies that documented a decrease in specialty referrals as a result of telemedicine, many individuals have mentioned this benefit anecdotally.

Additionally, the correctional physician can provide information to the specialist concerning the patient's history and some of the special considerations accompanying the care of inmate patients. Although most prison healthcare programs hire some healthcare practitioners within the prison system, many specialty physicians are often contracted from academic medical centers, urban hospitals, and other healthcare organizations. As a result, many times the individual treating the inmate is not familiar with the prison context. As certain treatments are prohibited within the prison setting (i.e., metal splints) and special protocols must be followed (i.e., inmates are not informed as to the exact time and date of their next appointment), it is important that correctional physicians have a means of communicating directly with healthcare practitioners outside of the prison system. Telemedicine can create this communication channel, thus improving the continuity of care offered to the patient.

Reduction of the Sense of Isolation Among Healthcare Practitioners

Another problem often facing prison systems is the sense of isolation experienced by healthcare practitioners. Not only are these institutions often located in rural areas, but the healthcare employees themselves are in isolated practice environments. Telemedicine can provide healthcare practitioners with access to colleagues and continuing education offerings at other medical centers. This access could improve recruitment of healthcare practitioners to correctional healthcare (3,6). Warisse and colleagues (9) noted one correctional provider as saying, "[t]his tool [telemedicine] has improved communication. We couldn't talk with specialists before, and now we can."

Multiple Medical Education and Administrative Uses

Many proponents of telemedicine argue that the key to making the technology efficient and cost-effective is by expanding use of the system from clinical uses to educational and administrative use (10,11). The corrections environment offers a number of administrative concerns that can be addressed by teleconferencing technology. Court hearings, parole hearings, and institution meetings are just a few of the uses that have been suggested (10). Florida is one of many states in which local jails are pioneering the use of videoconferencing systems to alleviate the costs, time, and expense involved in first appearance or arraignment hearings (2). Captain Robert Walla, jail administrator for the Charlotte County, Florida, sheriff's office, has found that using the videoconferencing system increases access for the disabled, making compliance with Americans with Disabilities Act requirements easier while allowing faster turnaround for cases in a secure, controlled environment (2). Walla has found that a judge can see 30 to 40 people in a morning using videoconferencing (2).

Continuing medical education has been found to be another important use of the technology by many institutions around the country. Healthcare practitioners are able to receive continuing education credits without having to take extended time off from work or incur expenses of travel to a distant location. In some situations, medical education has been tailored to the specific needs of certain inmate patients. In Ohio, custom in-service programs have been created and tailored to educating healthcare practitioners caring for inmates with special care concerns.

CHALLENGES TO IMPLEMENTATION

Although a strong argument can be made for the viability of telemedicine within the corrections environment, many challenges still prevent successful implementation. In fact, some programs have investigated telemedicine and ultimately decided against it.

Some of the primary challenges to implementation can be traced to a lack of incentives to participation. As telemedicine constitutes the implementation of a new technology and new work practices, use of this technology requires that organizational members take extra time to learn how to use it. Additionally, as it is a communication tool, it requires collaboration and coordination among individuals from distinct organizations that are not always accustomed to working with one another (8). Many individuals must coordinate and work together to create new procedures and practices for delivering healthcare. Nurses, physicians, security officers, and administrators must create new methods of scheduling, processing, and treatment.

Another challenge that can stem from lack of incentives is in the distribution of cost savings. As stated in Decreased Costs Associated with Inmate Travel, telemedicine can alleviate some costs of inmate transportation to healthcare facilities. However, it is important that the organization that exerts the effort also realizes the savings (9). For example, in the OSUMC/ODRC system, transportation savings are recuperated by the individual institutions that are participating. Therefore, there are considerable incentives to each institution to cooperate and work toward successful implementation, as dollars saved in transportation are realized in the institution's bottom line. In other prison programs, transportation may be handled by an overall administrative system that does not come through the budget of individual institutions. Therefore, efforts to implement the technology would not be compensated through savings to the institution, thus removing many of the incentives to implementation (9).

In some situations, prison systems do not want to invest in telemedicine until they can identify the total cost savings. However, a long-term and short-term evaluation of telemedicine must be made in assessing its ability to contribute to the bottom line, and these numbers are not always accessible. Increased continuity of care and improved communication among healthcare practitioners, though not readily quantifiable in specific dollars saved, contribute significantly to the total cost of delivering healthcare to inmate patients.

SUGGESTIONS FOR CREATING USE

Although implementation of new technology and processes can be overwhelming, several suggestions can be offered to potentially increase use. Obviously, many programs can be successful without following the suggestions provided; however, they may prove helpful.

First, before telemedicine can be attempted, it is important to have a commitment from the highest levels of the organization. Telemedicine requires collaboration and coordination from organizations with very different goals and objectives (8). In prison telemedicine, often a prison system must coordinate with an academic medical center. Therefore, it is important that the organizations involved share similar objectives and goals and that these goals are in line with the organizations' overall missions. Roles and responsibilities of various members within the program should be identified and described.

Second, some kind of needs assessment should be conducted among each of the organizations involved. In doing so, each organization can provide input into the pros and cons associated with telemedicine implementation so that problems can be addressed. In addition, a needs assessment can create a strong rationale for implementation and assist in persuading individuals from each of the organizations involved to participate.

Third, it is important to create an implementation team made up of members of each of the organizations involved. This team can develop a plan for coordinating implementation. The key individuals who are influential in carrying out the plan need to be informed of the implementation and the role that they will be playing. Incentives should be developed that provide additional motivation for participation. These incentives do not necessarily have to be in the form of economic rewards, as recognition and positive reinforcement can also be effective.

Fourth, it is important to develop evaluation tools for monitoring the success of telemedicine within a particular program. Each program is unique. Initially, a program should identify key factors that will indicate the success of the program and then develop measures for those. For example, if avoiding an inmate transport is important, evaluation tools can be created that enable transportation to be monitored. Some programs make the mistake of trying to measure too many things, creating long and complicated forms that are difficult to complete.

Finally, it is important to instigate a research feedback loop. Merely collecting the data is not helpful. A system should be put in place that shows organizational members how the telemedicine program is contributing to the healthcare of inmate patients. Therefore, report of evaluation findings should be distributed to organizational members on a regular basis so that changes can be made to the program when necessary.

CONCLUSION

There are as many reasons for justifying telemedicine within the correctional system, as there are challenges and obstacles that may impede its implementation. However, many programs have found telemedicine to be a successful method for augmenting the traditional method of healthcare for the inmate population. As corrections telemedicine applications continue to grow, a better understanding of the programmatic issues involved in the implementation of telemedicine across all system types can be achieved.

Acknowledgments

The authors wish to thank Heidi Bowers, telemedicine coordinator, Ohio State University Medical Center, for her help with the interview data gathered for the national survey.

REFERENCES

1. Brecht B, Gray C, Peterson C, Youngblood B. University of Texas Medical Branch-Texas Department of Criminal Justice telemedicine project: findings from the first year of operation. *Telemed J* 1996;2:2541.
2. Gailiun M. *National survey of telemedicine activity in correctional organizations*. Columbus, OH: Ohio State University, 1997.
3. Engleman L. Take two prisoners and call me in the morning. *Correctional Commun Q* 1995;April: 12–14.
4. Allen A, Scarbrough M. Third annual program review. *Telemed Today* 1996;4:10–17.
5. Allen A. UTMB-Galveston: in a league of its own. *Telemed Today* 1995;3:15–16.
6. Mekhjian H, Warisse J, Gailiun M, McCain T. An Ohio telemedicine system for prison inmates: a case report. *Telemed J* 1996;2:17–24.
7. Mekhjian H, Turner J, Gailiun M, McCain T. Patient evaluation of telemedicine consultations. Paper presented at the Western Speech Communication Association, Monterey, CA, February 1997.
8. Warisse J. *Communicative implications of implementing telemedicine technology: a framework of telecompetence*. Ph.D. diss., Ohio State University. Dissertation Abstracts International 57-10A. Columbus, OH: University Microfilms no. 9710679, 1996:4180.
9. Warisse J, Mekhjian H, Gailiun M. Interactive consults and practical benefits: measures of success extend beyond economics. *Telemed Telehealth Networks* 1996;2:44–45, 49.
10. Gilliland D, Liles R. *Report of evaluation study: telemedicine pilot project for the Michigan Department of Corrections*. East Lansing, MI: Office of Information Technology, Department of Management and Budget, 1996.
11. Dakins D. Innovative solutions propel program operations. *Telemed Telehealth Networks* 1996; 2:14–17.

Telemedicine: Practicing in the Information Age,
edited by Steven F. Viegas and Kim Dunn.
Lippincott–Raven Publishers, Philadelphia © 1998.

10

Military Initiatives in Telemedicine

Betsey S. Blakeslee and Richard M. Satava

Center for Total Access, Fort Gordon, Georgia 30905; and Department of Surgery, Yale University School of Medicine, New Haven, Connecticut 06510

The U.S. Military is recognized as the leader in telemedicine applications worldwide. Supported by substantial capital and human resources in research and development (1), a broad array of telemedicine tools have been developed from commercial off-the-shelf (COTS) technologies used in the Gulf War to Defense Advanced Research Project Agency (DARPA) telepresence surgery initiatives. From the simple use of electronic mail (e-mail) and the transmission of store-and-forward images using the plain old telephone system (POTS) to the development of systems that allow physicians to operate on patients at a distance, the military has explored initiatives that improve access to healthcare through the use of communications and information systems technologies. Reduction in capital and human resources and the realities of a changing overall military focus create a new context for the application of telecommunications, information systems, and bioengineering technologies in military healthcare systems. Three focus areas in military healthcare are undergoing dramatic restructuring and are driving applications in these technologies. These areas include (a) combat care for deployed soldiers, (b) day-to-day healthcare delivery services to soldiers and other eligible beneficiaries, and (c) operations other than war (OOTW).

The military faces the same challenges as the civilian sector in accomplishing long-term sustainability of these new healthcare technologies. Because of its early lead and substantial government investment in these technologies, the military can be viewed as a testbed for the civilian sector. The military provides the opportunity to learn from successes and continuing challenges. These challenges include the following:

1. Defining roles and responsibilities within the merging technical areas of telecommunications, informatics, multimedia, and bioengineering technologies
2. Bringing together the army, navy, air force, and marines into an integrated system
3. Integrating with civilian partners under triservice medical care (TRICARE) to provide day-to-day care for soldiers and beneficiaries
4. Operating under the constraints of reduced resources, resulting in the downsizing and merging of clinical resources

CHALLENGE OF INTEGRATION

Just as hospitals and providers in the civilian sector are consolidating and merging to create more cost-effective and efficient means for the delivery of healthcare, the military is bringing together the resources of the army, navy, air force, and marines into joint healthcare provider networks. Although the organizational cultural barriers to this integrated model remain significant, information and communications technologies are helping to provide the linkages necessary for successful long-term integration. Examples of programs developed to implement the integrated model include the following:

- Military Health Services System developed under the Office of Health Affairs of the U.S. Department of Defense (DoD)
- Theater Medical Information Program (TMIP)
- DoD Telemedicine Testbed
- TRICARE
- DARPA initiatives

Each of these programs attempts to bring disparate initiatives into an integrated system supported by a robust technical architecture. This architecture provides guidelines for interoperability that accommodates choice in the selection of various products and services. The architecture is compatible with the common operating environment (COE) of the overall military to assure seamless communications in the battlefield and sustain base operations. The need for the COE was underscored in the Gulf War when hospital ships could not communicate with evacuation aircraft or mobile army surgical hospital (MASH) units in the field. Each service developed its own proprietary communications and information systems, which is being restructured to achieve interoperability.

Problems with interoperability are not unique to the military. As the healthcare industry in the United States continues to consolidate in the wake of healthcare reform and increased competition, merged and acquired entities face the daunting task of achieving integration of their communications and information systems technologies. As the military moves toward seamless integration, it will likely set standards for the civilian sector. This is due to the sheer mass of its technical resources and the investment required by suppliers to meet military requirements. As the military continues to use more and more civilian sector healthcare entities for the day-to-day care of its beneficiaries, guidelines provided by a common technical architecture will be necessary to achieve a seamless military-civilian sector healthcare system. This underscores the need for more closely linked initiatives between the military and civilian sectors.

MILITARY HEALTH SERVICES SYSTEM

The Office of Health Affairs of the DoD has developed a strategic plan to achieve the interoperability of communications and information systems for military healthcare. This strategic plan includes the systems of the army, navy, and air force compatible with the COE. Known within Health Affairs as *Emerald City*, the strategic principles serve as the framework for the overall plan and include the following:

- Uniform data sets, processes, and standards
- Validation of process through prototyping
- Acceptable capabilities and ease of use, consistently presented
- Recognition of best value
- Centralized policy development and decentralized execution
- Incremental deployments that afford quick benefits
- Efficiency achieved by integrating common functionality
- Off-the-shelf products versus new development when possible
- Data entered once
- Infrastructure acknowledgments: interchangeable, interoperable, and transparent
- Comparable performance measurements across military and private sectors

These strategic principles support a structure that incorporates four major functional divisions: (a) executive information/decision support, (b) clinical, (c) logistics, and (d) resources (2). Coordination, consistency, and interoperability among these four functional areas are needed to provide the highest quality of healthcare to military personnel in times of war and peace.

Theater Medical Information Program

In support of readiness, the task of integrating healthcare information and communications systems is daunting. Not only must military medicine be compatible with the overall technologies used by the three services in times of war, the very nature of war itself is changing. In a post–Cold War era, the American military will be called on to provide for the national interest in a variety of geographic, climatic, coalition, political, and threat circumstances. In a paper published by the Association of the U.S. Army Institute for Land Warfare, Dubik (3) made a strong case for accommodating military strategy to accommodate a changing reality. He noted that U.S. strategic thinking has congealed around four concepts: Prevent and deter conflicts and win support in the international and domestic arenas. Current thinking suggests that the military may be involved less in traditional wars and more in OOTW. Often, OOTW require joint operations with troops from other countries, which presents another highly complex area for potential integration of systems.

To realize the vision of Health Affairs to support readiness within an evolving and dynamic environment, the TMIP office was established to focus on the specific actions required to achieve a fully interoperable communications and information healthcare system across all services. Representatives from each of the services lead integrated process teams in an effort to break the formidable challenge of integrating healthcare systems into manageable components.

Practical testing of integrated systems occurs at the designated TMIP testbed, the Center for Total Access (CTA) at Fort Gordon, Georgia. The testbed's primary purpose is to test the technical and functional efficacy of integrated systems to improve patient visibility and accountability, minimize evacuations, respond to trauma, leverage specialty care, and improve Command and Control (C2) situation awareness. The TMIP testbed uses the assets of CTA, Battle Command Battle Lab (Ft. Gordon, GA), the Regional Training Site-Medical, Dwight David Eisenhower Army Medical Center, 249th Combat Surgical Hospital, and the U.S. Army Signal Center and School. The Signal Center and School at Fort Gordon is responsible for establishing the Warrior Information Network and works closely with CTA to assure interoperability throughout the battlefield.

The first assessment of TMIP integration efforts took place in October 1996 and brought together systems developed by five entities across the joint services. The Electronic Theater Medical Record project, Version 1 (ETMR#1) demonstrated the ability to capture data at the point of injury and record it on an electronic dog tag, capturing the data as the patient moved through echelons of care. The ETMR interfaces with a patient-tracking system to track the patient at land and in the air during evacuation and placement in a military hospital in the United States (4). The plan is for TMIP to layer on existing and new applications over time, eventually building to a fully integrated system that is technically sound and meets the functional needs of providers charged with care of soldiers in war.

Department of Defense Telemedicine Testbed

The DoD Telemedicine Testbed was established to coordinate telemedicine efforts across the army, navy, and air force and to collaborate with other efforts of the public sector at the state and federal levels, as well as initiatives in academia, civilian healthcare networks, and industry. The testbed is composed of various sites that include the Center for Total Access at Fort Gordon; Akamai and the Pacific Medical Network at Tacoma, Washington; and Walter Reed Army Medical Center in Washington, D.C. The navy has funded 21 pilot projects from 1994 through 1997 and hopes to fund an additional $900 million for future telemedicine initiatives for connectivity from ship to shore. The air force initiative at Wilford Hall is focused on sustaining base desktop networking systems for providers. In addition, the air force is responsible for TRACES, the global patient tracking system. Additional research and development takes place at the Military Advanced Technology Management Office in Fort Detrick, Maryland, originally charged with overall management responsibility for the telemedicine testbed (5).

The activities being undertaken in telemedicine throughout the services include low-end store and forward systems and high-bandwidth systems for transmitting high-resolution images in real time. Some of these applications have been tested in deployed situations in Somalia, Honduras, Korea, Croatia, Macedonia, and Bosnia, providing valuable lessons. The deployment in Bosnia resulted in the transmission of more than 800 x-rays from the deployed MASH unit during the first 4 months of the operation. Lower use of telemedicine consultative services (28 in the same 4-month period) was due to three factors: Deployed troops were generally healthy and did not engage in hostile action, training and operational support was not adequate, and the systems experienced significant end-to-end downtime because of insufficient technical support and slow delivery of repair parts (6). Bosnia also provided lessons in the evaluation process of telemedicine as the military attempted close scrutiny of its systems and operations using evaluators in the field. As in the private sector, behavioral, training, and support issues were cited as in need of significant improvement and contributed to a lack of use of the systems.

In the military, there is a blurring of the distinction between telemedicine and medical informatics. Both technologies will be tested for compliance and efficacy under TMIP to ensure comparability and seamless integration of deployed and sustaining base operations. Focusing research, development, and acquisition into a cohesive plan between the three services remains an enormous challenge. To help ensure this integration, the management of the telemedicine testbed rotates between services.

Triservice Medical Care

To maximize use of the civilian sector to provide healthcare to beneficiaries, Health Affairs established TRICARE, a worldwide, health management organization-based, integrated healthcare system intended to serve beneficiaries in close partnership with the military. Contracts with major insurance providers have been established throughout various regions of the military and have highlighted the need for interoperability, not only between military and military entities but also between major carriers. Military providers, unlike their civilian counterparts, are allowed to provide telemedicine services across state lines and international boundaries. Some projects are happening with the civilian sector under TRICARE to test interoperability within states. The full realization of the potential efficiencies of the partnership will not be realized until the civilian sector can resolve the restrictive constraints of licensing and liability.

In anticipation of a fully integrated system throughout the military compatible with the civilian sector, the military has embarked on a triservice system to bring high-resolution video teleconferencing to the desktop of all military providers. The Medical Center (MED CEN) initiatives are being deployed throughout three major regions of the United States using COTS-based technology. The MED CEN network provides the backbone for telemedicine applications for military healthcare for the sustaining base and deployments. It is expected that TRICARE partnerships in the future will integrate with this system.

Defense Advanced Research Projects Agency

The DARPA mission is to develop imaginative, innovative, and often high-risk research ideas offering significant technological impact that goes well beyond the normal project development cycle and to pursue these ideas from the demonstration of technical feasibility through the development of prototype systems (6,7).

The systems that are being developed are setting the stage for the next generation of telemedicine. Based on the core principle that information is the key element for the practice of medicine in the twenty-first century, the technologies that are emerging are those that acquire information (sensors and imagers) for diagnosis, process information (medical informatics), and distribute the information (displays, teleconsultations) for therapeutic options. In addition, medical education is becoming information intensive (computer-assisted instruction, virtual reality). Thus, by reducing the practice of medicine to information handling, devices have been developed with the purpose of reducing casualties on the battlefield, as depicted in the following scenario.

> When a soldier is wounded, the body sensors, called the *personnel status monitor system* (which has global positioning satellite location, communications, and a suite of vital-sign monitors) alert the closest medic. Because the medic can see the casualty's location and vital signs on his or her hand-held medic unit, he or she can go immediately to the exact site. If numerous soldiers are wounded, by reviewing the vital signs, the medic can perform "enroute triage" and go to the most critically injured. The soldier can have an accurate diagnosis of internal injuries using a portable, handheld, three-dimensional teleultrasound unit (medical ultrasound and telemedicine package), which both displays the image for the medic and immediately relays it back to the MASH unit for physician interpretation. If the soldier can be stabilized, he or she will be placed in a life support for trauma and transport (LSTAT), which is a North Atlantic Treaty Organization stretcher that has an entire intensive care unit system embedded (i.e., ventilator, intravenous fluid administration, oxygen, suction, monitors, computerized medical record, and communication system). During evacuation, the soldier can be monitored, and, if necessary, remote instructions for change in ventilator, intravenous fluids, and so on can be given. If the soldier will hemorrhage to death before he or she can be evacuated, the medic can place the soldier in a mobile medical forward area surgical telepresence unit (an armored ambulance with an operating room and robotic hands with a controlling surgical workstation located in the rear echelon MASH unit). Together, the medic and remote surgeon will do just enough surgery to stop the hemorrhage ("damage control" surgery). The casualty will then be placed into the LSTAT and safely evacuated back to the MASH unit, where the surgeon can complete the operation. All of this far-forward care (for civilians, it is point-of-care) is only possible by and is totally dependent on the flow of information under the guidance of a sophisticated computerized medical record and telemedicine communications system.

The systems described in the preceding paragraph exist in the beta prototype phases, being completely validated during military field training exercises. The systems are undergoing stringent evaluation through animal and then appropriate human-use testing as U.S. Food and Drug Administration (FDA) approval is sought. Technically, the systems are being refined into final products, and manufacturing processes are being developed, completing the technology-transfer process. It is anticipated that commercial products will be available in 1999 to 2002, depending principally on the speed of the FDA approval process. Other even more advanced systems are under exploratory development.

DISCUSSION

Telemedicine and medical informatics are merging in medicine as in every other industry. The mainframe model of computers has given way to a networked model contributing to an artificial construct between telemedicine and information systems. The military has major integration challenges associated with having viewed telemedicine and information systems as separate entities with their own organizational constructs, funding, and methodologies. Less time is being spent on *defining* these technologies, and more time on actually *using* them as inseparable and integrated tools for the delivery of healthcare. Once again, the merger of the technologies is happening faster than the organizational entities' capacity to transform the organizational culture, a challenge shared in both the military and civilian sectors.

The military is committed to reengineering healthcare systems through the use of telecommunications and information technologies. Significant challenges lie ahead as outlined in a U.S. General Accounting Office (GAO) report (1). The key goals identified by the GAO to ensure that substantial government investments in military telemedicine and informatics result in increased access to healthcare, improved quality of healthcare, and reduced costs of healthcare for the military, include the following:

- Clearly define the scope of telemedicine in the DoD.
- Establish DoD-wide goals and objectives and identify actions and appropriate milestones for achieving them.
- Prioritize and target near- and long-term investments, especially for goals related to combat-casualty care and OOTW.
- Clarify roles of DoD oversight organizations.

To achieve these goals, specific objectives have been established resulting in assigned deliverables to the various entities involved in telemedicine throughout the military. These deliverables include the following:

- Identify a federal strategy to establish near- and long-term goals and objectives for military telemedicine.
- Establish a means to formally exchange information or technology among the federal government, state organizations, and private sector.
- Identify needed technologies that are not being developed in the public or private sector.
- Promote interoperable system designs that would enable telemedicine technologies to be compatible, regardless of where they are developed.
- Encourage adoption of appropriate standardized medical records and data systems so that information can be exchanged among sectors.
- Overcome barriers so that investments lead to better healthcare.
- Encourage federal agencies and departments to develop and implement individual strategic plans to support national goals and objectives.

There is much work to be done within the federal government and the military to bring together initiatives in telemedicine, medical informatics, and bioengineering to capitalize on significant capital and human resource expenditures. Structures exist to make this integration happen. Although the military has made progress in integration, organizational-cultural issues between military entities remain the greatest barrier to successful accomplishment of the mission.

REFERENCES

1. US General Accounting Office. *Telemedicine: federal strategy is needed to guide investments.* GAO/NSIAD/HEH, 1997:97–67;3.
2. Office of Health Affairs, US Department of Defense. *Military Health Services System information management/information technology strategic plan.* Defense Technical Information Center, 1996.
3. Dubik J. Sacred cows make good shoes: changing the way we think about military force structure. *AUSA Landpower Essay Series* 1997;Feb(#97–1):7.
4. Office of Health Affairs, US Department of Defense. *Theater Medical Information Project management plan. Version 2.1.* Defense Technical Information Center, 30 May 1996.
5. Zajtchuk J, Zajtchuk R. Strategy for medical readiness: transition to the digital age. *Telemed J* 1996; 2:179–186.
6. Satava RM. Surgery 2001: a technologic framework for the future. *Surg Endosc* 1993;7:111–113.
7. Satava RM. Speculation on future technology. In: Hunter JG, Sackier JE, eds. *High tech surgery. New approaches to old diseases.* New York: McGraw-Hill, 1993:339–347.

Telemedicine: Practicing in the Information Age,
edited by Steven F. Viegas and Kim Dunn.
Lippincott–Raven Publishers, Philadelphia © 1998.

11

Aerospace Medicine

Jeffrey R. Davis

Departments of Preventive, Occupational, and Environmental Medicine, University of Texas Medical Branch at Galveston, Galveston, Texas 77555

Aerospace medicine is one of three specialty areas of preventive medicine that is concerned with the health, safety, and performance of pilots, crew members, and ground support personnel for a variety of aircraft and spacecraft. The field of aerospace medicine is diverse and covers a broad spectrum of health concerns from toxic exposures due to the aerial application of pesticides to the dramatic changes in human physiology associated with long-term exposure to microgravity or weightlessness.

Aerospace medicine is practiced in multiple environments such as civil aviation, military aviation, and space flight. These environments have very different missions and subsequent health risks that lead to very different demands for telemedicine services. This chapter highlights examples of the uses of telemedicine in all of these environments.

CIVIL AEROSPACE MEDICINE

Civil aerospace medicine covers the environments of general, corporate, and commercial aviation and aeromedical evacuation services. The topics that are addressed include pilot medical certification and electronic medical records, passenger health and in-flight medical emergencies, and aeromedical evacuation.

Pilot Medical Certification and Electronic Medical Records

Licensed pilots must carry either a first-, second-, or third-class medical certificate from the U.S. Federal Aviation Administration (FAA) to be permitted to pilot an aircraft (1). This certificate is obtained after a medical examination by a certified aviation medical examiner (AME). Since 1996, the FAA has required the electronic transfer of electrocardiograms (ECGs) and is phasing in electronic medical records.

Pilots who must carry a first-class medical certificate (i.e., airline transport pilot) and who are older than the age of 35 years must have an ECG performed at age 35 years and annually after age 40 years (1). The FAA requires the electronic transmission of the

ECG; therefore, the physician who performs the examination must have access to appropriate equipment. The FAA reviews the ECG along with the physical examination to determine any need for additional testing or medical evaluation. This system was developed to improve the quality of the ECGs submitted to the FAA and to enhance the accuracy of review and diagnosis when determining a pilot's medical qualifications.

At one time, there were more than 6,000 physicians who performed aviation medical examinations for the FAA as AMEs. Many of these examiners performed fewer than 25 examinations each year, and, of the 25 examinations, many did not require an ECG. When the FAA introduced the requirement for the electronic transmission of ECGs, many AMEs did not purchase the necessary equipment as the cost could not be recovered by performing so few examinations; this reduced the number of AMEs performing aviation medicine examinations.

The FAA also implemented the electronic transmission of medical records through the Aeromedical Certification Subsystem (AMCS). This requirement was gradually phased in until the electronic transmission of most examinations was required. Only examinations that require detailed specialty examinations for certification, called *special issuance examinations*, are transmitted with paper files. The AMCS requires an IBM-compatible computer and software, as well as a modem.

The AMCS system replicates Form 8500, the FAA-required medical history and physical form. The form accepts only certain default limits in some fields (such as vision and hearing) and will not permit the transmission of a record with obviously incorrect information. This system has significantly reduced the errors committed in the history and physical forms that had previously required manual checking to ensure accuracy and quality. Overall, this system has improved the accuracy of the examinations, speed of transmission, and review by the FAA. The FAA focuses on cases that need special attention rather than manually reviewing thousands of essentially normal history and physical examinations.

Passenger Health and In-flight Medical Emergencies

The number of in-flight medical emergencies on commercial aircraft has been steadily growing since the early 1990s through data reported by several domestic and international carriers at a meeting of the Airlines Medical Directors, May 1997. Contributing factors have included the rapid expansion of commercial airline service during the 1980s and a growing number of international passengers. International airline traffic is projected to grow at a 5% to 6% annual rate (2). It is estimated that eight to ten medical emergencies occur every day on U.S. airlines; two to three emergencies each day require the aircraft to declare an emergency and land at the first available airport to evacuate the passengers (3). In-flight deaths have been estimated to occur at rates from 0.5 to 1.0 per 1 million passengers (4). Using U.S. Department of Transportation (DOT) data from 1995, 540 million passengers were carried on U.S. airlines. The estimated number of in-flight deaths may be as high as 250 to 500 per year using the in-flight death rate (4) and the DOT data. The medical director of Qantas Airlines estimates that 500 to 1,000 deaths may occur worldwide (5).

These statistics are leading to a growing awareness that the available level of in-flight medical care may be inadequate. The FAA reviewed the reported types and numbers of in-flight medical emergencies and is currently determining the need for any changes in required medical services.

The FAA established requirements for in-flight medical kits in 1986 and required the airlines to report in-flight medical emergencies from 1986 to 1988. The summary data by Hordinsky (6) showed that cardiovascular emergencies were the most common emergency. The most frequently used medical kit items were the blood pressure cuff, stethoscope, and nitroglycerin tablets. Independent data reported by several airlines at a scientific meeting of the Airlines Medical Directors, May 1997, confirmed that cardiovascular emergencies are the most common and account for slightly more than 50% of all in-flight medical emergencies. Published data from Qantas and United Airlines further support the assertion that cardiovascular emergencies are the most common (2,3).

The FAA-required medical kit on commercial aircraft does not include a defibrillator nor does it include medications and equipment to conduct advanced cardiac life support (ACLS) protocols. One international carrier, Qantas, began flying semiautomatic defibrillators in 1992 and has reported several successful conversions (2). The defibrillators have also been used to monitor the cardiac status of patients on Qantas flights. In late 1996, American Airlines announced that they would equip their long-haul aircraft with semiautomatic defibrillators, becoming the first U.S. domestic airline to do so.

Telemedicine support of in-flight medical emergencies has been limited to voice-only consultations with a physician. Some airlines provide this real-time consultation through internal medical departments, whereas others use services that provide voice consultations with emergency department physicians. These services are often supplemented by a database that includes the location of airports near appropriate emergency medical facilities should the aircraft need to make an emergency landing for medical reasons. Results have been reported by Med Aire, Inc., a medical contract service, that indicate the service lowered the rate of diversions for medical reasons by providing real-time emergency medical advice (7). These reports have not been methodically studied, yet it seems likely that the provision of real-time telemedicine consultation and monitoring should be able to reduce the number of medical diversions and possibly the number of in-flight deaths.

Some U.S. airlines are evaluating portable devices that downlink basic vital signs and ECGs via existing air-to-ground phone service (air phones). These trials are in development at the time of this writing and are not in operational use.

Future developments for the commercial airline industry may include expanding the basic medical kit to include ACLS medications and equipment; semiautomatic defibrillators; and some complement of telemedicine monitoring equipment for vital signs, arterial oxygen saturation, and ECGs. The debate in the commercial airline industry involves the cost of the equipment and services versus the perceived improvement in care and medical outcomes. Equipment that provides treatment and monitoring capability for vital signs, arterial oxygen saturation, and ECGs is in use or under flight development in military aviation.

Aeromedical Evacuation

There are many air ambulance services providing aeromedical evacuation in the United States. One provider, the Mayo Clinic, is highlighted as an example of the expanding use of telemedicine services. Mayo Medical Air Services provides aeromedical evacuation services for the Mayo clinics located in Rochester, Minnesota. This system is a comprehensive network of ambulances, helicopters, and fixed-wing aircraft established to transport serious medical emergencies to the Mayo clinics for treatment. To support this medical transportation system, the Mayo clinics implemented an extensive T1 network with more than 90 T1 lines.

The Mayo Clinic has several developmental projects in telemedicine, as reported by Dr. David Claywood during the U.S. Air Force Aeromedical Evacuation Telemedicine Technology Exposition in January 1997. These projects include the Asinc Project-2 that evaluates the feasibility of physiologic data transmission, digital photography, and information management via a 900-MHz radio system. To facilitate transmission of data, future broad-band satellite communications will be required. Evaluation of the quality and effectiveness of care, as well as the costs, will be a part of this study. For commercial aviation, a demonstration project is planned with a U.S. domestic airline.

Licensing and Malpractice

With the rapid spread of telemedicine services into commercial and corporate aviation and aeromedical evacuation services, issues of licensing, malpractice, and liability need to be addressed. In commercial aviation, industry practice has been to page for a physician in the event of a medical emergency. The flight may or may not successfully establish voice or other communications capability with ground medical services. For the on-board physician, there is no federal Good Samaritan act, and it is unclear which state law, if any, would apply to the medical emergency. If communication is established with a ground-based consulting medical service, the law is unclear if a physician in one state may provide care and accept liability for a patient flying over another state. Some states have passed laws prohibiting the provision of medical care to a patient in one state by a provider in another state via telemedicine services (8). There are no provisions for determining the appropriate state licensure that a physician must obtain to provide medical consultations for in-flight medical emergencies. The issues of licensure, malpractice insurance, and patient treatment across state borders will need to be resolved before widespread acceptance of in-flight medical care via telemedicine is possible.

MILITARY AEROSPACE MEDICINE

The U.S. Army flies UH-60 Blackhawk helicopters that are equipped with defibrillators and telemedicine monitoring equipment. No interference with aircraft avionics has been demonstrated with either the monitoring equipment or in-flight defibrillation. Monitoring equipment is flown that can monitor a five-lead ECG, blood pressure, pulse oximeter, end-tidal carbon dioxide, and temperature.

The U.S. Air Force has pursued a demonstration project for fixed-wing aeromedical evacuation aircraft called *Global Yankee* (reported by Dan Hague at the U.S. Air Force Aeromedical Evacuation Telemedicine Technology Exposition in January 1997). A suite of telemonitoring equipment has been evaluated that transmits ECG tracings, blood pressure, pulse oximeter and temperature readings, and electronic records. The Global Yankee project used low-bandwidth, line-of-site UHF transmission at 4,800 bits per second. In a 1-hour period, successful transmission occurred of two ECGs (one-lead), 47 sets of vital signs, and two electronic forms. The automatic integration and downlink of this information required three laptop computers to coordinate. A next generation study will evaluate the use of satellite transmission technology and more ECG leads.

The U.S. Navy has experimented with telesurgery to reduce the required number of aeromedical evacuations from ships deployed at sea. In 1996, seven operations were successfully carried out with teleconsultation, none of which required subsequent aeromedical evacuation (reported at the U.S. Air Force Aeromedical Evacuation Telemedicine Technology Exposition in January 1997). Further developments of this type will improve the operational capability of the fleet and reduce the operational impact of on-board medical emergencies.

SPACE MEDICINE

Telemedicine has been practiced in the U.S. Space Program since the inception of the program. The first Mercury flights in the 1960s provided telemetry of the ECG to the ground to monitor the cardiac stress level of the astronauts. In the intervening years, however, little emphasis was placed on real-time telemetry capability for providing medical care to astronauts in flight, in part due to the concern for privacy of the medical data. From the surface of the moon, telemetry of the ECG signal was monitored during extravehicular activities (EVAs), or space walks. During Apollo XV, one of the astronauts developed a cardiac dysrhythmia that heightened concern about the effects of spaceflight on the cardiovascular system (9).

In the Space Shuttle program, ECG data were routinely monitored during launch and landing and during EVAs. Monitoring of the ECG during launch and landing was discontinued before the Challenger accident in 1986, but EVA monitoring continued. Several types of dysrhythmias were noted during EVAs, most notably an episode of ventricular bigeminy; however, no monitored dysrhythmia has caused the termination of an EVA (9).

Medical care has been provided to astronauts via private air-to-ground links during all spaceflight missions. During the private medical conferences (PMCs), the astronauts can report their medical condition and seek advice from a physician (flight surgeon) in mission control (9). The majority of conferences during short-duration flights dealt with treatment of space motion sickness (SMS) as 70% of first-time Shuttle astronauts experienced some symptoms (10). The PMC is used to advise treatment and monitor its effectiveness. The availability of the PMC resulted in the successful treatment of SMS via intramuscular injections with promethazine (11).

More extensive telemedicine capabilities are being explored for future space station and planetary missions. The medical care systems for space stations have been designed to include an array of in-flight emergency and ambulatory medical equipment. Examination, laboratory, and physiologic data are all planned for downlink via satellite technology (9). Monitoring of physiologic data via satellite will continue during the performance of EVAs. Telepresence for diagnosis, surgery, or both is also in planning to back up the onboard medical officer with the goal of avoiding mission termination and aeromedical transport to earth (9). Much greater in-flight capability is envisioned, since aeromedical transport may take up to 24 hours from the space station, 3 days from the moon, and is impossible from Mars. The transit time of radio waves from Mars makes real-time telemedicine impossible, and the crew of a planetary mission will have to provide initial medical care followed by medical review and consultation from earth-based physicians.

CONCLUSION

This chapter provides a brief overview of the applications of telemedicine technology and services in aerospace medicine. Many applications are developmental, with quality, value, cost, and liability issues to be resolved. Commercial applications are likely to benefit from spaceflight and military development as these missions will drive technology and service solutions. Solutions from spaceflight and military environments may well provide the developmental testbed for commercial applications, permitting a faster entry of telemedicine services into the practice of commercial and private aerospace medicine.

REFERENCES

1. Federal Aviation Regulations. Medical Standards and Certification. *Code of Federal Regulations* 1996 August:Title 14(Pt 67).
2. Donaldson E, Peran J. First aid in the air. *Aust N Z J Surg* 1996;66:431–434.
3. Cottrel JJ, Callaghan JT, Kohn GM, Hensler EC, Rogers RM. In-flight medical emergencies. One year of experience with the enhanced medical kit. *JAMA* 1989;262:1653–1656.
4. Speizer C, Rennie CJ, Breton H. Prevalence of in-flight medical emergencies on commercial airlines. *Ann Emerg Med* 1989;18:26–29.
5. O'Rourke M, Donaldson E. Management of ventricular fibrillation in commercial airliners [Letter]. *Lancet* 1995;345:515–516.
6. Hordinsky JR, George MH. Response capability during civil air carrier in-flight medical emergencies. *Aviat Space Environ Med* 1989;60:1211–1214.
7. Garrett, JS. Southwest, Hawaiian airlines are now flying with MedLink. *Healthwatch, Med Aire, Inc. Newsletter* 1997;Fall:5.
8. Jones TL. Don't cross that line. Texas telemedicine law stirs up national debate. *Tex Med* 1996; 92:28–32.
9. Nicogossian AE, Huntoon CL, Pool SL. *Space physiology and medicine*, 3rd ed. Philadelphia: Lea & Febiger, 1994.
10. Davis JR, Vanderploeg JM, Santy PA, Jennings RT, Stewart DF. Space motion sickness during 24 flights of the space shuttle. *Aviat Space Environ Med* 1988;59:1185–1189.
11. Davis JR, Jennings RT, Beck BG, Bagian JP. Treatment efficacy of intramuscular promethazine for space motion sickness. *Aviat Space Environ Med* 1993;64(3 Pt 1):230–233.

Telemedicine: Practicing in the Information Age,
edited by Steven F. Viegas and Kim Dunn.
Lippincott–Raven Publishers, Philadelphia © 1998.

12

Evolutionary Design of the University of Texas Medical Branch Telemedicine System

*Jake G. Angelo, Michael B. Moore, *Tom K. Epley, III,
*Oliver M. Black, William S. Crump, and Rosa A. Tang

**Department of Information Services, University of Texas Medical Branch at Galveston, Galveston, Texas 77555; Department of Cardiovascular and Thoracic Surgery, Abilene Regional Medical Center, Abilene, Texas 79606; Department of Family Medicine, University of Texas Medical Branch at Galveston, Galveston, Texas 77555; and Department of Ophthalmology and Visual Sciences, University of Texas Medical Branch at Galveston, Galveston, Texas 77555*

The basic system used in the University of Texas Medical Branch (UTMB) at Galveston/Texas Department of Criminal Justice (TDCJ) telemedicine program is based on Compression Labs, Inc.'s (CLI) San Jose, California, Radiance conferencing system. The decision to use the radiance conferencing system was based on two test projects.

FIRST TEST PROJECT

Setup

In the first project, a testbed was set up for a 3-month test period. The testbed was a third-party integrator system specially developed for telemedicine. The system was subject to being moved once a month to three testbed sites: a public health clinic, a rural hospital, and another university. The network was a direct connect with manual patching via an RJ45 patch panel.

Results

Physicians were pleased with the video and audio quality; however, connect time from site to site took far too long and reliability of the system was not the greatest. The integrator's use of inferior equipment and poor construction made system breakdown a common occurrence. More reliability and a faster switching network were needed.

SECOND TEST PROJECT

The second testbed was the first TDCJ test. Requests were sent to several vendors to supply UTMB with five systems for a 90-day trial. One consultant site and four remote sites were designated.

Setup

The system installed consisted of the CLI radiance system with a computer integrated to the AMX for control. Video was fed to capture cards and captured in the computer and displayed on a 21-in. video monitor. Additionally, two 27-in. monitors displayed local and far-end video. A stethoscope was provided with an equalizer and an audio digitizer to convert the audio to data to be sent to the consultant site via a high-speed internal data port. The system used a fully remote control, three-chip camera for high-resolution color accurate imaging and a 16× lens for tight-zoom capability. There was also a document camera provided for sharing of documents and x-rays via video. A dial-up modem provided technicians with access for diagnostics and remote programming.

All telemedicine rooms were painted a light bluish-gray, as this lends itself to a color-accurate image with good definition. Additionally, light fixtures were added with special fluorescent tubes with a 3,500-degree color temperature to match the cameras. The network was again direct connect, but with a multipoint control system to switch from site to site. A terminal program was used with five one-touch buttons to select either single sites or a five-way multipoint. Control was from the consultant room or from UTMB's Technical Operations Center.

Results

Again, the physicians were satisfied with the video and audio. The network was fast, providing switching in less than 30 seconds, but the system was unreliable. Typically, the system had to be completely rebooted at least twice daily. The major benefit of this was exercise for the attending technicians who had to walk across campus to reboot the systems. The problems turned out to be caused by software in the personal computers (PCs) incorrectly controlling the AMX system. Revisions were made, but to no avail. Finally, the PCs were disconnected, the original touch panels were installed, and the system began operating reliably. Minor modifications were made to the touch panels to make them physician friendly (e.g., the designation "Aux. Cam." was changed to "Patient Cam." and "Aux. Input" was changed to "Medical Scopes").

There were still problems. The size of the system was a headache. Two 27-in. monitors on carts and a computer system typically filled up the remote-site examination room. With the removal of the computer system, some space was saved, and finally one of the 27-in. monitors was removed and replaced with a 13-in. monitor mounted on top of the Radiance system.

Additionally, the physicians did not like the document camera for x-rays. The physicians did not like having to direct someone to "move the x-ray," "zoom in," and so on. They wanted control. One of the simplest ideas was born out of the physicians' desire for control. The physicians requested that an x-ray viewer be mounted on the wall opposite the cameras. The x-ray was placed on the viewer, and the physician could pan, tilt, and zoom the x-ray to his or her heart's content, remotely. All UTMB telemedicine rooms have this "room modification."

SYSTEM ADOPTION

After 180 days, UTMB decided to purchase the systems used for the pilot project. The operation continued until UTMB decided to expand the systems to include new sites. At that point, a problem was realized.

Expansion Needs

The multipoint control unit used for switching sites would only allow eight systems. Expansion would either be limited to three more sites or another option would have to be sought. Manual switching was far too slow. Even digital access cross-connect–based systems require someone to switch sites manually, albeit via a computer. Speed in switching from site to site was deemed critical to the program—such speeds would be possible with an integrated services digital network (ISDN) system. ISDN is a system of direct-connect circuits with intelligent hubs at each end and all connections between. Each site is assigned a number for easy access through dialing. In other words, ISDN is a digital version of the telephone system. Local ISDN from telephone companies is becoming a reality in most of rural Texas. When the Texas Department of Information Resources announced an effort to institute a statewide ISDN network, UTMB decided to test the network for 3 months. As with any new system, the network had problems and connections were intermittent. Finally, the network was deemed usable, equipment was purchased, and the entire UTMB video network was changed to ISDN. It worked. Expansion sites were no longer a problem.

Medical Instrumentation Needs

Medical instrumentation was another problem. Stethoscopes usually did not function or functioned poorly. Part of the problem was the vendor's use of equalizers in line with the stethoscope audio. The equalizers allowed the physician to unknowingly "color" the sound and thus obtain inaccurate data. Additionally, the pickups used were not true stethoscope chest pieces but simply microphones mounted in a conical base. No diaphragm was present. The otoscope and ophthalmoscope also provided a small picture and were hard to hold and harder to operate. Better instruments that were easy to change were needed.

One of the challenges with telemedicine is that usually there is one room for all the medical practices. So all the instrumentation for all the practices should be on-

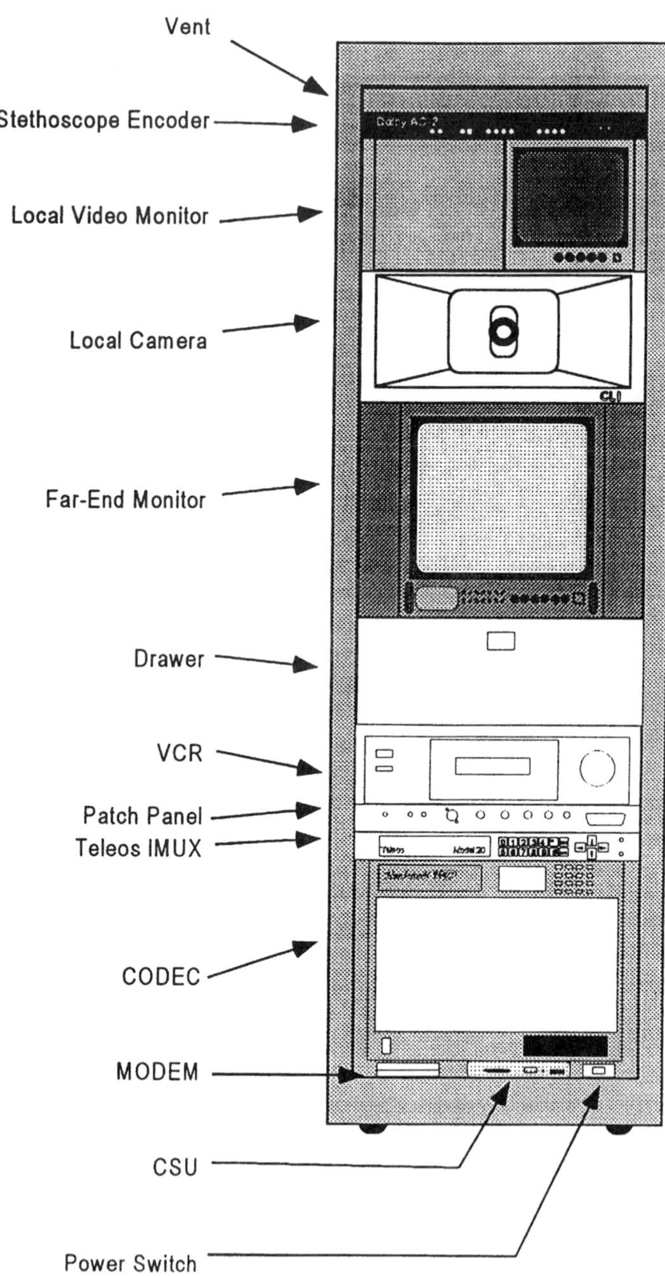

FIG. 12-1. University of Texas Medical Branch telemedicine unit front layout. VCR, videocassette recorder; Teleos IMUX, an integrated services digital network swtich; CODEC, compression and decompression device; CSU, customer service unit.

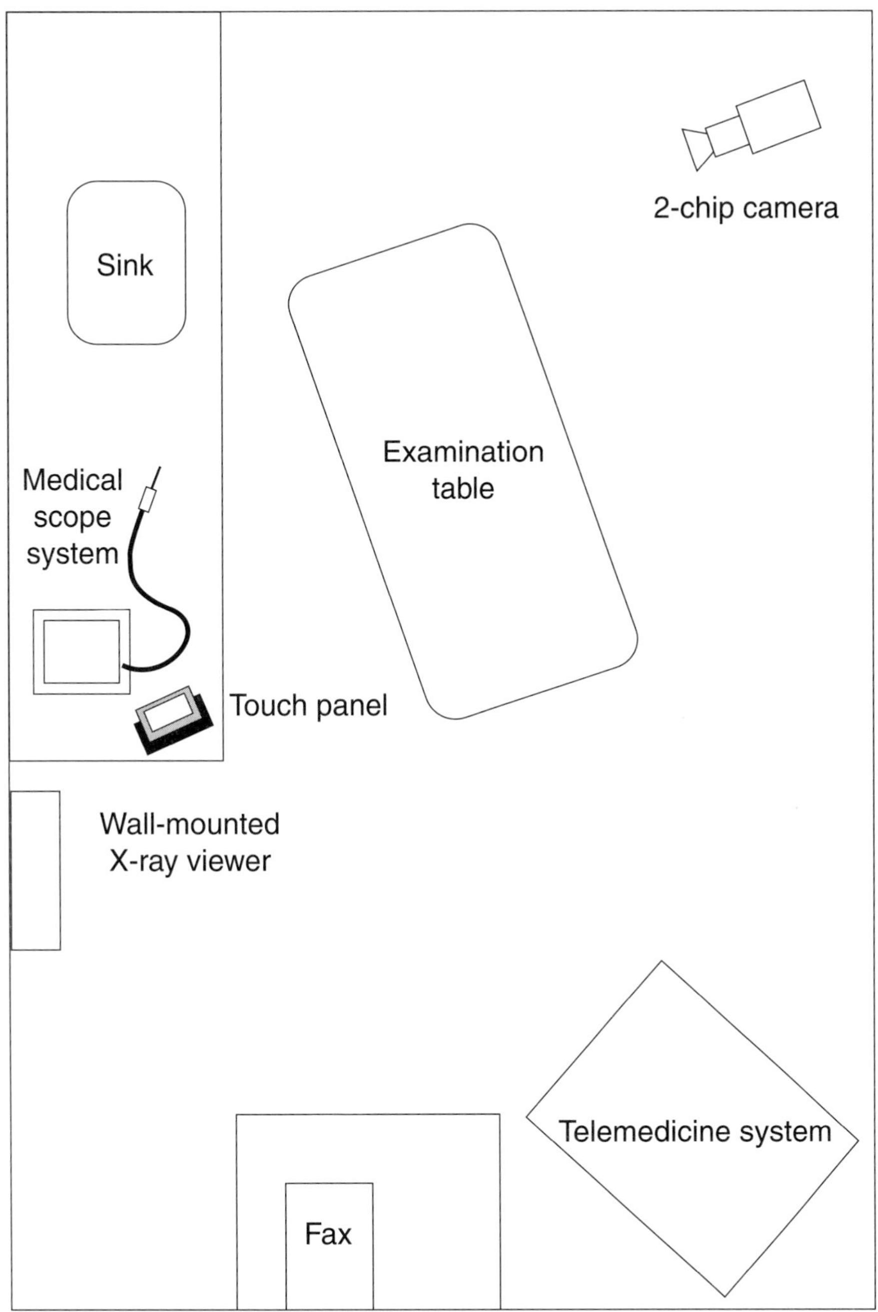

FIG. 12-2. Typical telemedicine examination room.

line in that one room. If traditional instruments are included, a room could be filled to the ceiling with specialized equipment. A plug-and-play medical camera system was also needed.

Security and Aesthetics Needs

One final challenge was the security and aesthetics of the system. The system was a room system with a 13-in. monitor stacked on top with a "whole bunch of wires" coming out of it. A decision was made to repackage the equipment into a modular 19-in. rack with steel sides and locking doors. Wheels were added to the rack for "pushability," and the rack was installed in the remote sites. Additionally, a patch panel was installed on the front of the unit to allow the stethoscope, touch panel, microphone, and so on to be plugged in without having to bring in a trained technician. This freed up a great deal of space and is the standard system used at the TDCJ sites. The UTMB system is shown in Fig. 12-1. A typical room setup is shown in Fig. 12-2.

The design is not really revolutionary as much as evolutionary. The system is not the prettiest but is designed to be as functionally efficient as possible. The system provides the operator with all the peripherals necessary to practice telemedicine in a prison environment.

FUTURE SYSTEMS DESIGN

As UTMB branches out into free-world telemedicine, there will be changes to the systems. The systems are modular and have expansion room for additional devices yet to be designated.

Systems on the market are available in a myriad of sizes and capabilities. Most systems feature International Telecommunication Union (ITU) standards compliance, which is a generic set of parameters set up by ITU that specifically lists parameters for manufacturers to adhere to so that different systems from different manufacturers can communicate with each other. Additionally, many vendors have their own proprietary video and audio software that may offer higher resolution, better audio, and so on. It is important to make sure that systems purchased have the ability to "talk" at ITU standards. Even if systems are proprietary software, all must be able to switch to the ITU standard for compatability. The best of both worlds would then be available—higher quality video and audio and the ability to talk to the outside world.

SYSTEMS STANDARDS

Standards are basically broken out into two video modes. These are known as *Full CIF* (FCIF) and *Quarter CIEF* (QCIEF). Table 12-1 compares the video resolution of these formats as well as a few manufacturers' proprietary algorithms.

TABLE 12-1. *Video resolution of International Telecommunication Union (ITU) video modes and manufacturers' proprietary algorithms*

Manufacturer	Format	Resolution
—	ITU FCIF	352×288
—	ITU QCIF	176×144
Compression Labs, Inc., San Jose, CA	CTXPLUS	480×368
V-TEL, Inc., Austin, TX	BLUE	352×288
Picturetel, Inc., Andover, MA	SG3/SG4	256×240

TABLE 12-2. *Digital bandwidth required and frequency response available for different audio formats*[a]

Format	Frequency response	Bandwidth required
ITU G711	50–3.4 kHz	64 Kbps
ITU G722	50–7 kHz	64 Kbps
ITU G728	50–3.4 kHz	16 Kbps
CLI VAPC/ADPCM[b]	50–3.5 kHz or 50–6.9 kHz	8–64 Kbps
V-TEL Proprietary[c]	50–3.4 kHz	32 Kbps or 12 Kbps
Picturetel SG3/4 and G724[d]	50–7 kHz	Figures not available

ITU, International Telecommunication Union.
[a] All specifications used are from printed sales documentation provided by each vendor or manufacturer.
[b] Compression Labs, Inc., San Jose, CA.
[c] V-TEL, Inc., Austin,TX.
[d] Picturetel, Inc., Andover, MA.

Video and Audio Specifications

It is important to examine a manufacturer's specifications carefully. Some companies have been known to advertise as "standards compliant," but a close look at their specifications reveals that they only communicate at QCIEF and cannot display the better video associated with FCIF. Resolution is perhaps the most important aspect of telemedicine videoconferencing.

There are also a plethora of audio versions available. Table 12-2 shows the different audio formats available via ITU standards and some proprietary formats. The digital bandwidth required and frequency response available for each format are also provided.

Echo

Echo is a primary factor when choosing a system. Echo is caused in a full duplex conversation when sound received and amplified over speakers in a conferencing system is reflected and picked up by microphones and rebroadcast back to the source. Most vendors have built-in echo cancellation. Two basic types of cancellation are semiduplex muting and digital-phase cancellation. Older cancellers rely on muting technology, whereby when audio is received, the audio being transmitted is either muted or cut back significantly. This type of cancellation leads to a bothersome cutting out of audio and frequently leads to conversations being repeated because the muting cut someone's comment off. Ideally, digital-phase cancellation is preferred. Digital-phase cancellation is when the audio coming in is compared to the audio going out. A digital "image" of the incoming audio is created and precisely mixed with the outgoing audio 180 degrees out of phase, thus completely canceling the echo going out. The result is a clean, full, duplex conversation with little or no echo or muting. Specifications on echo cancellers vary, but one of the most important parameters is length (in milliseconds) of echo cancellation. A larger room will take longer for the echo to return, thus a longer echo cancellation factor is needed. This echo return factor or echo cancellation factor can vary from 100 ms to 300 ms. In a larger room, a canceller with a 100-ms capability will not be able to stop an echo effectively. So, again, check the specifications. Also, make sure the frequency response of the echo canceller system matches the response of the conferencing system. Demonstrations of equipment are an excellent way to be sure the chosen systems will work.

Cameras

Cameras are another important peripheral for telemedicine. UTMB uses two cameras with its systems. A single chip is included and built into the rack with each system and is fine for general-purpose viewing. For a more accurate color image and high resolution, three charged coupled device cameras (CCD) are used. These units feature 750 lines of resolution and a 16× zoom lens. They are mounted on tripods remotely from the main system and allow the physician a different view of the patient. Some may argue that the cost does not justify the means, but of primary importance is the physician's perspective. Most physicians are sophisticated about what they want visually and can tell the difference between 750 lines of resolution and 350 lines from a less expensive single CCD camera. Again, demonstrate both cameras and allow the physicians to see both technologies and make the decision based on an actual use test, not specifications on paper.

A document camera is another device that is included with UTMB's telemedicine systems. These have specifications similar to cameras. UTMB uses simple, single CCD units and specifies a unit with overhead lights as well as back lighting. Auto focus is a handy feature, making the unit much simpler to operate.

CONCLUSION

UTMB continuously looks for new technologies to apply to telemedicine systems and distance-learning efforts. Other future technologies include asynchronous transfer mode–based technology and high-definition television. Costs are too prohibitive, and technology is not as widespread as needed to allow these new technologies to be used on a day-to-day basis, but just wait until tomorrow!

Whether through mounting an x-ray box or changing the text on touch panels, evolution has provided UTMB with a viable telemedicine platform that serves well. It is hoped that readers will learn from UTMB's experiences and make wise decisions regarding their telemedicine systems.

Telemedicine: Practicing in the Information Age,
edited by Steven F. Viegas and Kim Dunn.
Lippincott–Raven Publishers, Philadelphia © 1998.

13

Desktop Units

Rosa A. Tang and Jake G. Angelo

Department of Ophthalmology and Visual Sciences, University of Texas Medical Branch at Galveston, Galveston, Texas 77555; and Department of Information Services, University of Texas Medical Branch at Galveston, Galveston, Texas 77555

I. Definition and types
  A. Definition: A definition is any system that allows personal computer (PC)-based or laptop collaboration between points. To turn a PC into a collaboration terminal costs from $2,000 to $8,000. For videoconferencing, for example, this transformation includes two add-in boards that fit into standard expansion slots, an audio system, Windows software (Microsoft Corp., Redmond, WA), and a camera.
  B. Types: Several types of desktop conferencing systems are available for teleconferencing, and they have been in a state of evolution and flux. A classification of types is as follows:
    1. Audioconference: Since 1986, a full-duplex audioconference bridge has been introduced to allow audio interaction with two or more simultaneous speakers. This multipoint audioconference system uses a telephone with several interactive features on a desktop-based unit. Bridges by which audioconference attendees can be automatically placed into the conference using a password are commonplace.
    2. Audiographics (or data conference)
      a. Whiteboarding: Desktop-based, shared workspace systems that allow conference attendees located at multipoints to annotate, discuss, edit, and modify simultaneously on a virtual chalkboard present in each attendee's PC.
      b. Document conferencing: Allows multipoint conference attendees to work on slides, databases, spreadsheets, graphics, and so on that are stored in the desktop PC unit while conference attendees exchange further ideas using the audioconference modality. Participants in different locations can view the same computer screens simultaneously. Data is distributed electronically to the participant's desktop. This requires participants to have the same software installed. The T.120 standards series generated by the International Telecommunication

Union (ITU) is being implemented for this data-sharing modality. With the advent of more cost-effective telephone lines, a single line can accommodate the simultaneous transfer of audio and high-speed data, which is less costly and more advantageous. Data conference is being used for teletraining, distance learning, editing and designing presentations and reviews, sharing data, collaborative writing, market research activity, and medical second opinions.

3. Desktop videoconferencing: Videoconferencing is communication involving video, audio, and a data-sharing, real-time computer environment between two or more locations. The future is the multipoint control unit (MCU), which provides multipoint exchange of visual, verbal, and electronic information bridging through the same PC, which needs to be powerful enough to accommodate these three modalities simultaneously. The MCU is to be standards-based per ITU. As of this writing, video protocols use H320 standards. Data standards available are T.123, T.122, and T.125.
   a. Types of videoconferencing.
      i. Television type: at any number of points, distance education, training satellite, network
      ii. Interactive videoconferencing: at any number of points, interactive distance education training, compression and decompression devices (CODECs), telephone lines
   b. Desktop products for videoconferencing: Using desktop products for telemedicine applications has not been easy. Among the challenges are limitations of available products, shaky video quality, network integration downfalls, and lack of interoperability. For telemedicine applications, an ideal PC-based desktop system is a networked PC with an internal CODEC. In telemedicine encounters, there may be desktop-to-desktop or desktop-to-room conferencing.
4. Another classification: Desktop video products operate in three telecommunications environments, with their own functionality and features:
   a. Plain old telephone system (POTS)
   b. Local area network (LAN)
   c. Wide area network (WAN)
5. Desktop (DT) POTS: Provides two-way video over regular analog telephone lines. Acquisition and operating costs are small. Quality of video picture is poor but adequate for "talking head" level of communication (e.g., home care, psychiatry). Standard is H-324 with modem running at 28.8 Kbps.
6. DT LAN: Provides two-way interactive videoconferencing data and application sharing over LAN. If DT LAN operates with the Ethernet network, transmission of high-quality audio and video is possible. Limited to short-distance connecting sites on campus; however, can be the way to distribute video that transmits on campus over a WAN. Packet video products are designed to work over LAN.

II. Issues related to designing a telemedicine workstation
   A. Needs assessment and start-up issues from the healthcare provider's point of view: Electronic healthcare delivery is just another tool to deliver healthcare and not a different type of medicine. As with any new tool, its use and effectiveness should be assessed through strategic planning, which includes the following:
      1. Needs assessment: target population, disease, education.
      2. Cost return on investment projections: benefits such as decreased transport cost and physician and patient travel time.
      3. Assessment of the participant's willingness to use the new tool, which includes training when needed.
      4. Assessment of the infrastructure at each point and between: accessibility, cost, functionality, downtime of lines, technical support availability.
      5. Assessment of funding: Projections over a period with expected milestones to be achieved sequentially at a specific calculated cost. Budget for downtime of equipment and retraining personnel due to turnover.
      6. Setting up goals at all levels: participants at each point, technical group, patients, managed care organizations.
      7. Keeping abreast of technology upgrades: Do not implement without planning, as the planning process will help choose the necessary technology for the applications identified in the needs assessment. The failure of many telemedicine start-ups has been choosing the wrong executor who subsequently used the wrong technology. *Physicians of all types and levels of training need to be integral parts of the needs assessment and start-up issues.* When not familiar with computers and new, evolving telecommunications technologies, some personnel may sabotage a program that demands increased effort (translated into extra time and energy without due training, compensation, or incentive).
   B. Improving the financial bottom line of a healthcare delivery system is what executives want but not necessarily what physicians want if compromising the quality of healthcare delivery to patients is at stake. Any program that does not take into account the important role of the healthcare provider (e.g., doctors, nurses, physician's assistants) in the decision-making process from needs assessment to implementation is doomed to failure.

      Telemedicine is a tool to extend services that a healthcare delivery system or practitioner provides to out-of-reach areas and as such should not attempt to replace or interrupt the day-to-day delivery of face-to-face conventional medicine.
   C. The most important start-up issues are
      1. Identify key in-house technical and telecommunications personnel familiar with the modality of telecommunications as well as the hardware and software to be used.
      2. Identify healthcare professionals at each point who are agreeable and enthusiastic about participating. Give them at least moral if not monetary support.

3. Training is one of the most important issues.
4. Creation or adoption of technical and clinical protocols is a must before implementation.

D. Pilot phase performance
1. Phase 1
   a. Define the project in relation to the healthcare delivery system expectations.
   b. Interview remote-site providers, identifying their targeted needs.
   c. Interview consultants and identify time and services they are willing to provide and their expectations regarding incentives, reimbursement, and other matters.
   d. Train points personnel: remote site providers and consultants.
   e. Identify a cost-effective communication modality that will fit the need and validate the conclusion through a cost-benefit study.
   f. Assess tangible factors, including savings in transportation costs, incidentals related to travel savings (e.g., guards in prison systems), increased productivity, and reduced cycle time.
   g. Engage equipment vendors to provide trial equipment for a period and participate in the cost-benefit study. A 60-day trial is adequate for most cases. Vendors should not be expected to bear all costs but to share in them. Beware of vendors who offer the opportunity of alpha or beta testing, especially those that want you to pay for the equipment or other costs. This is not a trial, this is the vendor expecting you to discover the things their equipment is supposed to do but does not or does but should not. Negotiate mutual benefits such as free equipment at the end of the trial, consulting fees, research funds, and so on.
   h. Identify the primary person in charge of the project, someone who is driven so as to reduce obstacles to success. Tell him or her what to expect: the good, the bad, and the ugly. Remember, people are hesitant to try new features.
   i. Establish time lines for termination of the project on time. Use two sites for the first project.
2. Phase 2
   a. Identify the scope of the pilot phase project.
   b. Begin the project on needs assessment and adherence to established time lines.
   c. Overcome healthcare providers' resistance and skepticism. This is of utmost importance at pilot time.
   d. Identify potential barriers to full implementation and try to overcome before deployment.
3. Remember
   a. LAN, WAN, switch 56, or other telecommunication systems are not available everywhere in your institution; you need to identify infrastructures. Additional problems include the following:

i. The network is not always stable.
ii. Training and installation are not always consistent.
iii. Not every site will want to use the equipment in the same way.

b. At this pilot phase, secure commitment from staff to use the technology once it is deployed. The commitment is universal: Management, technical, and healthcare personnel need to be attuned as a team.
c. The promise to provide adequate and ongoing training is a managerial commitment; becoming proficient with the new technology is part of the staff commitment. The usability but also the limitations of the technology and the determination of the appropriate uses of it must be addressed by the needs assessment.
d. Plan to introduce the technology in phases, with the final goal being that of total implementation.
e. Cross training for equipment setup and testing is of utmost importance at both sites.
f. At the pilot phase, the program should accomplish the following, with data storage as the initial goal:
   i. Electronic information storage
   ii. Creation of images and documents in landscape orientation

III. Product evaluation during pilot phase
   A. Users should evaluate products as they comply with application needs. The product should support the PC platform and standards if available.
   B. Each product should be analyzed systematically with carefully chosen parameters. For example, video picture quality, motion handling, window size, frame rate, audio clarity, user friendliness of the application software, and its capabilities such as pointers, annotation tools, screen, and applications sharing.
   C. Test the product using at least two workstations to check how information would appear after transmission across a network. Do not buy a product after seeing a demonstration in a booth exhibit not knowing how transmission is to happen unless it is demonstrated in the booth.
   D. Ask vendors to provide statistics about their customer base. How many systems have they sold? Since when? How many are operational? Ask for references and check them out personally.
   E. In essence, given the lack of predetermined specification for telemedicine solutions in general, it is imperative that the user know what constitutes good quality, how to decide with certainty that it is good quality, how to assess the vendor's technical support and upgradability, and how user friendly the system is.
   F. Acquiring only the necessary telemedicine technology for compliance with the needs assessment can reserve funds for acquiring better systems as the user's needs expand, the technology improves, or both.
   G. The more sophisticated the system, the higher the support costs (e.g., transmission bandwidth, maintenance, personnel, training).

H. Evaluation of the system's performance should be ongoing throughout the pilot phase. Comparison of your data to those of other users should be built directly into the pilot phase cost and later into the operating cost of every project.

IV. CODECs and standards for videoconferencing
  A. Definition
    1. Video is a big signal requiring a large bandwidth pipe for transmission from one place to another. This requirement drives up the telecommunication cost. To avoid the cost increase, the video is compressed, requiring less bandwidth. However, there is a price to pay: The increased compression leads to decreased quality, which decreases cost. The device that performs the *co*mpression and *dec*ompression is called a *CODEC*.
    2. The CODEC is also the interface device between all the equipment in the room and the network. Video, audio, and data connect into the CODEC, which transmits a single digital signal over the network to the remote site(s).
  B. Uses of CODECs
    1. A CODEC must be located at each site to perform compression and decompression and act as the interface. The quality of the video will be degraded. The more compression, the more degradation. Video quality should be selected based on the intended application.
    2. CODECs use a variety of methods to compress a motion video signal.
    3. Since 1990, an internationally accepted standard H.320 CODEC allows different vendors' products to intercommunicate (P×64 or H.261 standard). CODECs have become less expensive and overall quality has increased. Desktop CODECs capable of providing bandwidths of up to 384 Kbps are common, and there are expectations of higher bandwidths.
  C. DT WAN
    1. Provides compressed and digital videoconferencing at bandwidths from 56 Kbps to 1,536 Kbps over switched (integrated services digital network, 56) and unswitched (fractional T1) networks
    2. Connects two or more sites
    3. Less expensive than room systems (i.e., $2,000 to $15,000)

V. Cost issues and facility options (cost versus quality): The old saying that "you get what you pay for" may hold true for telemedicine equipment as the traditional, full-motion, high-bandwidth systems (768 to 1,536 Kbps) provide the best resolution and motion, and the lower speed units (128 to 769 Kbps) generally offer lower resolution and less motion quality. The higher bandwidth units can cost from $40,000 to $50,000, whereas a simple 384-Kbps desktop system costs from $4,000 to $10,000. Again, quality costs money, and the task at hand determines a level of quality that is within the budget. Without knowing the quality to be achieved or knowing budget limits, a platform decision cannot be determined.

VI. Factors affecting final vendor selection from the healthcare provider's point of view
  A. Salesman ethics: whether he or she tells the truth about the customer base and connects healthcare professionals to exchange ideas regarding equipment.
  B. Performance during pilot phase: agreeable to work within healthcare professional schedule and availability for questions or to act as the remote site.
  C. Cooperation: Provide equipment and training to the healthcare professional on a trial basis and stand by the team while the trial period is ongoing.

Telemedicine: Practicing in the Information Age,
edited by Steven F. Viegas and Kim Dunn.
Lippincott–Raven Publishers, Philadelphia © 1998.

14

Network Design for Telemedicine Programs

Tom K. Epley, III

Department of Information Services, University of Texas Medical Branch at Galveston, Galveston, Texas 77555

This chapter provides a high-level overview of the network-design process, including issues to be considered in making design decisions, identifying a number of network designs, and identifying their relative strengths and weaknesses. Some recommendations and items for consideration in supporting a telemedicine network are also provided.

DEFINE THE REQUIREMENTS

When designing a video network, it is very important to understand how it will be used. Just as there are many types of computing equipment and applications, there are many technical solutions and system requirements. The time spent in design and analysis not only helps assure an appropriate solution but will save effort later during implementation and ongoing support.

One way to determine the requirements may be to use the information provided in this chapter, as well as other specific requirements. You may have to create a checklist to use when interviewing various customers, groups, or service providers to obtain information and organize it in a format that will allow design considerations to be reviewed.

Identify Applications

Identifying the type of video applications should be a first step. These include

- Full interactive telemedicine in which both ends of the connection have simultaneous voice and image transmission.
- One-way video and two-way sound in which only one end can view the other, but both ends have the ability to hear and talk to each other.
- Store-and-forward video applications in which the video is stored for later transmission and viewing between sites with no real-time interaction between the two ends.
- Fixed image transmission in which a fixed image, such as a photograph or x-ray, is transmitted from one site to another.

- Multipoint video in which more than two sites are simultaneously connected. These vary from full interaction between sites to a video origination site with multiple reception sites with or without interactive sound.

Store-and-forward and fixed-image applications transmission requirements can generally be called *data applications* as they are actually moving data files across a network. However, the other video applications described in the preceding list are quite different. In designing a network, it is very important to identify any data application requirements. Examples might include electronic medical records, electronic mail (e-mail), automated scheduling systems, order entry and result reporting medical systems, and billing systems. Each of these may have very specific requirements that will impact the network design. One of the most important considerations will be to determine when the connectivity must be active. If the network connectivity assumes the data application will be using the same network as the video, will connectivity only be available during telemedicine sessions or must it be provided at all times?

Identify Users

To develop a design meeting the needs of everyone who uses the system, it is necessary to identify as much as possible what specialties and groups will be users. The type of specialty will determine the quality of the video and sound required. For example, we at the University of Texas Medical Branch (UTMB) at Galveston have found that the psychiatry department requires the highest possible quality due to the importance of small movements and changes in voice. This quality translates into higher bandwidth requirements for the network. However, the orthopedics department generally requires less bandwidth and is more interested in providing adequate quality in viewing x-rays. The specialties identified will also determine what medical peripherals will be used. The medical peripherals may include otoscopes, endoscopes, dermascopes, stethoscopes, interfaces to microscopes, digital radiology images, and slit-lamps and will have to be supported by the network design.

Other groups can include continuing education. In some cases, with instructors who rely heavily on remote viewing of fixed images, such as slides or overheads, network speed is not a critical issue. However, teaching by a very enthusiastic instructor who uses animated gestures and moves about the room will require additional speed to provide an acceptable level of quality.

Identify Equipment

Identify what additional equipment may be required, such as fax machines for paper medical records, laboratory results, and so on. Is a telephone required that can be used for private conversations, reporting trouble with the system, and even remote diagnostics and setup using a modem from a support location?

Identify Locations

To design the network, it is necessary to identify the locations of all of the known initial and planned locations to be supported. Identifying the locations is especially important for nonsatellite design. It is also important to understand the future growth plans and associated areas. It may not be possible to determine the cities to be connected; however, it may be possible to identify an area such as "the eastern third of Texas"; "metropolitan Houston"; or "a three-state area, including Louisiana, Mississippi, and Florida." Area identification will help guide the decision as to what technologies will be used, the cost projections, and support requirements.

Estimate Use

Use of the system should be estimated in several ways, including gathering answers to the following questions:

- Will more than one consultant be communicating with a patient site at a time?
- Will one site be communicating with multiple sites simultaneously?
- How many hours per day will each site be communicating through the network?

There are also data issues, including

- Is there a requirement for an immediate, unscheduled connection without interrupting a scheduled connection?
- What are the hours of operation for each site? Will support be required 24 hours a day, 7 days a week?

In some environments, telemedicine sessions are conducted at regularly scheduled times. Physicians, patients, consultants, and applications allow a network connection at a predetermined time and duration. However, many operations are highly dynamic and need a network design that provides a great deal of flexibility in availability and capacity. It is important to understand the scheduling issues before developing a network design.

Identify Budgetary Objectives

It is important to identify the budgetary objectives relative to the network cost. Networks can vary widely in cost based on the issues discussed in the preceding sections, as well as the communication speed (bandwidth) provided. Network costs can be identified as one-time installation costs and ongoing monthly costs. Depending on the technology selected, costs may be usage sensitive (amount of time connected) or fixed.

Considerations for funding should also include determining if a central organization will fund the network or if a billing process will have to be developed. Will a process have to be developed to track use by user or location? Other issues may include leasing to spread the initial costs over time or up-front purchase.

IDENTIFY THE NETWORK OPTIONS

After gathering and understanding information gained in the previous sections, the next step in network design is to identify the available options and to identify the strengths and weaknesses of each. It is at this point that careful consideration must be given to stability and performance relative to user requirements. Hopefully, at this stage you will also have an idea of scheduling flexibility and possible future growth and application requirements. You should also know if there are other requirements that may not be used initially but must be considered in the design process. For example, should the network provide dial-up connectivity to other networks in other states or countries?

Not all types of communication technology are available everywhere. In Texas, there are more than 50 operating telephone companies providing service, and there is no requirement that they provide the same services or "all services." It is very likely that with state and federal legislation some of these obstacles will be eliminated. As of this writing, however, options are available based on your location and the location of your desired connection. It will be necessary to verify at each site the method chosen or a compatible alternative that is available for connection to the network.

Available options can be identified as those provided internally within your organization; those provided by carriers such as Hughes Satellite, GTE, Southwestern Bell Telephone Company, MCI, or AT&T; those provided by groups creating, operating, and sharing a network, such as consortiums; and those provided by state networks.

Dedicated Digital Networks

Dedicated digital networks are networks composed of digital T1 or fractional T1 circuits. A T1 circuit is composed of 24 channels of 64-Kbps circuits, which when combined into a single circuit can provide up to 1.54 Kbps. These circuits are usually land based and can be leased from telephone operating companies or provided by internal networks and others. The circuits may be transmitted through the air by microwave or digital radio, or they may be ground based, using private or public networks on copper or fiberoptic circuits. Fractional circuits are often described as ¼, ½, or ¼ T1 and represent 6, 12, or 18 channels. It is also possible to purchase 56-Kbps digital services in some areas.

Dedicated networks are connections that are installed and remain connected at all times. These are not dynamic and require each site in the network to have a permanent connection, which is usually provided at a set bandwidth.

Advantages of a dedicated digital network include flexible scheduling, excellent opportunities for data networking, and not having to share with others. The primary disadvantage is the high cost for a link 24 hours a day, 7 days a week, which may only be needed a few hours a day. It is also possible that without an expensive video bridge that connects sites to each other, this design may not connect all sites to each other but only to a central location.

Integrated Services Digital Network

Integrated services digital network (ISDN) services continue to gain popularity as they become more widely available and less costly. ISDN services are commonly described in two ways: basic rate interface, a 128-Kbps circuit, and primary rate interface, a 1.4-Kbps circuit. ISDN services are often constructed using ISDN switches, allowing sites to actually dial each other across either a public or private network. Basic rate interface circuits are becoming common in homes and small offices for data connectivity and desktop video applications.

The advantages of ISDN include flexibility in scheduling, the ability for each site in the network to connect to each other, network charges that are often based only on the time the network is used, and fairly simple access to worldwide networks that use ISDN technology.

Satellite Networks

Satellite networks are usually composed of a large central satellite facility with more bandwidth and local satellite facilities. The ability to use newer, smaller dishes and less expensive network equipment continues to make satellite networks less costly and easier to install. Design decisions include identifying the bandwidth required for each site and the total bandwidth required at any one time. It is possible to have fully interactive sessions at a very high bandwidth or compressed video sessions using up to T1 speeds. Usually, a customer contracts with a satellite provider for a set amount of bandwidth during a set period. This may be 24 hours or an 8-hour window. During this time, the customer can request that the provider connect sites (usually at predetermined times).

The cost of satellite networks is directly related to the speed the customer requests and the amount of time contracted. Speed and time costs are high relative to other options over shorter distances. If the network is to span the country or even several states, however, satellite networks should be investigated.

Another advantage of satellite networks is a "one-to-many" distribution of programming. When a central site distributes video and many sites are receiving, it can be very cost-effective. The satellite bandwidth is only used to distribute the signal once and not for each site. Distribution of the signal once is used widely by educational and public broadcast networks and can also be used for videoconferences with one-way video and a telephone dial-in system to ask questions.

The primary disadvantages include the cost of providing multiple, simultaneous, interactive video sessions and the limited ability to provide high-speed data circuits over long periods at reasonable cost.

Internal Networks

Internal networks are usually communications systems built by an organization or consortium to meet its needs. Internal networks may include one or more of the technologies described in the preceding paragraphs. The benefit of these networks is that they are often built to share the cost of providing a service and often cover wide geographic areas. Additionally, the networks are usually managed by a central organization that either performs the work or contracts to meet the service requirements.

If a network is very large, it has increased ability to buy services at a reduced cost but, if small, it is at a significant disadvantage. It is always expensive to build a small network and provide management and support. Additionally, small networks generally have limitations for connectivity.

Just as e-mail is becoming productive because large numbers of individuals are using the system, video networks are effective because they are able to reach large numbers of sites at reasonable costs, very reliably, and with as few scheduling constraints as possible.

Hybrid Networks

Hybrid networks are simply a combination of the various technologies as appropriate to meet the application requirements with the most cost-effective solution. It is very likely that large networks will combine satellite, leased digital circuits, and internal networks to build an integrated functioning solution.

New Technologies

New technologies for both networks and video systems continue to be developed at a rapid rate. The ability to attain high quality at lower speeds (and lower cost) continues to help expand telemedicine and other video networks. The newer generation of desktop video systems achieves more than 20 frames per second and may achieve 30 frames per second by 1999. Asynchronous transfer mode networks will become more readily available and less costly. Telecommunications legislation will continue to encourage network providers to provide new services, and increased competition will help drive the cost down.

HOW SHOULD TECHNICAL SUPPORT BE ORGANIZED?

Technical support includes the staff providing maintenance and management of the network, scheduling of the network (including bandwidth management), coordination with network service providers, and coordination of installation. In some organizations, technical support may also include video technology, user training, technology research and design, and billing. It is important that each organization determine which of these functions is required and which organization is to provide the service.

The decision to provide maintenance and network management is dependent on the geographic distribution of the sites. If the sites are widely distributed and a quick response is required for maintenance issues, outsourcing the support to a vendor who has a distributed staff and can respond in the required time should be considered.

Technical support is an important issue; however, keep in mind that this equipment, if installed properly, is very reliable. It is also important not to overlook installation of remote support tools to provide programming and diagnostics from a central location.

Another component of this decision is the availability of internal staff and their current skills. Most maintenance of network and video equipment is done by component replacement and customer diagnostics. If you are going to be in the internal-support business, it is important to provide adequate, ongoing training for the staff and spare parts for maintenance. Also, keep in mind that video technology support is not simply fixing equipment. Video support requires knowledge of room design for lighting and sound, camera design, as well as some awareness of the telemedicine application to ensure that the technology is installed in a manner consistent with the customer's environment.

If network support for data applications is required, it is important that this support be done by or in a coordinated manner with the organization's current data network support organization. There are many issues that can limit the performance and compatibility of network support functions if improperly designed. It is important that coordination starts with the design of the network and continues as it becomes operational.

To minimize failure and reduce the difficulties in providing technical support, it is important to develop a working model for delivering telemedicine support. The working model should include a standardized method of building the networks, equipment configurations, and programming. The model may have to vary slightly but should always strive to be as consistent as possible. Consistency allows evaluation of components that work well and elimination of any that does not; it simplifies training requirements (for both support staff and customers), spare parts inventories, and vendor disputes; and it also reduces the difficulties and time spent in getting systems to work together.

UTMB's experience has shown that a properly designed and installed system often operates for more than 1 year without maintenance. Additionally, network reliability can be increased by considering redundant communication links, alternate paths, and optional high-availability commitments purchased from communications vendors.

It is up to each organization to determine the reliability required. Also, remember that in many cases a new network installation requires time to attain a high level of stability. During this time, the support staff, customers, and possibly the vendor will be developing and refining their operating processes to diagnose and resolve problems. System users will be learning how the equipment works and what the buttons do. During this period, it is best to define the installation as a pilot project. Most users expect pilot projects to be testing and learning experiences, and expectations will not be the same as with systems that are production ready.

It is important to achieve a high level of reliability and performance. Reliability and performance should be approximately 99% or better to attract and keep physicians and patients satisfied that telemedicine is a viable process for delivering medical care. It is difficult to regain credibility with either physicians or patients if the systems or networks perform unreliably.

CONCLUSION

UTMB has found that one organization can provide all of the support. A group composed of a manager, scheduler, two video engineers, a part-time training specialist, and one telecommunications specialist is able to support UTMB telemedicine project, as well as approximately 100 hours per month of distance learning and 25 hours per month of videoconferencing. The support process includes coordination of a state video network operation that provides the network, management of the video equipment and peripherals, scheduling, training, technology research, and billing.

The UTMB support process is made possible in part by providing training to all team members and cross training in other specialties. For example, the telecommunications specialist is also trained to maintain the video equipment.

Telemedicine: Practicing in the Information Age,
edited by Steven F. Viegas and Kim Dunn.
Lippincott–Raven Publishers, Philadelphia © 1998.

15

Telerobotics in Surgery

Jon C. Bowersox

Department of Surgery, Stanford University School of Medicine/Santa Clara Valley Medical Center, San Jose, California 95128

The ultimate goal of telesurgery is to project surgical expertise to a remote location, enabling operations to be performed on patients who are inaccessible because of distance, hazardous environments, or other physical barriers. To some, telesurgery means robots wielding scalpels and other instruments in an automated operating room. To others, telesurgery is merely looking over the shoulder of a less-experienced surgeon, providing advice from afar. No matter how the future is interpreted, however, delivering surgical care to remotely located patients introduces challenges not faced by other physicians using telemedicine.

Remote consultation can be readily applied to preoperative and recuperative care, but the craft of operative surgery requires the skilled manipulation of tissues by surgeons using their hands or other instruments. Even for a master surgeon, a fundamental set of conditions must exist for surgery to be performed successfully. Simply stated, sensory input to the surgeon must be accurate and adequate; it must be presented in real time, without detectable delay; and the surgeon must be able to effect changes based on the data presented. For a surgeon removed from the patient's side, satisfying these conditions presents a formidable challenge.

FOUNDATIONS OF TELESURGERY

Although seemingly a novel concept, remote teleoperation began in the early 1950s. At the end of World War II, the U.S. Atomic Energy Commission rapidly scaled up nuclear reactor development and construction. A method was needed to safely handle the highly radioactive materials that would be used daily, frequently in tasks requiring dexterous manipulations. Consequently, the Argonne Laboratory began developing control devices that could precisely translate human arm motions to remote locations (1). The first electromechanical teleoperator was demonstrated by Goertz and Thompson in 1954 (2). Over the next decade, a variety of electrical, hydraulic, and pneumatic telemanipulators were developed, allowing operators to safely and precisely assemble reactor components and conduct experiments with radioactive materials, even on a microscopic scale. Operators were separated from contaminated environments by leaded walls or thick glass. They controlled manipulator arms by directly viewing them through windows or indirectly by using closed-circuit cameras and video-display screens. Although crude by today's standards, telemanipulators handled tasks as precise as pouring small quantities of isotopes or as challenging as moving waste-laden drums.

Extending remote handling capabilities to surgery was first proposed by Alexander in 1972 (3). At the time, the U.S. National Aeronautics and Space Administration was exploring methods for providing surgical care to astronauts, particularly those who would be fabricating the planned orbital space station. The high costs of computation (one megabyte of memory cost $550,000 in 1970; the cost today is less than 0.001% of that amount), slow processor speeds, bulky components, and limited telecommunications capabilities relegated these dreams to the realm of science fiction. In the 1990s, however, explosive growth in computing power, component miniaturization, and the proliferation of powerful telecommunications networks have provided the enabling technologies necessary for developing telesurgery systems. Coupled with the recognition by minimally invasive surgeons that complex operative procedures could be safely performed using indirect video visualization and limited tissue manipulation, widespread interest in the potential of operating on remotely located patients has emerged.

SYSTEMS FOR TELESURGERY

The term *telesurgery* describes a spectrum of possibilities for delivering procedure-based healthcare to remotely located patients through an electronic interface. All possibilities are based on the premise of digital devices being used to transfer multisensory data to and from a remote surgeon. The least costly and complex application of telesurgery is the passive display of visual information to a remote observer, as in videoendoscopy. Adding two-way video and audio communications and a shared whiteboard requires greater resources but is feasible. Actually operating on patients from a distance using telemanipulators remains a developmental challenge, only possible in the laboratory as of this writing.

Telesurgical systems require a patient and a surgeon separated by distance, interface devices, and digital data encoders and decoders. Video, audio, and haptic subsystems are configured for specific applications. Video components include high-resolution, charge-coupled device cameras (laparoscope and operating room scene cameras), video displays, and whiteboard overlays for image annotation. Standard audio devices include stereophonic microphones and speakers or headphones (Fig. 15-1).

Special-purpose robots, devices that follow a programmed sequence of instructions, may be used as components of telesurgical systems. Robotic arms were first developed to enable surgeons to more precisely control camera position during laparoscopic surgery (4–6). With minor modifications, the same devices could be controlled by a surgeon from a remote location (7), and could be used to position

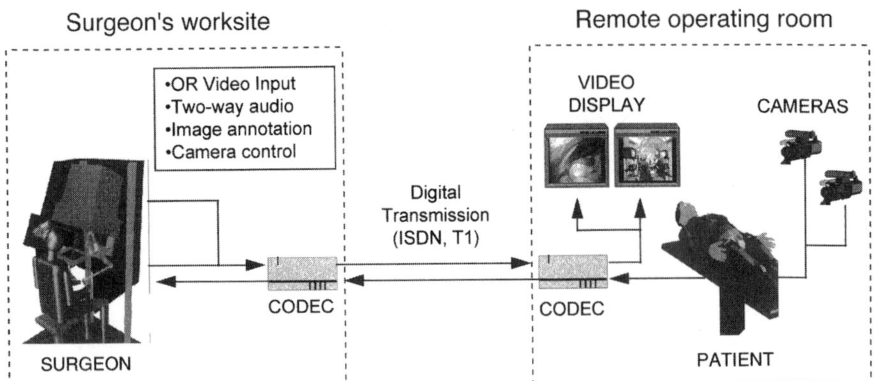

FIG. 15-1. Telesurgery systems include video and audio sensors at the remote site, encoders and decoders to convert signals from analog to digital format (compression and decompression devices [CODECs]), transmission devices, and video displays. Remote camera control and the image annotation (shared whiteboard) add value to passive systems but increase costs and complexity. OR, operating room; ISDN, integrated services digital network.

retractors as well as laparoscopes (8). The robotic devices remain passive adjuncts to surgery, with actual operative procedures still performed by surgeons who are present in the operating room.

Robots have also been developed for specialized surgical applications requiring precision and reproducibility, such as stereotactic tissue biopsy (9,10) and femoral canal preparation for hip arthroplasty (11). In these specialized applications, the location of the surgeon is not as critical as the need for attaining accuracy and reproducibility. Surgeons provide supervisory control to the computers actually planning and executing the procedures. Current technology limits use to structures that can be rigidly fixed, such as skeletal structures and the brain. Although telesurgical robots are feasible, the need for control from a remote location has not been established.

The most complex systems for telesurgery use electromechanical telemanipulators, which provide a haptic interface to the remote environment through which touch or feel can be perceived and hand motions can be transmitted. Telemanipulators act as a bridge, connecting an operator's hands to surgical instruments at the remote site. Although generally configured as master-slave robotic systems, surgical telemanipulators are directly controlled by hand motions rather than through autonomous computer instructions.

TELESURGERY TODAY

The most frequently reported use of telesurgery has been for operative videoconferencing. A remotely located surgeon can observe a procedure through one or more cameras and provide visual and auditory feedback to the operative site. Although

remote control of camera or retractor position is possible, the operative procedure is actually performed by a surgeon at the patient's side. Consultative telesurgery can be used for advising, mentoring, or proctoring for competency. Almost all applications described have been in the field of minimally invasive surgery in which indirect viewing and manipulation of the operative field are standard.

Demonstrations of operative videoconferencing have established the feasibility of transmitting videoendoscopic images in real time over commercial communications channels. In one report, a laparoscopic cholecystectomy was observed over a distance of 16,000 Km (12). Limitations observed in this test included a 950-ms delay in image display at the remote site, resulting in a perceptible discontinuity between audio and video feed. Also, the image resolution (352×288 pixels) and frame rate (15 frames per second) were only half those normally viewed by a laparoscopic surgeon in the operating room (12). The acceptability of video compression and reduced frame rate for observing laparoscopic surgery has been reported in a pilot study, but the conclusions were based on limited, prerecorded image sets (13).

Case reports have described the successful use of commercially available, off-the-shelf products in telesurgical systems used for proctoring students learning laparoscopic surgery (14,15). The system configurations have included standard laparoscopic surgery equipment, as well as a robotic positioning arm that holds the laparoscope. The robotic arm was modified to allow touchpad control by the remotely located proctor. Thus, the camera could be precisely steered to the desired position by the expert surgeon. The proctor viewed procedures from a separate room and communicated to the inexperienced surgeon through an audio link by annotating the operating-room video display and by positioning the camera in the desired location. In pilot studies, cases were completed successfully, and satisfaction was reported by proctors and trainees (14–16).

Kavoussi and colleagues have performed a controlled trial of telementoring in patients undergoing endourologic surgery (7). Surgical residents were mentored by an experienced urologist located 300 meters away from the operating room. Procedures performed included nephrectomies and retroperitoneal lymph node dissections in 23 patients. Emphasis was placed on patient safety, with an experienced surgeon present in the operating room if needed. The overall success rate was 95.6%, and no operative complications occurred. In general, remote mentoring increased times required for completing procedures but not significantly.

A surgical telemanipulator system was first described by Green and coworkers in 1991 (17) (Fig. 15-2). Developed for military use in treating combat casualties, Green's telepresence surgery system focused on performing conventional (not laparoscopic) surgery through an intuitive interface. In telepresence surgery, high-fidelity visual, auditory, and haptic cues are presented to the remotely located surgeon, creating the perception that the operator is physically present at the patient's side (18,19).

Immersion in the remote environment is facilitated by a high-resolution, stereoscopic video display, full-frame rate, and by maintaining the integrity of the eye-hand (oculovestibular) axis. A surgeon grasps conventional surgical instrument handles attached to servocontrolled manipulators. The remote site, linked by coaxial

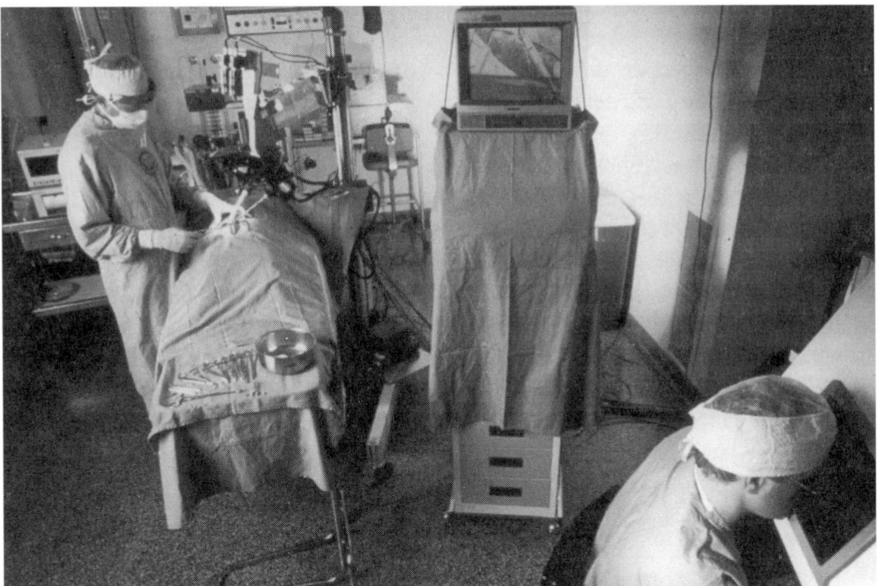

FIG. 15-2. A prototype telepresence surgery system has been used successfully in preclinical studies. The system includes a surgeon's workstation **(left)**, computer controller **(center)**, and remote surgical unit **(right)**. The surgeon views the operative field on a high-resolution, stereoscopic video display and uses four-degree-of-freedom, servocontrolled manipulators to control surgical instrument tips at the remote site. The two sites are connected by coaxial cables at a distance of up to 200 miles.

cables, has identical manipulators with standard surgical instrument tips. The surgeon's hand motions are precisely replicated at the remote end, thus enabling the instruments to be manipulated as deftly as if they were attached to the instrument handles. The system provides force feedback to the surgeon's hands, allowing tissue characteristics to be accurately sensed (20,21).

Telepresence surgery has been used in a feasibility study to suture blood vessels in anesthetized swine (19). Arteriotomy closures performed with the telepresence system took 2.5 to 2.8 times longer than conventional suturing but were completed with identical accuracy. The telepresence surgery system has also been used to perform cholecystectomies, nephrectomies, and gastrostomy closures; to repair liver lacerations; and to accomplish remote endoscopic manipulations in 14 animals (21).

The prototype system used in feasibility studies had four degrees of freedom (similar to operating with a fused wrist). Systems are reportedly in development that will provide six degrees of freedom, as well as the capability of working through a minimal access aperture. The potential advantage for laparoscopic surgery is in restoring the manual dexterity that is lost by operating through 512-mm skin ports. Prototype systems have been described for laparoscopic telemanipulator systems; however, no preclinical or clinical results have been reported (22,23).

TELESURGERY'S FUTURE

There is no question that telesurgery will open new vistas for surgeons in the twenty-first century. However, several key issues must be addressed before telesurgical systems move into operating rooms. As with other telemedicine disciplines, a real need must be established for applications to migrate from testbed environments to direct-care delivery. Currently, the ability to mentor or proctor surgeons is not limiting the diffusion of minimally invasive surgery through the surgical community. As medical education changes, such a need may develop.

Other regulatory issues to be addressed include safety, particularly when manipulating tissues with robotic components, and the capability to sterilize delicate electronic components. Standards for the security, integrity, and reliability of broadband network connections must be established and validated before the responsibility for patient care can be transferred to a remotely located surgeon. Although commercial aircraft have been certified to "fly-by-wire," multiple hardware and software redundancies have been engineered into the control systems. The U.S. Food and Drug Administration, as well as risk managers and healthcare insurers, will likely require similar standards for telesurgery before systems are approved for clinical use.

Laparoscopic surgery gained rapid acceptance among surgeons who were reluctant to leave their traditional tools and techniques. Laparoscopy is a technology that has been driven by user need, not by developer push. Lasers for laparoscopic cholecystectomies, although aggressively marketed, were not needed, and their use has vanished. Telesurgery must be developed with these analogies in mind. When systems are available that safely offer distinct advantages, telesurgery will become part of the surgeon's armamentarium.

CONCLUSION

The performance characteristics of available telesurgery interfaces reflect the lack of understanding of human factors in surgery. Surgery is a highly complex skill, yet it is taught and practiced as a craft. To develop truly intuitive telesurgery interfaces will require task decomposition and analysis, similar to those performed in aviation and nuclear power industries. As more research effort is directed to this area, questions about the applicability of virtual environments, head-mounted displays, and other components can be addressed scientifically. Telesurgery must offer clear benefits over other options to become widely accepted. Surgeon capabilities and performance will be major criteria by which success is measured.

GLOSSARY

Haptic pertaining to the sensations of touch and feel (tactile), motion (kinesthesia), and position (proprioception)

Robot a reprogrammable, multifunctional manipulator designed to move parts, tools, or specialized devices through programmed motions for the performance of a variety of tasks

Telemanipulator (teleoperator) a device with sensors (e.g., cameras, force sensors) and actuators (i.e., grasping tools and handles) under the direct control of a human operator

REFERENCES

1. Hull HL. Remote control engineering: an introduction. *Nucleonics* 1952;10:34–35.
2. Goertz RC, Thompson WM. Electronically controlled manipulator. *Nucleonics* 1954;12:46–47.
3. Alexander AD. Impacts of telemation on modern society. In: *Proceedings of the first CISM-ITOMM symposium*. 1972:121–136.
4. Gagner M, Beglin E, Hurteau R, Pomp A. Robotic interactive laparoscopic cholecystectomy. *Lancet* 1994;343:596–597.
5. Sackier JM, Wang Y. Robotically assisted laparoscopic surgery. From concept to development. *Surg Endosc* 1994;8:63–66.
6. Finlay PA, Omstein MH. Controlling the movement of a surgical laparoscope. *IEEE Eng Med Biol Mag* 1995;14:289–291.
7. Moore RG, Adams JB, Partin AW, Docimo SG, Kavoussi LR. Telementoring of laparoscopic procedures: initial clinical experience. *Surg Endosc* 1996;10:107–110.
8. Partin AW, Adams JB, Moore RG, Kavoussi LR. Complete robot-assisted laparoscopic urologic surgery: a preliminary report. *J Am Coll Surg* 1995;181:552–557.
9. Rovetta A, Sala R, Cosmi F, et al. Telerobotics surgery in a transatlantic experiment: application in laparoscopy. *SPIE J* 1993;2057:337–341.
10. Kall BA. Computer-assisted surgical planning and robotics in stereotactic neurosurgery. In: Taylor RH, Lavallee S, Burdea GC, Mösges R, eds. *Computer integrated surgery: technology and clinical applications*. Cambridge, MA: MIT Press, 1996:353–361.
11. Stuberg SD, Kienzle TC III. Computer- and robot-assisted orthopaedic surgery. In: Taylor RH, Lavallee S, Burdea GC, Mösges R, eds. *Computer integrated surgery: technology and clinical applications*. Cambridge, MA: MIT Press, 1996:373–378.
12. Go PMNYH, Payne JH Jr. Endoscopic surgery teleconferencing. *Int Surg* 1996;81:18–20.
13. Hiatt JR, Shabot M, Phillips EH, Haines RF, Grant TL. Telesurgery: acceptability of compressed video for remote surgical proctoring. *Arch Surg* 1996;131:396–400.
14. Luttman DR, Jones DB, Soper NJ. Teleproctoring laparoscopic operations with off the shelf technology. *Stud Health Technol Informatics* 1996;29:313–318.
15. Kavoussi LR, Moore RG, Partin AW, Bender JS, Zenilman ME, Satava RM. Telerobotic assisted laparoscopic surgery: initial laboratory and clinical experience. *Urology* 1994;44:15–19.
16. Schulam PG, Docimo SG, Saleh W, Breitenbach C, Moore RG, Kavoussi L. Telesurgical mentoring: initial clinical experience. *Surg Endosc* 1997;11:1001–1005.
17. Green PS, Piantanida TA, Hill JW, Simon IB, Satava RM. Telepresence: dexterous procedures in a virtual operating field (Abstract). *Am Surg* 1991;57:192.
18. Bowersox JC. Telepresence surgery. *Br J Surg* 1996;83:433–434.
19. Green PS, Hill JW, Jensen JF, Shah A. Telepresence surgery. *IEEE Eng Med Biol Mag* 1995;14: 324–329.
20. Bowersox JC, Shah A, Jensen J, Hill J, Cordts PR, Green PS. Vascular applications of telepresence surgery: initial feasibility studies in swine. *J Vasc Surg* 1996;23:281–287.
21. Bowersox JC, LaPorta AJ, Cordts PR, Bhoyrul S, Shah A. Complex task performance in cyberspace: surgical procedures in a telepresence environment. *Stud Health Technol Informatics* 1996;29:320–326.
22. Taylor RH, Funda J, Eldridge B, et al. A telerobotic assistant for laparoscopic surgery. *IEEE Eng Med Biol Mag* 1995;14:279–288.
23. Schurr MO, Breitwieser H, Melzer A, et al. Experimental telemanipulation in endoscopic surgery. *Surg Laparosc Endosc* 1996;6:167–175.

Telemedicine: Practicing in the Information Age,
edited by Steven F. Viegas and Kim Dunn.
Lippincott–Raven Publishers, Philadelphia © 1998.

16

Teledermatology

Mark H. Lowitt

Department of Dermatology, University of Maryland School of Medicine, Baltimore, Maryland 21201

Dermatology was one of the first medical specialties to embrace telemedicine, doing so as early as the 1960s (1), and has remained near the forefront of telemedicine research and implementation. It is not yet possible to firmly define technical or methodological standards for most elements of teledermatology, but examination of some active teledermatology programs and research to date yields some early insights into the directions teledermatology will take in the future.

The information in this chapter derives from (a) the small body of scientific literature devoted to teledermatology issues, (b) telemedicine system descriptions with a dermatology component listed on the telemedicine information exchange (http://www.telemed.org), (c) a draft document of proposed teledermatology standards created by the standards subcommittee of the American Academy of Dermatology's Telemedicine Task Force, and (d) discussions with teledermatologists and telemedicine system administrators from programs in the United States and abroad. These remarks are not intended to be all-inclusive or to represent all current programs but rather to provide an overview and sampling of the practical impressions of many active members of this rapidly expanding field.

WHAT IS THE CURRENT STATUS OF TELEDERMATOLOGY?

Dermatology provides an excellent testbed for telemedicine for several reasons. First, as dermatology is a visually oriented specialty, telemedicine lends itself well to transmission of its most critical element—visual inspection of the skin. Second, the majority of dermatologists practice in or near urban areas, leaving large areas of the country suboptimally served by traditional means of specialty-care delivery (2). Third, dermatology can serve as a model for other telemedicine specialties because it involves important elements from a range of disciplines, including (a) talking with the patient to elicit a history (important in internal medicine, pediatrics, and psychiatry, for example), (b) visual pattern recognition (radiology, pathology), and (c) surgical treatment and pre- and postoperative management (surgery and surgical subspecialties).

Most telemedicine programs are still in early phases of implementation or development. Although legislation allowing reimbursement for telemedicine services is slowly appearing on a state-by-state basis, most current programs remain operational due to the following (3):

1. Internal or external grant support
2. Donated equipment or transmission costs or both
3. Underwriting by military or U.S. Veterans Administration funding
4. Contracts with large entities, such as prison networks
5. Private sources (e.g., foreign governments or royalty)

A range of high- and low-bandwidth systems for teledermatology are in use in the United States and internationally. No standards defining optimal systems for teledermatology have yet been established. For such standards to emerge, progress must be made in three areas: (a) Further research is required to objectively define the key technical and operational parameters necessary for teledermatology examination; (b) the telemedicine industry will need to continue movement toward more unified standards of image compression, transmission, and unification of currently proprietary system elements (e.g., distant camera control); and (c) financial obstacles to long-term maintenance of telemedicine programs, including reimbursement issues and equipment transmission costs, will have to be resolved because of their direct impact on the types and costs of the systems.

WHAT TECHNOLOGIES ARE BEING USED FOR APPLICATIONS?

Most active telemedicine programs involving teledermatology use a combination of live-interactive video (IATV) with store-and-forward (S&F) technology (77% of programs). IATV is used alone in 15% of programs, and S&F is used alone in 8% of programs. A striking feature of national telemedicine programs is that among approximately 40 teledermatology programs, more than 30 different companies have provided hardware, software, or peripheral equipment. In many cases, a given vendor has been used by only one or two programs. This observation confirms the suspicion that industry-wide standards are still far afield.

A major controversy in the approach to teledermatology development lies in the enigmatic dichotomy of IATV versus S&F technologies. The following advantages to live, two-way, IATV transmission are apparent:

- The dermatologist can directly interface with the patient, allowing for direct questioning to gather historical information.
- The dermatologist can examine the body regions and specific lesions of his or her own choosing rather than relying on the primary care provider's (PCP's) selection of still images.
- The patient has the opportunity to meet and interact directly with the dermatologist and to ask questions.
- The entire experience more closely replicates the familiar, in-person, doctor-patient examination.

- Financial reimbursement for IATV examinations may be more easily deduced from current practice.

Some disadvantages of IATV include persistent difficulties with reliability of the equipment and connections, extremely high costs of setup and maintenance of a network, the necessity that parties at both ends of the transmission be simultaneously available, and slow pace. Visits by IATV generally take longer than in-person examinations (4).

The following are advantages of S&F systems:

- Dramatically reduced equipment and transmission costs (compared with IATV).
- Asynchronous transmission of information, allowing both sender and recipient to perform their roles on their own schedules.
- Images can be collected with portable digital cameras and interpreted on office personal computers (PCs), obviating the need for costly telemedicine rooms.
- Transfer of data can occur over plain old telephone system lines.

Disadvantages of S&F for dermatology include loss of direct contact between dermatologist and patient and limitations on the data set available for review: Dermatologists often ask different questions of patients than do PCPs, and the dermatologist may wish to examine lesions or regions other than those presented.

Framed most concisely, the chief advantages of S&F technology are lower costs and diminished technical complexities. A major objection to S&F, from the dermatologist's standpoint, is that care of patients by examination of their cutaneous images alone represents a substantial departure from the method of traditional, in-person evaluation taught to physicians for thousands of years. The practice of radiology translates relatively easily into an S&F telemedicine framework, because the evaluation of a standard series of still, two-dimensional images is the modus operandi of the specialty and the standard taught in radiology training programs. In radiology, the major difference from standard care rests in where the image is displayed (i.e., on a computer monitor at work or at home as opposed to a radiographic film on a light box). Although identification of dermatologic disease with still images (35-mm slides) is routinely taught in dermatology residency programs, the use of such images for the treatment of actual patients is not a feature of current training. A standard series of cutaneous images, such as one expects when ordering a chest radiograph, has not yet been established. S&F technology for dermatologic applications may therefore offer much to both patient and physician in certain circumstances; however, continued work toward establishment of standards for S&F examinations will be critical for its long-term success.

An additional use of digital imaging technology in dermatology, which has been gaining momentum, has been the incorporation of digital imaging systems into surgical and cosmetic surgical dermatology practices. Such systems, now more accessibly priced, enable rapid viewing of pre- and postoperative images (5) and even image morphing capabilities to project potential outcomes of cosmetic procedures for patients. Digital archiving can also be used for sequential follow-up of patients with multiple or atypical moles who are at risk for developing malignant melanoma. Sequential or alternating comparisons of previous photographs can lead to early detection of new or newly changed suspicious lesions that may otherwise have been overlooked. As public awareness of melanoma rises and the incidence of the disease has continued to rise, several off-the-shelf systems have been introduced. More complex uses of computers and digital images are used in computerized image analysis in which active research is pursuing more effective means of computer-assisted diagnosis (6).

WHAT ARE THE TECHNICAL STANDARDS NECESSARY FOR TELEDERMATOLOGY?

Inquiry into the technical standards for teledermatology yields more questions than answers. Many different standards should be established, including the appropriate clinical setting, equipment, and transmission parameters, among others. Because of the rapid changes in these areas and because standards for dermatology have not yet been established, this section presents what I see as some of the critical decision points for each proposed standard. Mention of specific vendors or products is avoided due to the rapid pace of changes in these areas. Discussion of elements of the clinical examination, such as patient selection and clinical personnel, are presented in Chapter 33.

Cameras

Digital Still Cameras

For strict S&F applications, digital still cameras offer the greatest convenience and portability. As these cameras are growing in popularity in the consumer marketplace, an avalanche of new units has become available. Because the requirements for image quality and color accuracy for teledermatology consultation exceed the needs of the general home user, many of the currently available lower-end digital cameras are not appropriate for medical application. Cameras providing greater pixel density (e.g., 1,024×768 or greater) are preferred; however, they tend to be more expensive. When dermatologists were asked to render diagnoses from projected slides (4,000 dots per sq in.) compared with digitized images using 24-bit color (17 million colors) (7), pixel resolution of 574×489, and 92 dots per sq in., the digitized images were found to be as informative as the slides (8). A comparison of diagnostic agreement between super video graphics array images (640×480 pixels, 8-bit color) and National Television Systems Committee video revealed no significant differences between the two (9). In one study using 24-bit color and 832×624 pixel resolution, images were considered acceptable overall: Variability in photographic expertise was blamed for some of the poorer quality images (10). Some experts contend that 640×480 pixel images and 8-bit color are acceptable: Although physician confidence declines with greater image compression, intraobserver diagnostic agreement is not greatly affected (11). Because images stored on the camera's disk drive must be downloaded to the user's PC or mainframe computer, the software enabling this transition should provide a simple and efficient user interface.

Video Cameras

Video cameras for use in IATV as room cameras are most convenient for the physician when remote camera control (e.g., pan, tilt, zoom) is available. Because industry-wide standards for these operations are not yet established and many current systems still operate under proprietary algorithms, it is difficult for two units of different origins to talk to each other. Although 3-charge coupled device (CCD) or "3-chip" cameras are touted for better image and color reproduction and head-to-head comparisons are not yet available, many experts find the less expensive 1-CCD cameras perfectly acceptable for dermatologic applications. As recommended by Schosser (12), important features for video cameras include a manual shutter, manual and automatic white balance, and automatic gain control defeat. Schosser also advocated the use of video camcorders because of their flexibility, low cost, and capability to record directly onto videotape. Color fidelity may be assessed with use of a color grid examined at both the proximal and distal sites compared to ascertain relative consistency and accuracy in color reproduction.

Peripheral Devices

Even when remote camera control is available, the limited space in most examination rooms precludes complete cutaneous examination with monitor-mounted cameras. An additional hand-held camera for closer examination and for access to hard-to-visualize areas is a critically important tool for dermatologic examinations. Early marketing efforts toward dermatologists by telemedicine equipment vendors offered variations on the dermatoscope, a hand-held 10× tool requiring direct skin contact. Although offering excellent detail and attractive images, the usefulness of the device is severely limited by the following:

- The majority of dermatologists do not use the dermatoscope during the course of in-person examinations and therefore are unaccustomed to the appearance of anything other than pigmented lesions with the device.
- The requirement that the lens be applied directly to the skin makes scanning of the cutaneous surface for abnormalities impossible.
- The instrument is not appropriate for areas of the skin that are not intact (e.g., ulcers).
- Interpatient sterility issues become paramount.

For these reasons, several small, handheld cameras (either palm-sized or on gooseneck stands) with close-up (macro) lenses have emerged as an excellent solution. These cameras, operated by an escort accompanying the patient, may be used (a) to visualize the feet, intertriginous areas, and other cutaneous locations not well served by the mounted camera; (b) to scan a designated region with detail surpassing that of the mounted camera; and (c) to zoom in on individual lesions for greater detail. Such a device allows the examining physician to follow the traditional diagnostic method used in in-person examinations: (a) screening for abnormalities, (b) examining lesions closely, and (c) choosing a diagnosis (13). The built-in light source of many of these units enables toggling to a polarized light, which can eliminate some surface reflectance and improve visualization of the cutaneous microvasculature. The ultimate role of the polarizing feature in the armamentarium of telemedicine peripherals remains to be seen.

Document Camera

A third camera that may be included in an IATV system is a document camera, a device resembling an overhead projector that enables live transmission of chart material, radiographs, and other documents. Although theoretically useful, many of the currently available products suffer from the technical problem that an entire 8½ in.×11 in. document (a page from a written medical record, for example) cannot be legibly transmitted in toto, necessitating the time-consuming and frustrating exercise of asking the remote presenter to "move the paper to the right, no, I mean left," and so on. Adding to the technical problem the fact that many physicians' handwritten notes are illegible leads to a generally unsatisfactory situation. Some solutions include faxing the record (time consuming and inconvenient if a bound chart must be entirely disassembled to allow faxing of individual sheets), scanning the document, then transmitting the image (expensive and time consuming), or using the other hand-held camera for documents (good quality but subject to distortion from movement of the presenter). A completely computerized medical record, integrated with the telemedicine system, would be an ideal solution to these problems, but such systems are difficult to implement and not yet ready for off-the-shelf use.

Bandwidth

What bandwidth is optimal for teledermatology examination? What is the minimum acceptable bandwidth? These deceptively simple questions are still not well answered. Although many users choose 384 Kbps (¼ T1) as a minimum acceptable bandwidth and others might select full T1, it becomes clear on comparison of many systems that (to paraphrase Gertrude Stein) ¼ T1 is not ¼ T1 is not ¼ T1. In other words, even when operating at the same bandwidth, significant variations exist between different systems.

Bandwidth requirements have been a major focal point of teledermatology research at our institution. Acceptability for bandwidth is dependent on both user impressions (patient and physician) and quality measures such as interphysician diagnostic agreement. In a study comparing user impressions at full T1 and at ¼ T1 bandwidths, patient satisfaction was very high and not appreciably different between the two groups (14). Although physician diagnostic confidence and satisfaction with image quality waned during ¼ T1 examinations, interphysician diagnostic agreement (when diagnoses were compared with those of in-person physicians examining the same patients on the same days) was similar (approximately 80%) for both bandwidths. (These values also match data demonstrating baseline diagnostic agreement between two in-person dermatologists as being in the range of 77%. [Unpublished data. MH Lowitt. Baltimore Veterans Affairs Medical Center, Baltimore, MD, 1998.]) We are currently collecting data on user impressions, diagnostic agreement, and cost and outcome measures for lower bandwidth applications in dermatology.

Lighting and Room Color

Without excellent lighting, even the most expensive telemedicine equipment fails to provide ideal images. Lighting should be of sufficient intensity (150 foot-candles) and the color temperature should approach 2,400K (tungsten) or 5,000K (daylight) (12). Additional lights for use with peripheral cameras are recommended, but different lights used in the same examination should be the same color. Representatives from several well-established teledermatology programs tend to agree that teledermatology examination operates most successfully when ceilings and walls are painted light, neutral colors (e.g., eggshell, gray).

Acknowledgments

I would like to thank the following people for their contributions to this chapter: Chris Barnard, Lennis Bensen, Anne Burdick, Michelle Gailiun, Lee Green, Sue Groves-Philips, David Haid, Robert Harrison, Joseph Kvedar, Douglas Perednia, Chuck Phillips, Marcia Rigby, Robert Schosser, and Ann Temkin.

REFERENCES

1. Murphy RLH, Fitzpatrick RB, Haynes HA, Bird KT, Sheridan TB. Accuracy of dermatologic diagnosis by television. *Arch Dermatol* 1972;105:833–835.
2. Perednia DA, Brown NA. Teledermatology: one application of telemedicine. *Bull Med Libr Assoc* 1995;83:42–47.
3. Perednia DA, Allen A. Telemedicine technology and clinical applications. *JAMA* 1995;273:483–488.
4. Burdick AE, Berman B. Teledermatology. *Adv Dermatol* 1997;12:19–44.
5. Price MA, Goldstein GD. The use of a digital imaging system in a dermatologic surgery practice. *Dermatol Surg* 1997;23:31–32.
6. Stoecker WV, Moss RH. Digital imaging in dermatology [Editorial]. *Comput Med Imaging Graph* 1992;16:145–150.
7. Perednia DA. What dermatologists should know about digital imaging. *J Am Acad Dermatol* 1991; 25:89–108.
8. Perednia DA, Gaines JA, Butruille TW. Comparison of the clinical informativeness of photographs and digital imaging media with multiple-choice receiver operating characteristic analysis. *Arch Dermatol* 1995;131:292–297.
9. Schosser RH, Sneiderman CA, Pearson TG. How dermatologists perceive CRT displays and silver halide prints of transparency-based images: a comparison study. *J Biol Photogr* 1994;62:135–137.
10. Kvedar JC, Edwards RA, Menn ER, et al. The substitution of digital images for dermatologic physical examination. *Arch Dermatol* 1997;133:161–167.
11. Sneiderman C, Schosser R, Pearson TG. A comparison of JPEG and FIF compression of color medical images for dermatology. *Comput Med Imaging Graph* 1994;18:339–342.
12. Schosser RH. Teledermatology: concepts and effective techniques [Seminar]. American Academy of Dermatology Annual Meeting, San Francisco, March 1997.
13. Perednia DA, Gaines JA, Rossum AC. Variability in physician assessment of lesions in cutaneous images and its implications for skin screening and computer-assisted diagnosis. *Arch Dermatol* 1992;128:357–364.
14. Lowitt MH, Kessler II, Kauffman CL, Hooper PJ, Siegel E, Burnett JW. Teledermatology and in-person examinations: a comparison of patient and physician perceptions and diagnostic agreement. *Arch Dermatol* 1998;134:471–476.

Telemedicine: Practicing in the Information Age,
edited by Steven F. Viegas and Kim Dunn.
Lippincott–Raven Publishers, Philadelphia © 1998.

17

Overview of Reengineering Process Using Telemedicine Implementation

Kim Dunn

Department of Internal Medicine, Texas Department of Criminal Justice, University of Texas Medical Branch at Galveston, Galveston, Texas 77555

Two major forces reshaping healthcare delivery are the financing of care and the expectation of accountability for the outcomes of that care. The need for information to measure and document value to healthcare customers (payors and patients) and accrediting organizations (e.g., the Joint Commission on Accreditation of Healthcare Organizations, National Committee on Quality Assurance, National Commission on Correctional Health Care) is paramount. However, clinicians, administrative structures, and information systems in healthcare delivery settings are not optimally prepared for these emerging expectations with ever-increasing demands for information. In a culture of uncertainty, a broadening lack of trust and understanding between the constituents of the care-delivery processes is growing. Much of this lack of trust stems from not understanding the frames of reference and expectations among payers, clinicians, administrators, and information system personnel. Although institutions feel pressed to buy the electronic patient record to meet documentation needs, an emerging consensus is that a comprehensive system does not currently exist and that the real problem is not the lack of technology but the fragmentation of communication.

A good starting point for restoring communication in the healthcare process lies in one of the most troubling arenas of healthcare: poor communication among patients, their primary care practitioners, and subspecialty practitioners. Therein lies the real opportunity for telemedicine implementation in the healthcare scenario: the examination of how communication technology (video and audio) can be implemented to support the patient, the primary caregiver, and the specialist by allowing them to see one another while they discuss the patient's problem together. Because of the many unknown issues regarding telemedicine, its implementation can serve as a unifying focus for these constituents to explore together its effective application to support and improve clinical care. Essentially, telemedicine implementation can be a starting point for reengineering the care process, particularly the automation of that process. Schematically, this is shown in Fig. 17-1.

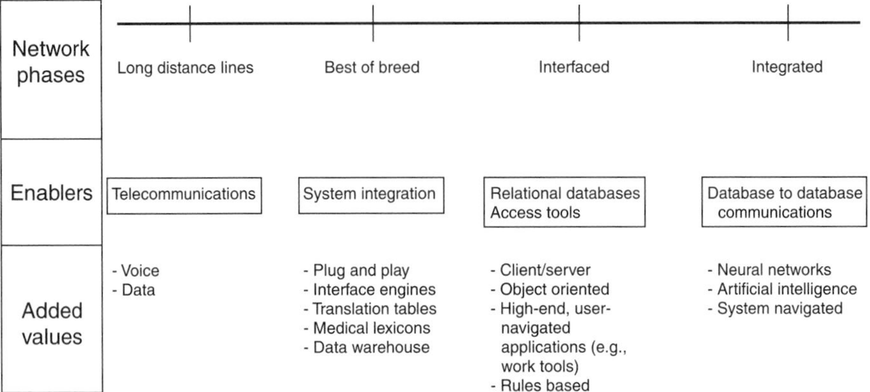

FIG. 17-1. Phases of network information system evolution in healthcare.

The reengineering process has two key components as it relates to telemedicine: physician leadership and the reorientation of information systems from an administrative focus to a clinical focus.

PHYSICIANS AND INSTITUTIONAL LEADERSHIP

Physician leadership is crucial to telemedicine implementation in a multidisciplinary environment. Physician leadership is necessary to work with administrators to define the operational needs for telemedicine application, ensure commitment to sustaining a program, develop clinical protocols and train remote site presenters, and implement an outcomes management program to ensure the quality of a program. Essentially, the physician issues related to implementation of telemedicine are the same needed for healthcare in general and can be seen as a definable subset of any given healthcare system. The biggest impediment to physician leadership is the lack of skills necessary for that leadership.

Clinicians are not trained in several key information arenas that would help make them effective leaders in contemporary practice: business principles, information system implementation and evaluation, and population disciplines relevant to outcomes management. Additionally, clinicians are trained in a hierarchical system with few role models for interdisciplinary interaction. This lack of training and role models provides a backdrop for understanding clinicians' recalcitrance to lead activities requested by administrators, information system personnel, and payers to change the delivery system. Clinicians are reluctant to engage in such business activities as resource use and billing documentation maximization. The lack of exposure to information system understanding underlies the reluctance to work with the process for new information technology systems. The lack of exposure also contributes to the difficulties extant in healthcare delivery systems: multiple, competing clinicians requesting information systems with separate software packages for their specialties. These specialty-specific information systems meet individual specialty needs but, in the main, do not work together as a comprehensive system for a given integrated delivery system. Just as there are courses in pharmacology to teach physicians how to determine optimal treatment for their patients, so too there is a need to understand information systems to meet both the physician's needs and the group practice's needs. The lack of population disciplines contributes to physicians' discomfort with accepting feedback on performance. The linear approach to clinical training contributes to physicians' lack of understanding about how to effectively work with mid-level practitioners and, to varying degrees, explains a sense of vulnerability from nonphysician participation in the decision-making processes.

Three strategies can be used to assist physicians to develop the leadership skills necessary for leading a reengineering effort such as telemedicine implementation. Each of the following strategies can be useful for addressing many of the cultural issues in an effort to migrate to a shared sense of responsibility for institutional performance.

- Telemedicine protocol development and training to improve communication and clinic efficiency
- Defining requirements (process flow and data elements) via prototyping work tools for multidisciplinary documentation
- Interdisciplinary faculty development in outcomes management

INFORMATION SYSTEMS

Institutions have invested in information systems that are principally for administrative purposes (e.g., billing and ancillary care processes such as pharmacy, radiology, and laboratory) with little attention to the congruence for system architecture. These systems are inadequate for the emerging model of accountability for clinical outcomes and their management. Realization of this has prompted institutions to critically examine their own information system processes and data needs and to ask a fundamental question: Who needs what data at what point in time for what purpose? This provides an institution and its caregivers the opportunity to then determine the best mix of external vendors and in-house information system infrastructure necessary to meet the clinical and administrative needs of the institution and patients.

Simply stated, reengineering involves clinicians and information system experts working together to define their information needs in the care process, and then having information systems experts develop automated work tools to provide that care. It must be fully appreciated that it is an iterative and long process. Schematically, the process is shown in Fig. 17-2.

This process represents a formidable and seemingly insurmountable task for institutions because of the overwhelming complexity and chaotic nature of healthcare delivery. The clinical information system reengineering strategy is to migrate from supporting the administrative functions of a healthcare system to supporting the clinical care functions of a system. Key data needed for administrative purposes (e.g., billing, quality assurance, resource use, accreditation requirements) can be abstracted

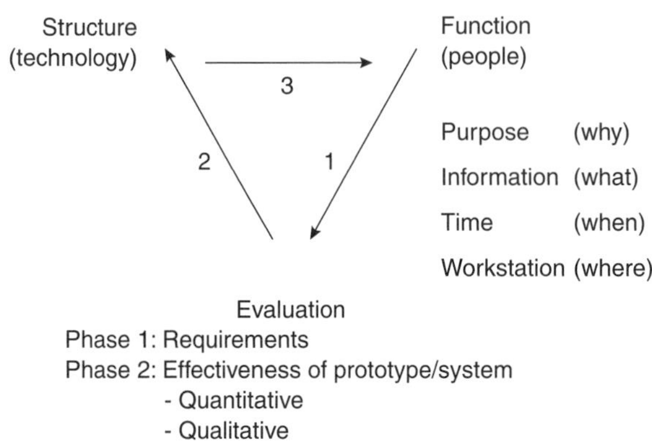

FIG. 17-2. The iterative process of information system development. (*1*) Define requirements; (*2*) define technology to meet those requirements; (*3*) prototype technology to determine if the selected technology meets user requirements.

or pulled from these clinical work tools as they develop greater sophistication. Returning to the starting point of why healthcare systems exist (i.e., providing care to patients) and focusing on using the interaction of one patient, one primary care practitioner, and one specialist to define the care processes can be a good starting point for an institution.

Telemedicine provides a testbed for experimentation to understand an institution's information needs and to evaluate the effectiveness of its care processes. Experimentation must be viewed as a continuous process and one that must be attended. The remainder of this book is organized into several sections to provide an overview of components for telemedicine implementation and an opportunity to examine institutional efforts to improve overall system functioning. Chapter 18 provides an overview of a process to develop communication protocols. Chapters 19–22 give an overview of the different ways in which an existing network can be used for both training current practitioners in the use of protocols and training nurses and physician's assistants at remote locations.

Chapters 23 and 24 provide one approach to automating the electronic patient record using a telemedicine clinic as a testbed. Chapters 25–27 provide perspective on the approaches for integrating ancillary support services, pharmacy, laboratory, and radiology for the telemedicine clinical encounter.

Chapter 28 provides an overview of how to approach developing a physician leadership program in outcomes management using telemedicine as a testbed. Chapter 29 explores how telemedicine can be a testbed to explore delivery system satisfaction from all participants—patients, subspecialists, and remote-site participants. Chapters 30 and 31 examine using telemedicine as a starting point for cost-based accounting in clinical care and assessing cost-effectiveness of telemedicine practice.

In Chapters 32–50, the perspectives of physicians and surgeons with telemedicine experience at the University of Texas Medical Branch at Galveston, who answered a series of questions over 6 months, are presented. The specific questions were meant to foster the development of telemedicine clinical protocols, to foster template generation for documentation of a clinical encounter, and to stimulate clinicians into defining and leading three key areas for reengineering: developing referral guidelines, prototyping an automated documentation tool, and defining measurable outcomes. This process can serve as one approach to getting information system requirements across the spectrum of clinical services to define the overall needs of an integrated delivery system.

Referral Guidelines

- Which patients could be seen via telemedicine?
- Which patients could not?
- Which patients could be seen in an emergency setting?

Documentation of the Clinical Encounter

- What information should be available to the physician before the patient is seen, while the patient is seen, and after the patient is seen?
- How does the physician want that information and where does the physician want that information?

Defining Clinically Relevant Outcomes

- How would the physician like to have feedback on the consultation?
- What clinical endpoints would the physician be interested in monitoring to document the effectiveness of the clinic?

CONCLUSION

Given that the future of healthcare is uncertain, the careful implementation of telemedicine with appropriate institutional support can allow improvements in the healthcare delivery process. Although it is not possible to predict the future, it is possible to invent it.

Telemedicine: Practicing in the Information Age,
edited by Steven F. Viegas and Kim Dunn.
Lippincott–Raven Publishers, Philadelphia © 1998.

18

Organization for Telemedicine Services: Developing Administrative, Clinical, and Technical Protocols

Michael B. Moore, Jade S. Schiffman, Beth L. Cory, Casey D. Peterson, and Kim Dunn

Department of Cardiovascular and Thoracic Surgery, Abilene Regional Medical Center, Abilene, Texas 79606; Department of Ophthalmology, University of Texas Medical Branch at Galveston, Galveston, Texas 77555; Department of Nursing Services, Texas Department of Criminal Justice Hospital, University of Texas Medical Branch at Galveston, Galveston, Texas 77555; Department of Clinical Affairs, Texas Department of Criminal Justice Hospital, Galveston, Texas 77555; and Department of Internal Medicine, Texas Department of Criminal Justice, University of Texas Medical Branch at Galveston, Galveston, Texas 77555

Because the telemedicine environment places certain limitations on patient interaction, the need to clearly define protocols that compensate for these limitations is great, especially for the individuals that are involved in the process of presenting remote-site patients for consultation. Additionally, quality-of-care and cost-containment issues must be addressed (1). Administrators and technical personnel must realize that activities in a telemedicine practice environment have a dramatic impact on patient care and that they must be involved in any meaningful protocol development effort. Finally, the acceptance of the telemedicine system by clinicians will be enhanced when the effectiveness and efficiency of the system is maximized (2). For this reason, the term *telemedicine protocol development* is used to describe this multidisciplinary process.

This chapter provides a generic mechanism for establishment of protocols dealing with clinical, administrative, and technical activities for telemedicine programs. Functionally, it may seem that these activities have little in common. A careful analysis, however, reveals that the characteristics of the telemedicine environment lend themselves to systematic approach to the provision of healthcare services through a variety of technical modalities.

The clinical encounter and its attendant interpersonal communications and sensory and cognitive tasks must form the starting point of clinical protocol development. Experienced clinicians that have independent decision-making responsibilities generally make decisions through iterative hypothesis testing, aided by personally developed heuristics that serve as "triggers" for hypothesis formation (2). Additionally, it must be realized that expert clinicians make decisions and form hypotheses immediately on beginning the clinical encounter that influence both the course of the clinical encounter and its final outcome. Certainly, these heuristics that form the basis of clinical decision making often depend on the type and quality of patient interaction. Conversely, clinicians that are relatively more dependent in their decision-making responsibilities may be more dependent on heuristics and use iterative hypothesis testing less than independent decision makers (3).

The level of independence in decision making is dependent on clinician role and experience. This forms a continuum from experienced clinicians with responsibilities for independent practice through a variety of other healthcare providers that exhibit lesser degrees of independence and greater degrees of interdependence with clinicians of more advanced training or greater experience. For obvious reasons, telemedicine encounters generally take place in an environment where these two types of decision makers must collaborate in the clinical encounter. In this way, the telemedicine environment creates a new type of clinical encounter that is fundamentally collaborative in nature (4). This contrasts to the traditional clinical encounter, in which role-specific activity, rather than collaboration, is the norm. For the purposes of this chapter, the interactive videoconferencing environment is assumed to be the telemedicine site in question, as it is the most common (5). However, a similar structure could be used to develop protocols for other environments, including store-and-forward technology.

FUNDAMENTALS OF CLINICAL PROTOCOL DEVELOPMENT

In an environment that differs radically in its communications techniques and technology from the previous generation, it is important to impose structure on the fluid situation that develops to reduce error and increase efficiency and satisfaction (6). To develop effective telemedicine protocols, it is helpful to define fundamentals of telemedicine protocol development that guide planning and protocol development activities. The objective of these fundamentals is to provide a starting point for telemedicine system planning founded on the experience of established programs as well as theoretical knowledge regarding the conduct of the clinical encounter.

Compensate for Telemedicine Environment's Structural Differences

Clinical protocols recognize and compensate for the structural differences of the telemedicine environment. The most obvious structural difference is the technology that comes between the patient and clinician. Therefore, clinical protocols must compensate for the inability of the consultant to directly interact with the patient. There are two other key differences that are introduced in this new paradigm of interaction, however, and these differences directly relate to management of health information and its availability to clinicians. First, the temporal relationship between clinical activities is changed from the traditional encounter. For example, within the telemedicine environment there is no waiting for the laboratory test, the fax from the radiologist, or the lost outpatient record to be found for the consult to go forward. The time-critical nature of the interactive videoconferencing environment forces a different temporal sequence on clinically related events. Second, the sharing of health information among multiple sites becomes a paramount issue within a system that is providing clinical services at multiple sites at the same time.

Consider Clinical, Technical, and Administrative Issues

Clinical protocols are fundamentally multidisciplinary efforts that consider the clinical, technical, and administrative issues surrounding telemedicine as a new mode of healthcare delivery. All of the individuals from the clinical, technical, and administrative areas that support the delivery of care should be involved at some point during both the initial protocol development efforts and the necessary review and revision processes.

Enhance Performance of the Remote-site Clinician

The telemedicine environment creates different roles and responsibilities that are fundamentally collaborative in nature. Collaboration can create a difficult environment for the remote-site clinician who is often placed into an unfamiliar clinical situation and required to perform clinical skills directly related to the consultant's area of clinical practice and for which he or she is unprepared. Consequently, these demands must be accounted for in any protocol developed.

Provide Specific and Clear Guidance for Clinical Activities

The telemedicine environment is one in which often one individual clinician provides services to a diverse patient population and facilitates care delivery from a wide variety of domain experts. Therefore, telemedicine protocols must provide specific and clear guidance for clinical activities that is both generalist oriented and multidisciplinary in focus. Ideally, these protocols are designed for a specific application and task. However, clinical protocols are not replacements for judgment or clinical skill and, if used as such, can lead to error in application and delivery of care.

A GENERIC TEMPLATE FOR CLINICAL PROTOCOLS

What clinical protocols are developed and implemented at a particular institution varies because of resources, clinical practice environment, and technical considerations. However, there are common issues that should be addressed by clinical protocols regardless of the institution. It is essential that clinical protocols are developed only after a complete process analysis of the functions being supplemented by telemedicine services. The core of this process analysis is to include the deconstruction of processes critical to the delivery of healthcare to the system's constituent population. The results of this process deconstruction form the basic components for the development of protocols. Protocols that have been developed in a vacuum, without this basic administrative, technical, or clinical input, are likely to fail. Additionally, protocols that do not complement existing processes for healthcare delivery introduce confusion and inefficiency into the delivery system's processes, including those dealing with telemedicine.

Although it is outside the scope of this text to provide a full discussion of process analysis, documentation, and reengineering, many of the techniques used in these activities are useful for the efforts required for successful clinical protocol development. The tools of qualitative research are also useful.

A useful hierarchy for clinical protocol development involves first dividing telemedicine activities geographically and then examining functional activities within each geographic division. The rationale for dividing activities geographically is to isolate those activities that are temporally or physically related or dependent. For example, the process required to support similar administrative activities may be different at geographically separated sites.

The basic division of telemedicine services geographically is into those that occur at the *consultant site* (provider of services) and those that occur at the *remote site* (receiver of services). Caution must be exercised in this geographic analysis. Many environments use remote sites that serve as delivery points of care for users of the healthcare delivery system that are used only for telemedicine services. In this case, an additional division of activities would also include a *referring site*, which would be the location where the healthcare consumer receives the bulk of his or her healthcare.

Activities can then be divided by function into two main areas. First, activities that support the administration and technical implementation of telemedicine services can be titled *administrative/health information tasks.* Second, activities that support the facilitation of individual telemedicine clinical events can be titled *clinical facilitation tasks.*

Consultant Site Operations

At a consultant site, administrative/health information tasks include the selection of patients for telemedicine services and providing clinical information services to support telemedicine activities. The process that identifies patients for telemedicine services should be developed with the clear leadership of the supervisory or consulting clinicians, with input from a multidisciplinary focus group of administrative, technical, and clinical personnel. Additionally, it should be recognized that although referral and selection of patients clearly involves clinical judgment and skill, it is in many managed-care focused systems primarily an administrative task. Technical leadership for telemedicine services should also be focused at the consultant site for both role or process definition and for clinician focus.

At a consultant site, clinical facilitation tasks would include, but not necessarily be limited to, providing technical support for telemedicine services and presenting clinical information to facilitate telemedicine services. Often, the focus of technical or health information support is on the remote sites. In many cases, however, the consultant sites have unique technical support requirements. Also the consultant site often must be prepared to support the individual consult with health information, as it is also often the site for advanced diagnostic services, the results of which must be incorporated into the care of the patient that is physically located at the referring site.

Remote-site Operations

At a remote site, administrative/health information tasks would include scheduling patients for telemedicine services, coordinating the execution of laboratory and diagnostic procedures, and providing clinical information services to facilitate telemedicine services.

At a remote site, clinical facilitation tasks would include, but would not necessarily be limited to, providing technical support for telemedicine services, executing physical examination activities to facilitate telemedicine services, and presenting clinical information to facilitate telemedicine services. These areas are expanded in the following sections to show the various activities that would be included.

Providing Technical Support

Providing technical support for telemedicine services would include functions related to the operation and troubleshooting of telecommunications equipment and any special procedures to clean and maintain telemedicine system peripherals.

Executing Physical Examination Activities

Executing physical examination activities to facilitate telemedicine services would include demonstrating an understanding of clinical terminology, the ability to perform cardiopulmonary examinations as required using the provided telemedicine peripherals, performing musculoskeletal examinations as required, and performing neurologic examinations as required. Other clinical skills, including wound examination or suture and staple removal, should also be considered.

Presenting Clinical Information

Presenting clinical information to facilitate telemedicine services would include the requirement to present a core element of patient information that might include patient identification and demographics, as well as other information needed for specific subspecialty environments. Clinical information presentation can take on critical importance in an environment that is still tied to separate paper records for the consultant and remote sites.

Training

Although the training of remote site presenters is outside the scope of this chapter, it should be obvious that process analysis, task deconstruction, and protocol development is the starting point for developing training programs for healthcare professionals engaged in telemedicine services. This can form the basis for more advanced training for providers as well (7). The acceptance of the telemedicine system is enhanced when remote-site presenters are trained in these skills (8).

Referring Site Operations

Because they are not involved in the delivery of telemedicine services, referring sites are often overlooked in telemedicine system planning. Until an integrated health information system is in place within the system, however, the collection and forwarding of health information to the patient's primary point of healthcare delivery is a task of critical importance (8). Obviously, administrative/health information tasks are paramount in this analysis and if not accounted for can prevent the entire system from being functional.

CONCLUSION

Clinical protocol development for telemedicine services is a systematic process that uses the tools of process analysis, documentation, and reengineering to create models of telemedicine service delivery that are complementary to existing service delivery models used for nontelemedicine services.

REFERENCES

1. Huston JL, Smith TA. Evaluating a telemedicine delivery system. *Top Health Inform Manag* 1996; 16:65–71.
2. Sox HC, Blatt MA, Higgins MC, Marton KI. *Medical decision making*. Boston: Butterworth–Heinemann, 1988.
3. Moore MB. Acceptance of information technology by health care providers. In: Huff C, ed. *The proceedings of the symposium on computers and the quality of life.* New York: Association of Computing Machinery Press, 1996:49–56.
4. Moore MB. An introduction to telemedicine: implications for clinical practice. *Phys Assist* 1996; 20:99–108.
5. Peredina DA, Allen A. Telemedicine technology and clinical applications. *JAMA* 1994;273:483–488.
6. Daft R, Lengel R. Organizational information requirements, media richness, and structural design. *Manag Sci* 1994;32:5, 554–571.
7. Lunin LF, Ball MJ, eds. Perspectives on information science and health informatics education. *J Am Soc Inform Sci* 1989;40:365–377.
8. Brecht B, Gray C, Peterson C, Youngblood B. The University of Texas Medical Branch–Texas Department of Criminal Justice Telemedicine Project: findings from the first year of operation. *Telemed J* 1996;2:25–41.

Telemedicine: Practicing in the Information Age,
edited by Steven F. Viegas and Kim Dunn.
Lippincott–Raven Publishers, Philadelphia © 1998.

19

Distance Education versus In-class Instruction

Alice L. Parker and Lorne A. Parker

Teletraining Systems, Inc., Stillwater, Oklahoma 74074; and
Teletraining Institute., Stillwater, Oklahoma 74074

The information age is not as easy to pinpoint as the twentieth century, which began with the first tick of the clock on January 1, 1900, and will end at midnight on December 31, 1999. Many different points in technological time can be identified. Inventions are the easiest benchmark: Gutenberg's press, the pony express, the telegraph, the telephone, the railroad, the automobile, the airplane, the radio, the television, the computer, the satellite, the Internet.

Each invention has facilitated, as well as made more difficult, the transfer of information from one location to another. The term "user-friendly" really did not come into play, however, until people began to shop around for personal computers for office and home use.

In the medical and corporate community, as well as the institutional arena, each electronic advance was quickly accepted as another medium for transferral of necessary data, methods, techniques, texts, and contexts. All have been based in the world of information exchange.

INTERACTIVE DISTANCE EDUCATION

The first use of distance education was probably in 1939 when an Iowa school started a project to meet the needs of homebound and hospitalized students. A few postsecondary institutions began experimental applications in the 1940s and 1950s. From the mid-1960s to mid-1970s, distance education gained momentum as many colleges and universities implemented large audio teleconferencing systems, many of them for continuing medical education. The teleconferencing systems linked from 20 to 200 locations, reaching thousands of people in their home communities. Toward the end of the 1970s, however, the growth rate of distance education began to taper.

The window of distance education can be as small as a telephone or as large as a giant television screen. The important dimension of the window is that it opens and closes. In other words, the window offers the ability to interact with others regarding whatever the message or the content of information may be.

Distance education does not pretend to be the ultimate solution to the corporate or institutional dilemma about contentment with the status quo regarding staff experience and expansion of intelligence, whether there are a variety of leaps of learning and understanding, or the expansion of personal horizons that quickly or ultimately benefit the corporate sponsor. On the other hand, distance education is a cost-effective, program-specific medium that can achieve a meaningful percentage of organizational goals and objectives.

Distance education is an integrated system for the delivery and management of corporate, institutional, or organizational training programs. This is achieved through the use of appropriate or advanced telecommunications services. Technically, distance education is the use and expansion of the earlier applications called *teleconferencing*.

The principle of connecting students in one location with a teacher in another still exists. Now, though, it is not only a matter of picking up the telephone. The same two-way concept is involved, to be sure. Sometimes it is actually a telephone. Sometimes it is a telephone that will, via a national and sophisticated network, still bring voices together. The technology of distance education has leapt beyond the actual telephone, though, and into the realms of two-way video, desktop conferencing with live video and graphics, global satellite up-link and down-link capabilities, the Internet, and asynchronous activities.

The tangible benefits of a well-planned, well-executed distance education program are many. Years of research prove that distance education achieves benefits that are real and measurable. The benefits, of course, vary from institution to institution, but some can be put in general terms.

1. Distance education provides timely instruction to a greater number of individuals. Organizations can deliver updated information or "refresher courses" as quickly as the need arises. Existing delivery methods may already be in place, but experience has too often proved Murphy's Law. Many trainees have been held back in a conventional training program simply because there were not enough chairs in the classroom. Distance education can relieve that sense of frustration, which also contributes to employee turnover or detours in the path of advancement, by opening training options to more individuals by creating a multiplicity of learning environments.
2. Distance education can greatly reduce training expenses. Each year, organizations commit billions of dollars to cover the costs of rounding up their "students" from all over the country, the region, or the state, or even a large city, just to bring them together to learn. Transportation, lodging, meals, and entertainment are traditional bullets that must be bitten to accomplish the basic task of education. And these costs never decrease, unless the organization decides to drop them altogether, which has its own price. Distance education does not promise to eliminate the need for people to gather, to share personal experiences, and to honor achievements and services rendered. When it comes to training people in the essential areas mandated by the market, by the institution, or by whatever agenda is deemed worthy, however, distance education can provide welcome relief to managers, department heads, and professionals who find themselves torn by having to decide whether to send their people to school or to control what is usually a diminishing budget item.

3. Distance education increases productivity. Many training programs require a student to spend more time coming and going than he or she actually spends in training. Although it is true that some hands-on situations require the physical presence of the individual being trained, many others can handle everything through distance education. So, travel days can be turned into workdays, not only providing the company with production continuity but also immediate application of the course's content. Most distance education programs are designed to be incorporated into part of the regular business day. Increased productivity also applies to the instructors or trainers, for they can double or triple, at least, the number of students in the class.
4. Distance education creates greater training flexibility. By using the in-place training environment, organizations can plug in or respond to new information to modify present training programs as the technology changes. Spontaneous, interactive classroom situations can be augmented by prerecorded materials, thus remaining flexible for day-to-day modification. In addition, there is also the increased availability of key speakers or experts, people who could not fit in their hour on the stage if it meant a day going or returning. In the distance education setting, it is feasible to link individuals to a multitude of scattered classrooms where not only instruction is possible but also student response is affordable. Similarly, distance education enables instructors to share resources from different locations, and this has proven to be a value-added benefit through the promotion of cooperation. It also mitigates the potential feeling of alienation.

Considering the educational applications and the institutional benefits, it is not difficult to recognize the increased involvement on all corporate and organizational levels in the realm of distance education.

If there is a stumbling block along the way to implementing distance education, it usually lies in the area of content development or course adaptation and instructor preparedness and confidence. The following section, Designing Content for the Distance Education Classroom, provides insights into various techniques and methods that can be used to deliver engaging, interesting, and effective instruction at a distance.

Although distance education and in-class instruction are similar, allowances must be made to transcend the geographic separation of distant classrooms. The techniques suggested in the following section explain how an instructor or presenter must prepare for teaching at a distance. The techniques are certainly applicable for in-class instruction and, for the most part, improve traditional instruction because they require planning ahead, provide for variety, and personalize the learning environment, no matter if instruction is in person or at a distance.

DESIGNING CONTENT FOR THE DISTANCE EDUCATION CLASSROOM

You may be questioning the feasibility of creating an effective distance education program and system. There are so many things to think about! Consider, though, that your telecommunications and educational or informational needs are unique.

Your first step, therefore, is to develop a set of basic design components or guidelines for your distance education program. Guidelines provide a framework in which you and others can build a training curriculum that uses one or more teleconferencing modes. Distance education is not a stand-alone element in any corporate or institutional agenda. Distance education always fits into an overall instructional or informational design sequence.

There is no magic to a systems approach, for it is simply a means or process of solving problems, but one that can be subdivided into practical, operational steps. Although the general goal may be the same for both face-to-face experiences and distance education, research and personal involvement prove that there are significant and meaningful differences when it comes to designing a distance education program. Some differences to consider include the following:

- Individuals are always physically distant from one another; even if there is a core group at the site of origination, there will be responses coming in from afar.
- Individuals are using telecommunications technologies to interact with one another; however, one may use audio only while others use compressed video, so course content should accommodate a spectrum of possibilities.
- Individuals may be intimidated by, frightened, embarrassed, or ignorant of the electronic technology involved: There is a need to overcome these discomforts when distance teaching systems are used.
- Individuals may be alone in a distant location, or they may be in a large group. The isolation or group camaraderie will put a different spin on the process that is designed to develop the most effective results.

There are few "givens" when it comes to distance education, and, although these are not to be considered negative elements, they are certainly different from the expectations of an instructor-trainer in a face-to-face environment. Consider the following parameters:

- When is a group not a group? You might think you have a class of 100 trainees or students, and it is only an accident of geography that they are divided among a dozen or so locations. You are no doubt familiar with the old "getting-to-know-you" exercises at seminars and workshops. Distance education strains the limits of even the most creative of facilitators when it comes to bringing participants' humanity out in the context of a widely dispersed class. It can be done, but you will have to work hard to bring it about.
- Meaningful discussion is no accidental occurrence. Only the most tedious or inept instructor can fail when it comes to generating responsive exchanges between participants. Meaningful discussion just does not happen, however, because it takes a dynamic trainer to elicit responses from the expressive person and the reluctant individual. In distance education, just as in "real life," there are those who think they are infringing on program time regardless of the meaningful nature of their response, or they are wary of taking up somebody else's time, or they may not have the right choice of words to spontaneously make a statement or ask a question.

- Guess what? It is not just preschoolers who have short attention spans. In the late 1800s, North Americans loved to listen to people make speeches or have debates that lasted for hours. It is no accident that orators were on the stump for approximately the length of one of today's movies. These events were a curious kind of entertainment at a time when there was not much to distract the crowds from their own short lives. Thanks to all the media input people "enjoy" today, the adult attention span has returned to one that is not so different from little tots who must have their eyes and ears shift points of view every few minutes. "Very long" is usually translated to approximately 15 minutes. Even with visual interruptions that are programmed periodically in a presentation, the audio message should be succinct and to the point.
- "It ain't over 'til it's over," Yogi Berra said. Did you know that Yogi Berra was the American League's most valuable player three times? It did not matter what he said, he played the game better than almost everybody else. And he was right about things being over. There are those who believe that a training session ends when the trainer and the charts and graphs exit the broadcast arena: Not so. The communications loop has not been completed until it can be seen that the message has been received and understood as intended. Distance education does not provide the nonverbal cues that face-to-face training can, even when two-way video is used. So, you have to include a feedback mechanism when you design a program.

Developing That Ideal Design for Your Needs

None of this is easy, but it is fundamental. There are five basic elements in the design process for any distance education program: (a) humanizing the approach, (b) fostering participation and interaction, (c) the delivery or presentation of the message, (d) the avenues for feedback, and (e) mechanisms for evaluation. These are almost universal, for they are part and parcel of any training situation or demand, they cut across the boundaries of subject matter, and they pertain to one single session as well as to a year's curriculum. They are applicable regardless of the length of the program, the types of learners, and the sizes of groups.

Thou Shalt Not Fly by the Seat of Thy Pants Unless Crashing Is the Goal

Regardless of the experience one has as an instructor, trainer, or communicator, the use of a systematic methodology is critical. In distance education, the critical path to achieving your goals has its required steps, as well as numerous obstacles. Following one's intuition about instructional design can create serious hazards that may not be recognized until *after* the learning moment has passed.

Instinct is no substitute for working within a prescribed structure or set of guidelines. Without a tried-and-true format or system, you will find it difficult to create a significantly effective distance education program on any level. Those trainers who have experience only in face-to-face, classroom programs have many things to learn about the methodologies of distance education.

HUMAN ELEMENTS

Believe it or not, there are communicators who consistently ignore the reality of people involved in the distance teaching and learning process. From the viewpoint of the teacher or trainer, the human factor may seem to be the most obvious, most important ingredient in any consideration of a learning environment. However ironic it may appear, though, this is often the last thing considered in the communications process, as the technology, the budget, and the message's design are deemed to be more important than the people involved in the learning experience.

The five main human elements of distance education are

1. Humanizing factors
2. Participation means
3. Message delivery
4. Feedback methods
5. Evaluation means

Humanizing Factors

In many situations, the word "humanize" is used to mean making something have human characteristics. In distance education, to humanize means focusing on the importance of the individual and overcoming distance and technology by creating a collegiate or community spirit or rapport.

Trainers and planners, teachers and instructors, healthcare professionals, chief executive officers, and departmental managers should remember what it was like to be alone in a room and be expected to either learn or to impart important information. It is not an odd experience to be part of a group of three in which no one is exactly sure how to operate the equipment or handle the various educational elements. Nor is it impossible to imagine someone in Nome, Alaska, talking in midwinter to a counterpart in Key West, Florida, by way of Oklahoma City. Geographic distance will become a moot consideration only after people are convinced that a shared experience will bring them closer together.

Hello, I'm . . .

Everyone has been in situations in which the name tag hastily written in felt-tip pen is the only means of identification. From the affixing of that sticky slip of paper to the chest, the rest is up to each person to draw conclusions, ask questions, become acquainted, and establish a basis for communication. "Getting to know you," the song goes, "getting to know all about you. . . ." If it is not an easy process in face-to-face meetings, then it is even more difficult in long-distance situations.

Many studies that examine the process of distance education find a direct link between making the participant feel comfortable with everyone involved and the actual degree of participation so crucial to the success of any distance learning situation. The sharing of concerns and problems and their possible solutions, the introduction of new policies or procedures, and the request for feedback all require willingness to participate that comes only when an individual feels at ease with the medium of exchange that welcomes his or her contributions and reactions. For example, when personal visits allow program designers or trainers to meet with forthcoming participants, there is measurable and progressive enthusiasm that extends to the actual program's presentation. Commentary increases, as do questions and hoped-for responses. People want to share more after they have allayed their individual fears of embarrassment, shyness, or reluctance to make that spontaneous, anonymous commitment on air to which they can be held accountable. Of course, this kind of preprogram contact is the ideal situation. It may seem impossible for the Nome–Key West–Oklahoma City network, but it is not, because a local supervisor or even a long-distance call can help pave the way toward effective distance learning.

There is a satisfaction quotient in distance education, just as there is in any tutorial or learning experience. In some cases, satisfaction is the feeling that the one-time participant has when the last word is said. For others, the meaningful first time out can mean that subsequent involvements can be more productive and rewarding. Distance education groups can include the novice and the veteran, the expert and the initiate; therefore, it is important that the distance educator be aware of how best to reach everyone in the participating group. Not only does this allow for the creation of realistic program goals, but the knowledge also allows for a range of examples that are relevant to different levels of involvement. The pace and the structure or style of the programming can also vary according to the makeup of the people who are participating.

You Were Expecting . . . ?

How many new places have you visited where the first response was, "you know, this looks a lot like . . ." or something equivalent that establishes contact between something familiar and something foreign or new? With this in mind, expectations should be humanized so the trainer can anticipate that equation, which generally involves having the same expectations of face-to-face educational situations as past experiences.

Although it is not always possible, distance education can, as Marshal McLuhan wrote in his book *The Medium is the Massage*, "make the medium the massage, as well as the message." It is important to concentrate on the positive qualities of the distance teaching media, which are many. To spend time apologizing for system limitations is to only reinforce possible disappointment with broadcast delays, one-way broadcast, compressed video, or whatever is different from television at home or the in-house seminar.

Attributes of a distance education system include the following:

- The system has its own informal, personally approachable quality that actually enhances a more conversational approach to the information being transmitted, thereby diminishing the possibilities of a tedious, formal lecture.
- Distance education is inherently interactive. In contrast to many media (e.g., memoranda, training manuals, videotape or audiotape lessons), distance education allows immediate interchange between individuals, participants and trainers, executives and managers. Everyone recalls those significant moments when the instructor responds

positively to a question we have asked, or when we suddenly see the light because we have heard another participant's revelation.

- Anonymity is an asset. Many individuals, separated either by long hallways, the distance between buildings, or miles, find the spatial difference to be a guarantee of a degree of anonymity. Therefore, they can ask that potentially embarrassing question without fear of seeing dismay on others' faces. Or they can hide behind the facade of distance, thus shielding age, physical appearance, or an infirmity that may inhibit responses by other participants. Plus, there are those who feel most comfortable in a setting that provides an atmosphere of greater concentration and focus without predictable distractions.

Clearly, the onus of effective distance teaching is borne by the trainer or the programmer who must bring all of these diverse elements into the final mix, the educational program itself.

Time, of course, is the governing factor in the institution or introduction of any of the means of humanizing the presentation that are presented in the list that follows. If there is an adequate span of time to incorporate all into your plans, then luck is with you. In many distance-teaching situations, however, the brevity of time is the way things happen: For example, "We need to get to our people before the weekend." At moments like that, one is lucky simply to have the correct contact numbers and the necessary technology in place. Consider the following accordingly.

- For personal, face-to-face contact with the enrolled participants, either on an individual basis or as a group conference, call before the actual program's transmission.
- Establish personal contact with everyone via electronic mail (e-mail), a Web page, or even fax or surface mail. This message is a welcoming one that lets all know how important it is for the program to succeed, and that success will be based on individual and group involvement. This communication should include the agenda, the program's goals, and preparation or suggestions for ways to make the first (only or successive) program significant. Questions may be asked or problems presented for solution. It does not hurt to let the participants know who you are and what your ideas for the class are: If possible, include a photograph so people have an idea of what the moderator or teacher looks like.
- Invite the participants to send their own biographies, so you can know more about each of them and you can, if time allows, extend to the others a brief biographical sketch, even if only titles and location, before the distance education session's commencement. This can be made part of the registration form easily.
- A master roster always works for the trainer. Having a quick-look listing of each participant's name, title, job, location, and so on can provide the moderator-mediator with the means to identify people as they respond. Such a device also allows you the means of directing questions or information needs to particular people and focusing on specific interests in the context of the course.
- It is more than name, rank, and serial number. When opening the program, ask for an informal roll call. As a trainer, it is important to identify voices with names, while

participants will use their own ears to try to picture counterparts and fit these to subsequent responses. The experienced trainer knows who to ask about the weather, who to say something to about the last time you visited them, and when it is important to reveal that the person is accompanied by others whose voices will be heard.

- "A participant by any other name. . . ." It is most important that each participant, when possible, be identified by name. Even those who are content to be anonymous take some pleasure in being identified by name.
- Be yourself. You are a trainer, a moderator, a facilitator, because it is what you do well. You have a talent for relating to others, as well as the critical ability to handle a learning experience and manage a learning environment. There is no reason for you to lack confidence, if you have all your ducks in a row before the beginning of the program. If there are possible problems to be encountered, be prepared to respond appropriately and not in panic. Be yourself: wise, kind, friendly, articulate, and someone in charge.

A Portfolio of Techniques to Add That Human Dimension

There are certainly other means of bringing the personalized element into the mixture that constitutes a distance education environment and experience. These require additional planning, some cost, and certainly time adequate for their design and development.

How Much Time Do We Have Left?

It should be stressed that "humanizing" a program or presentation takes time. There is the danger of spending a major portion of class time making people feel comfortable in the distance education environment or generating the desired rapport. Then suddenly it dawns on everybody that there is no way, short of speed-speaking, to get through the agenda and provide all the planned materials. So the trainer must establish a well-balanced approach, one that takes into consideration the desired effects and still achieves learning.

Participation Means

If distance education only meant the use of telecommunications technology, then this would be a chapter about one-way audio or video, use of videotapes or audiotapes, or the transmission of information electronically. Active participation is vital in distance education. Distance education studies parallel those in other disciplines, such as educational psychology, communications, and group dynamics. They show that the chance to participate directly is central to the success of any learning or communication process.

Two fundamental guidelines can be noted in a consideration of distance education participation.

1. Participation opportunities and strategies should be carefully planned in advance of the program's presentation.
2. Participation not only involves encouraging group members to contribute to the program but also having people interact with the content itself as you present it or as it is included in predistributed support materials.

Interactive involvement is not something that just happens. There are those who think that is why church protocol does not encourage applause after the parson's sermon: Only rarely do parishioners feel so moved as to acknowledge their spiritual participation. Studies suggest that there is an automatic training in which, over time, individuals consciously or unconsciously adapt their particular ways of communicating to become more interactive. Interaction is not a uniform response, however, for there are those who want to jump into the pool immediately, while others only put their toes in the water. This lack of uniformity is why building in participation formats as part of the overall program and asking some individuals to be responsible for taking the lead are among the ways of ensuring interaction will take place.

The second guideline concerns the preconception most have that participation always involves some kind of active response: asking a question, expressing a concern, asking for something to be repeated so notation may be made, and so on. These activities are means of self-expression that reveal people are listening and responding to what is happening.

Remember, though, that distance educators are involved in *distant* education, that they cannot always see, hear, or observe responsiveness. There is something called "active listening," which is also called "anticipatory alertness." Not that distance educators see that light bulb go off in someone's mind or watch the mental gears shift; call it a trainer's intuition, but distance educators know when what is being presented is being ingested and being chewed on even without witnessing verbal or visual reactions. The skillful distance educator will use questions, written and oral, or guide the group with mental exercises, both of which are designed to stimulate this internally active participation that is so important to listening and learning.

To help facilitate all forms of participation, other than the enrollee's walking out the door or turning off the receiver and microphone, the following ideas are on participation techniques.

Plant Questions

Planting questions, a quick-pick idea, is not unethical. Distance education is not a White House press conference in which certain correspondents are offered the opportunity to ask politically prepared questions. Distance education does involve both rhythm and pacing, however, as well as an abhorrence of silence. So, it is important to consider calling a few participants first, establishing contacts, and asking a select few to agree to asking pertinent questions, should the discussion lag. There are some cautionary notes in this prebroadcast preparation: It is best to avoid the "most-favored student" syndrome (i.e., the use of the skilled associate who may assume a familiarity you are not ready to deal with on-air), and there is the danger that the same question will be asked twice or will come at an inopportune time.

Questions Are Tools

You as the trainer know the most appropriate questions to ask. These are questions that provide pivotal answers that move the discussion forward and remind learners what is to be learned, how best to summarize what has been said, and to anticipate what is to come. If there is any doubt in your mind that these questions may not be forthcoming, for whatever reasons, then it would not be inappropriate to send them out in advance as part of the preparatory materials, such as the agenda or syllabus. Depending on how you wish to handle these questions, you may wish to suggest that people pick those questions that interest them most. Watch out, though, for this can backfire on air if no one wants to ask any of your questions.

What Do You Do When . . . ?

Just in case nobody noticed along the way: Distance education is 99.99% adult education. Therefore, the proven, effective, participatory methods used in all mature education programs can most likely be used. These could include role playing, a case-study presentation, a panel discussion, or an interview with an expert who is not one of the participants.

The true test of the trainer, therefore, is to create interesting case studies, not just someone reading a report. Actually, some interesting case studies can be handled through the interview process or set up prebroadcast as different group activities and presentations. Role playing takes on a very human dimension when played across the miles, such as in a telephone conversation with somebody who knows something you do not understand. A panel discussion involving individuals from four states, each with different laws or requirements, can generate considerable interest from participants in other locations.

Why Is Everybody Always Pickin' on Me?

The suggestion of a four-state panel discussion leads into another suggestion to keep in mind. Say that in your group of participants you can locate four distinct groups, each of which can augment or amplify a single concept or idea of a four-program series. So, you go to each group in advance and invite them to talk together, such as by e-mail, before the particular segment germane to one of the programs. Let them know you are building into that section their response and behold what responsibility for group action can do for a broader audience. As witnesses to such demonstrations of interest and opinions, we heartily endorse this method if it fits your specific needs.

Do Not Forget What Goes on Before and What Can Happen After

Pre- and postactivities are always useful tools in stimulating responses and activities and participation at the different locations of any distant education program. These activities include more than starting the discussion on air, for they include what direct or indirect effects can be anticipated on-site for each participant or group of participants. Is one of your goals to help individuals immediately apply what they have learned? Is it to prepare the person for something coming down the line soon? Is it to inform others about significant changes in policy that can affect their workforce? Is the message a warning? Whatever the objectives, it is possible to expand, enhance, or extend the value of the program by using the introduction of preprogram or postprogram inputs or materials.

If there are sensitive issues involved, it is best to deal with them before the fact. Springing surprises on the day of the broadcast is a sure way of disengaging a major portion of the participants who immediately begin that process of "anticipatory alertness" as to their potential involvement in the program or session.

Message Delivery

Everyone has had experience as a communicator. That is perhaps the most critical dimension of human existence: communicating particular messages to other human beings. Many have spent time communicating long messages in the form of speeches and lectures. All have spent time listening and seeing others present their messages, long or short. It is safe to say that a comparatively smaller number have spent time analyzing how messages are designed.

Why are some messages remembered and understood better than others? Message delivery is the way the communication is presented so it will be received, understood, remembered, and responded to.

Listener Attention

One important guideline in designing a presentation is the difference between the rate at which one speaks and the rate at which one thinks or absorbs what is spoken. The average rate of speech for most people is approximately 125 words per minute, whereas the brain processes data at much higher rates (one estimate is upwards of 300 words per minute). Inherently, this provides a gap, one which can lead minds to wander when listening to a speaker. Distractions fill the gap (e.g., personal thoughts, visual observations, sounds nearby, daydreaming) so it is important that distance educators recognize that little can be done to bridge that gap except by making the presentations as interesting and engaging as possible, so the mental space can be filled with related images. Visuals, repetition, and summaries can help provide cues, however, for those whose minds have strayed occasionally or momentarily.

Listener Fatigue

Another aspect to consider about presentations is boredom and restlessness. There are those times when the shuffling of papers, the twitching in seats, and the coughs or clearing of throats signal that people are drifting away, inexorably almost, on the retreating tides of interest in what is happening. Distance educators have to fight this.

Distance educators may not equal the latest Stephen King novel when it comes to avoiding those boring moments, but they can do things to create changes of pace and style to keep people interested. Messages can be designed to incorporate variety, such as using shorter segments or interspersed question-and-answer times. As a rule of thumb, lecture segments should be no longer than 20 minutes. Longer sessions can be programmed to accommodate an interesting menu of actions and exercises.

Presentation

Verbal cues help emphasize the important ideas that the speaker wants to be remembered and recollected. Use the tried and true announcements, such as "Now, this is important . . . ," or, "I want you to remember this point. . . ." When messages such as these begin a paragraph or a section, participants' ears perk up and pens are poised above paper.

Support from the Electronic Sector

Electronic support materials placed at a Web site (e.g., outlines, word lists and glossaries, supplementary articles, bibliographies, graphics) can be enlisted to support your presentation and keep people in the ball game. The Internet and Web pages are a marvelous way to provide a secondary channel for information, because they can be called on as evidence of what is being presented and can be referred to and referenced at a learner's convenience.

In general, the more interesting a speaker can make the message, the more attentive each individual will be and the more information will be remembered. Speakers who use illustrations and examples relevant to the discussion and to the learners' experiences and needs and who punctuate their messages with vivid and meaningful detail and imagery will be the most successful presenters.

Variety Is the Spice of Distance Education

Plan short segments. If you have a very, very, very long segment, break it up with some related or semirelated elements to keep people on their ears, then come back to the main topic. Variety has long proven a viable means of keeping interest levels high, thereby increasing attention span and concentration. The idea of a fast-paced program does not imply that it should be like a Disney-produced feature film. Segments of 5 to 15 minutes, alternated with activities, are at a quick pace.

Repeat and Summarize

It is a natural tendency to avoid repetition; however, there is a need to repeat and summarize far beyond apparent comprehension. Why do speakers want to avoid this? The best guess is that speakers know what the message means, but "Just how many times do I have to repeat myself?" is not the correct approach. Teaching is repetition: How else did you reach where you are today? Important information, necessary news, and critical facts should be offered more than once, otherwise students may believe they are not all that important. Remember, too, that participants have long participated in an educational style that requires redundancy, that things are only crucial to their "passing the course" if it is said more than once. So, expert distance educators recommend repeating new words, phrases, concepts, and theories at least three times during an hour's program.

Back to Print

Do not forsake the printed word, ever, not in our lifetimes anyway. You should never avoid the opportunity to back up what your program is going to present or is presenting via the medium of ink, whether it be outlines, brochures, or even a detailed workbook or text. Although the Internet and sharing information asynchronously have a vital place in modern life, print will always offer a permanent record for review and recollection.

Summarize

At the end of a session or a program sequence, nearly all presenters use some form of bringing together the key points of what has been offered to the participants. Although most trainers depend on the participants being quick enough to record the words that come after "Now, let me summarize . . . ," it is possible that there are those who do not have the stenographic skills to record this synopsis. So, it would not be inappropriate for the trainer to say *after the presenter's summary* something such as, "Now, if you didn't get everything, we'll be sending you a short summarizing document." Friends are won on all sides with that action.

Feedback Methods

Feedback—providing a response to learner performance—is the fourth essential ingredient in the communications process. As students perform new tasks or use information in new ways, they need feedback on their "degree of correctness." This information helps reinforce learning while providing an opportunity to clear up misunderstandings and fill in gaps.

There are two basic types of feedback: internal and external. Internal feedback comes from within the learner. For instance, the answer to an examination question or the release of a free-throw shot may just "feel right." External feedback, on the other hand, comes from outside the learner. External feedback can come from an instructor or some type of training aid. For example, an instructor may provide feedback on pronunciation of a foreign language. Or students may consult solutions in the back of a book for feedback.

For distance educators, many techniques can be used to provide external feedback. However, feedback can be a touchy subject. Although most people say they welcome feedback, few people truly enjoy being "corrected." The following feedback guidelines should help ensure that feedback is valued by learners.

1. Timing is important. The learner must be able to relate the feedback to the associated behavior. If too much time elapses between the behavior and the feedback, the feedback is not effective.
2. Positive feedback is more easily accepted than negative feedback. As any communication, feedback must be "received" by the learner to be useful. Because most learners have a high self-image, they are more likely to receive positive feedback about their performance. This does not mean you cannot provide "corrective" feedback; just be sure to emphasize what was done right as much as possible.
3. Feedback should be specific. Telling someone, "Good job," when he or she swings a golf club is not nearly as effective as saying, "Good, your left elbow was nice and straight."

So, what does one do with feedback? As you can see, feedback has a complexity all its own as far as completing the communications loop.

Aid Students in Forming Correct Responses

When you have asked a question and received an incorrect or incomplete response, do not immediately provide the right answer: Prompt the student for another response. You can do this by asking a diagnostic question (e.g., "How can we get more participation from students?"), describing what the student has just said (e.g., "So, you are suggesting that timeliness is not important when providing feedback?"), or suggesting a missing idea (e.g., "What role should the site facilitator play in providing feedback?").

Use Objective Criteria to Evaluate Performance

At the end of each major learning segment, you should provide learners with a formal evaluation of their work. First, set up a criteria sheet related to your learning objectives and share the criteria with the learners. Then have learners perform an appropriate task and rate them according to the criteria. For example, after a segment on memo writing, you may have students write a memo on a specific topic. You would then evaluate the memos based on the criteria you had established (e.g., clarity, grammar, format). Of course, evaluating individual performance takes time, so use your site facilitators. If possible, have them evaluate student assignments from their site. For psychomotor learning or learning that must be demonstrated by physically performing some task, it will probably be necessary to use site facilitators to assist in the evaluation. If you will be evaluating written assignments, have students or site facilitators e-mail assignments to you. Remember to always provide timely feedback.

Have Students Evaluate Their Own Performance

For many tasks, students have "intrinsic" knowledge of their performance. However, they frequently focus on the negative aspects of their performance unless encouraged to do otherwise. To help learners acknowledge strengths (thus improving the chances that the strengths will be repeated in the future), ask them to list two things they did well. Then help the learner focus on areas for improvement by asking for two things they would do differently if they could do the task again. By asking for only two points, there is just enough to feel good about and just enough for the student to work on.

Incorporation of feedback mechanisms is not a last-resort kind of activity. It should be a natural progression of the educational process. If trainers simply wanted to deliver a message or a body of information involving no response, they could set up a mailing system; read their material in front of a plain, gray, concrete block wall; and then go to lunch. As professional communicators, distance educators are enlisted exactly because they avoid that approach. The duty is to make the learning process as full a circle of human communication as possible, which includes growth for all involved, including distance educators.

Evaluation Means

Message delivery concerns how information is communicated to learners. How well a message is received still must be determined. Just as learners need feedback on their performance, instructors need feedback as well. This type of feedback is frequently called *evaluation*.

Basically, evaluation also completes the communication loop—you communicate a message, which is received by students, who then let you know what they heard. Thus, ongoing evaluation helps take the pulse of the group.

Evaluation can help answer such questions as: Is what I am saying interesting or boring? Does everyone understand what I am saying? Did I leave out any important details? Immediate feedback then becomes a stimulus to help decide on an action. That is, instructors can decide whether to continue in the way they have been or to make adjustments. Evaluation helps eliminate the tendency to "overtalk"—to continue an explanation longer than necessary because instructors do not know if the audience received the message.

When instructors interact with a class in a traditional setting, they receive subtle feedback in the form of nonverbal cues that constantly helps them gain information about how the message is being received. Yawns or bored expressions are forms of negative feedback that stimulate instructors to change what they are saying or how they are saying it. Erect postures and looks of interest are forms of positive feedback that reinforce what instructors are doing and saying. Thus, nonverbal cues form a part of the corrective information called *feedback*. Although this kind of information is not present in all forms of distance education, it should be used when it is present.

An easy way to incorporate evaluation in a distance course is to plan for verbal feedback from the group. After each natural division in the material, you can ask questions such as, "Was the message too fast? too complex? clearly explained?" You can also use less-structured feedback by suggesting that learners interrupt with questions at any time. When using this method, remember to be sensitive to attempts by class members to interrupt. Your choice depends a great deal on your delivery style, the content, and the type of group.

Evaluation centers around building in mechanisms that can help complete the communications loop between you and learners. With students physically separated from you, you will want to plan ways to obtain evaluative feedback during the session as well as off-the-air. If you think that the group is hesitant to provide feedback, you may wish to ask several individuals in advance of the session to provide it for you.

Evaluation as a Motivating Factor

Evaluation also serves as a motivating factor for an instructor. The reactions instructors receive from learners help them maintain their enthusiasm. That is why it is important to reach out to students using the network's two-way capability. Because instructors are more accustomed to feedback from traditional classes, they tend to seek feedback primarily from local audiences. But remember, classes at remote sites are in a different environment and receive your message in a different format than local classes. So, make sure you seek feedback from multiple sources. Remember, promoting the feeling that every participant in the session, whether that individual is sitting right next to you or is joining you from a location hundreds of miles away, is important to the success of the course.

Use On-the-spot Application of Information

Find out if the material presented is relevant to students' situations. Pause several times during the presentation to ask for individual feedback. Ask one or two students to briefly comment on the value of the information to him or her. Would the person use it? If so, how? Application-of-information feedback stimulates others to think creatively.

Review Recorded Sessions

Self-feedback is another excellent tool for improving next week's or next year's course. Many times, educators miss an important ingredient because there was no time to stand back and be an observer. Reviewing a recorded session can be a valuable feedback tool. What were the strengths and weaknesses of that session? What might be changed in time for the next session? Were opportunities provided for participation? Did individuals take advantage of those opportunities? Did the message come across with enthusiasm? Did it come across in a natural, spontaneous delivery? This type of self-feedback can be as important as that from students.

Use Written Forms of Evaluation

Encourage written feedback to determine whether your course is meeting its objectives. Either paper or electronic forms can be used. If you choose to use a paper form, design it for easy mailing and faxing: Use only one side of the page for feedback, design a header that serves as a fax transmittal, and use the back for your mailing address to allow the form to be folded and placed in the mail. Include the forms in your printed materials. If you are conducting several sessions, color code the forms. This way you can easily identify the "yellow" form as dealing with a particular session or topic. Electronic forms can be provided via a Web page or e-mail. By providing forms or discussing paperless feedback in your printed materials, you are conveying the message that you are sincerely interested in obtaining feedback. No matter which method you use, make sure the form has a simple, easy-to-fill-out design. You should also make the feedback anonymous to encourage honest feedback.

Get on the Information Superhighway Map as Soon as Possible

Although there is some benefit to continuing your contact with the participants along the route of the simple postage stamp, it is up to you to determine your time frame. Our modern postal system goes farther than metered mail. The U.S. Postal Service, as with so many other communication enterprises, has great deals when it comes to shipping information quickly.

If hourly responses are a factor, then e-mail is the answer. Technology is at such a point that if you do not use it, you do not lose it, but you actually postpone your own ability to use feedback. The network is what you yourself create. What you want, you can make it become. Linkages are what you build. The response mechanism is what you construct. You set the limits, the dimensions, and the parameters, so the program can reach its maximum potential.

CONCLUSION

This chapter describes distance education and its practical application. It also presents methods for designing, delivering, and evaluating distance courses along with the research that supports the importance of building them into any distance education program or course. By using these tips and techniques, you will increase student satisfaction and learning. How do we know? Because the five components are based on sound research and because thousands of educators have been successful using them!

Although researchers continue to study distance education, we are confident that using the five design components—humanizing, participation, message delivery, feedback, and evaluation—help us be effective as distance educators.

Telemedicine: Practicing in the Information Age,
edited by Steven F. Viegas and Kim Dunn.
Lippincott–Raven Publishers, Philadelphia

20

Training for Effective Telemedicine

David J. Solomon, *Paula D. Townley, Casey D. Peterson, Kleanthe C. Caruso, *Casi T. Doughty, Kim Dunn, Sterling A. North, Lorne A. Parker, and Owen J. Murray

*Department of Internal Medicine and Office of Educational Development, University of Texas Medical Branch at Galveston, Galveston, Texas 77555; *Department of Education and Professional Development, University of Texas Medical Branch at Galveston, Correctional Managed Care, Galveston, Texas 77555; Department of Clinical Affairs, Texas Department of Criminal Justice Hospital, Galveston, Texas 77555; University of Texas Medical Branch at Galveston/Texas Department of Criminal Justice System Nursing Services, Galveston, Texas 77555; Department of Internal Medicine, Texas Department of Criminal Justice, University of Texas Medical Branch at Galveston, Galveston, Texas 77555; Office of Continuing Education, University of Texas Medical Branch at Galveston, Galveston, Texas 77555; Teletraining Institute, Stillwater, Oklahoma 74074; and Department of Correctional Managed Health Care, University of Texas Medical Branch at Galveston, Galveston, Texas 77555*

The University of Texas Medical Branch (UTMB) at Galveston relies heavily on telemedicine to provide healthcare for inmates in the Texas Department of Criminal Justice (TDCJ). After conducting more than 5,500 telemedicine consults from 1995 to 1997, it became clear that lack of training and written protocols for conducting telemedicine was inhibiting the program's effectiveness. As a first step in addressing the lack of training and protocols, UTMB conducted a rudimentary training needs assessment through a set of focus groups. The training and protocol issues outlined by the members of the focus groups provide the basis for this chapter.

The focus groups were conducted during a 2-hour session as part of the *Telemedicine: Practicing in the Information Age First Annual Conference* held at UTMB's Open Gates Conference Facility on April 24–26, 1997. The conference attendees were divided into four groups of approximately 30 participants. Each group had a moderator and a recorder who took notes. In addition, the sessions were audiotaped.

The focus groups included designated physicians from several different specialties. Many of these physicians had extensive experience providing consultative and surgical follow-up care for inmates at outlying prison units via telemedicine. Each group also included four or five health professionals who had extensive experience presenting patients at the outlying prison units. The groups also contained health administrators from the prison units, health educators, and several primary care physicians employed by the UTMB/TDCJ healthcare network who were based at outlying prison units and who referred patients to UTMB physicians through telemedicine consults.

The sessions began with short presentations by the specialist physicians outlining their view of training and patient data needs for conducting telemedicine sessions within their particular specialty. Moderators then presented a series of structured interview questions to ascertain more general training needs from the physician's point of view. Structured questions to ascertain the training needs from the patient presenter's point of view followed. The last portion of the session was devoted to questions posed to the group as a whole concerning how best to structure a comprehensive training program and develop a set of protocols for conducting telemedicine sessions.

After completing the focus group sessions, the moderators and recorders met and consolidated the information that was gathered. The findings were organized and presented back to the conference attendees on the following day.

Participants identified a number of training and documentation issues that they thought would improve telemedicine as it is practiced within the UTMB/TDCJ system. Participants also thought the effectiveness and efficiency of the telemedicine sessions would be increased with the development of protocols for presenting patients and for the collection and flow of patient information between the referring physician, presenter, and physician specialist consultant before, during, and after the telemedicine session. Although many of the training needs and protocols were generic, it was also clear that additional information and presenter skills were needed for telemedicine sessions within specific specialty areas. Participants also identified systems and information flow issues that should be addressed for a telemedicine program to function efficiently.

The UTMB/TDCJ healthcare system is large and provides care to a prison inmate population that is distributed over a large geographic area. Some aspects of the training issues and protocols outlined by the focus groups are specific to the UTMB/TDCJ system. Much of the material, however, is relevant to other telemedicine programs.

The focus groups provided information on training, protocol development, and system changes in five areas. These include required presenter skills, necessary patient data, preparing and orienting the patient, physician skills, and structuring a training program.

PRESENTER SKILLS

Presenters need a variety of skills and knowledge. These include (a) understanding how to use and troubleshoot the telecommunication equipment; (b) appropriate medical terminology; (c) history, physical examination, and presentation skills; and (d) familiarity with telemedicine protocols for orienting, preparing, and presenting patients to the consulting physician. Specific specialty areas may also require the presenter to have additional data collection skills or may require that patient data be presented in a specific format.

Conference participants thought that an adequate understanding of how to use telecommunication equipment and the ability to troubleshoot at least rudimentary equipment problems was a key skill for presenters. Telemedicine sessions are frequently canceled or terminated prematurely due to equipment problems. Participants thought these could often be solved, allowing the consultation to continue, if the presenters had appropriate training. The presenter also should know how to position the patient and camera so that the physician can adequately observe the patient. There are a whole range of sensing devices that can be attached to telecommunication equipment to provide consulting physicians with additional data. Presenters should know how to operate and position commonly used devices, such as stethoscopes and otoscopes, and in the case of specific specialties, other, more specialized devices, such as slit-lamps and endoscopes.

Presenters should be well trained in physical diagnosis and capable of performing correct and consistent physical examinations. Although presenters are generally licensed health professionals with formal training in physical diagnosis, conference participants thought that additional training and refresher courses should be created to help ensure that data collection is done appropriately and is consistent across presenters. These training sessions would also provide a mechanism for instructing presenters on performing less common physical examination maneuvers, such as specialized joint or neurologic examinations, that are required for some specialty consultations. The knowledge that presenters are adequately trained in physical diagnosis, particularly when the consulting physician has been involved in the training process, greatly increases confidence in the information provided by presenters. Training for presenters in turn facilitates the acceptance of telemedicine as a viable alternative to having a patient travel from the remote site to the medical center.

Physicians thought that the use of a standardized format for presenting patients and the use of appropriate medical terminology would facilitate telemedicine sessions. Such a format should be developed and included in the presenter training program. The program should also include a review of common medical terminology.

An important aspect of the presenter's role is orienting and preparing the patient for the telemedicine consultation. This includes informing him or her of the purpose of the visit and who the consulting physician will be and describing what will happen during the consultation. The presenter should see that the patient is properly gowned (if necessary) and that any other physical preparation that is needed for the consult is completed. This process should be emphasized in the presenter training and orientation program.

PHYSICIAN ORIENTATION FOR TELEMEDICINE

As with presenters, an orientation would facilitate physicians who practice telemedicine. Physicians need a basic orientation on how to operate telecommunication equipment. Although technical support may be more readily available at the central site where the consulting physicians are located, having the physician capable of operating the camera sound equipment and peripheral devices facilitates the encounter. The physician must also be oriented to the patient information system, whether it be electronic or paper. The appropriate flow of information among the referring physicians, presenters, and consulting physicians is key to an effective telemedicine program.

Consulting physicians should learn to communicate effectively with patients and presenters at a distance. There are subtle differences in communicating via telecommunication equipment, such as how to face the camera. Mastery of these techniques can improve the physician-patient relationship that is critical for effective healthcare.

An extremely important issue that was brought out in the focus groups was the need for the consulting physician to be cognizant of the situation at the remote site. There was a strong feeling among the presenters that a great deal of frustration and miscommunication can be avoided if the consulting physicians are more aware of issues in providing healthcare in the prison environment. They suggested that physicians who regularly consult via telemedicine at some point visit a remote prison unit. The lack of understanding and miscommunication probably ran in both directions. The presenters and referring physicians at the outlying prison units were also unaware of the pressures and constraints under which the hospital-based specialists must operate and how these limit their ability to provide optimal telemedical support to the outlying prison units. Visits, such as by the specialists to the outlying prison units and by the health professionals at the remote units to Hospital Galveston, and face-to-face discussion, such as in the focus groups this chapter is based on, are essential for facilitating the mutual understanding and respect that are necessary for a telemedicine healthcare system to function effectively.

KEY PATIENT DATA AND APPROPRIATE INFORMATION FLOW

Lack of key patient data and problems in the flow of patient information were identified as significant problems. Patients often arrive for a telemedicine consultation without any clear goal documented for the session. Sessions are regularly canceled because critical laboratory tests were not performed or the results were unavailable at the time of the consult. Referring physicians complained that they often do not receive adequate feedback, or their goals for the telemedicine consult are not met. Consultations are handwritten and often not legible. Consulting physicians complained that telemedicine consultation requests are not screened as closely as face-to-face consults and are sometimes inappropriate.

To a large extent, these problems can be traced to the way information flows among telemedicine participants and the administrative protocols for telemedical consults. Figure 20-1 outlines the flow of information among healthcare members involved in a typical telemedicine consult in the UTMB/TDCJ system. A telemedicine consultation is requested via a referral from the primary care physician at the inmate's home prison unit. If the inmate is not at a unit that contains a remote telemedicine site, the inmate travels to a telemedicine site with his or her chart. The presenter must obtain the necessary history, physical examination information, and prior medical history information from the patient and the patient's chart. In many

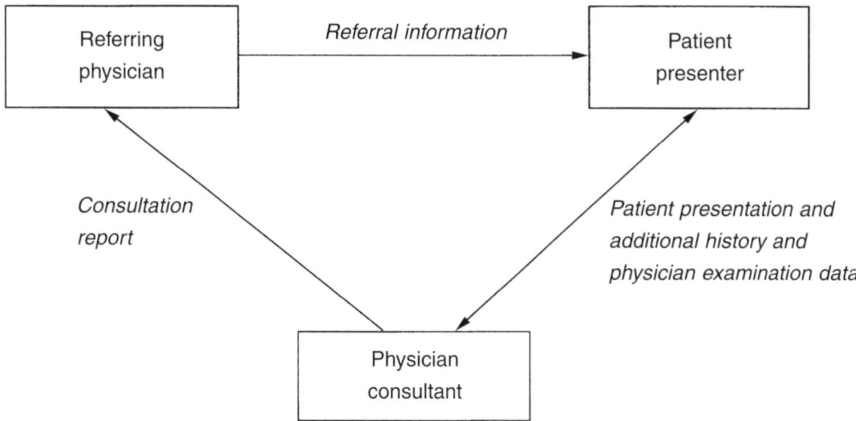

FIG. 20-1. Information flow in a telemedicine consult.

cases, the health professional presenting the patient has never seen the patient before. The current electronic information system distributes the information concerning the referral from the referring physician to the presenter, and the consulting physician limits the consult request to two lines. With such limited information, the presenter and consulting physician often have great difficulty determining the purpose of the consult. Clearly, a better information system and more clearly defined protocols for requesting, reviewing, and processing telemedicine consults was warranted.

SUGGESTIONS FOR AN IMPROVED INFORMATION SYSTEM

Health professionals at the prison unit where the inmate is housed have the most comprehensive understanding of the nature of the inmate's health status and specific medical problem(s). For this reason, conference participants decided the consultation request form should describe the reason for the telemedicine referral and the intended goals, requests for information from the consulting physician, or both. The form should also contain information that would help the consultant physician in providing a successful consultation. This information would include but not be limited to current medications, adherence issues, strategies tried in the past to address the complaint, social history, and past medical history.

As telemedicine consults are often canceled because required laboratory or radiologic results are not available, the form should also contain a checklist of key test data that are required for the consult. This information is to some extent specialty-specific and should be developed with consultation from the specialty physicians. Under the revised system suggested by the conference participants, unless these data are contained in the patient record and checked off, the inmate would not be transferred to the remote site telemedicine unit for the consult. The exception would be tests that are normally performed at the remote telemedicine unit.

This form, along with the inmate's medical chart, would travel with the inmate to the remote telemedicine site and be provided to the presenter. The presenter would perform a baseline history and physical examination and add the information to the form. The form would be faxed to the consulting physician at Hospital Galveston before or at the beginning of the telemedicine consult. After the consult, the consulting physician at Hospital Galveston would append his or her findings and plan for the inmate, and the complete record of the consultation would be forwarded to the referring physician.

DEVELOPING A TRAINING PROGRAM

Developing a comprehensive telemedicine training program and appropriate documentation for a large, decentralized healthcare system, such as UTMB/TDCJ, is a major undertaking. The preceding sections describe the training needs outlined by the four focus groups at the conference. This section presents some thoughts on how a training program could be devised to address these needs.

A number of characteristics of the UTMB/TDCJ system impact the design of a training program. First, the system is highly decentralized, with more than 100 prison units spanning a large portion of Texas. Second, physicians from more than 22 subspecialties provide telemedical consultations via the system. Each subspecialty has different information requirements, and many require patient presenters to have specific skills. Third, the UTMB/TDCJ system is a correctional healthcare system, in which security is a major concern that can impact both the delivery of care and training. In developing a telemedicine training program for a correctional institution, such as TDCJ, it is important to include security personnel to ensure the program is consistent with the institution's security needs.

Given the range of people needing training and the variety of training needs, a number of different instructional modalities are likely to be required. These include written documentation such as manuals, reminder cards, and data collection forms.* Training tapes and other audiovisual aids also play a role. The telecommunications equipment used for telemedicine can provide a means of delivering interactive instruction in a geographically decentralized system such as UTMB/TDCJ. Hands-on instruction and evaluation at regularly scheduled, quarterly training meetings may be included as part of the training program.

Written documentation is clearly going to be a major component of the educational program. Instructional manuals can provide both initial training and reference material for many aspects of the telemedicine system. Pocket-size cards can be extremely helpful for outlining the data to be collected for a specific problem or storing key reference information or a brief description of how to perform a physical examination maneuver. Data collection forms, though also key to the flow and collection of information, can serve as reminders, prompting both presenters and physicians to collect and record key medical information.

*Although not intuitively obvious, data collection forms can serve an instructional role, prompting presenters to collect or present key data in a telemedicine encounter.

TABLE 20-1. *Potential evaluation modalities for different components of a telemedicine training program*

Skill and knowledge	Trainee evaluation	Program evaluation	
		Process	Product or outcome
Cognitive knowledge (i.e., use of equipment, procedures)	Written test performance	Written feedback forms Trainee interviews	Aggregate written test performance Question and answer measures of telemedicine practice
Physical examination skills	Standardized patient examinations Physician observation of presenters performing examinations	Written feedback forms Debriefing standardized patients Trainees and physician observers	Feedback from physicians and specialists about the presenter Physical examination Skills in telemedicine sessions
"Telemedicine presence" and the ability to communicate with patients	Feedback from patients and standardized patients	Written feedback forms Trainee interviews	Aggregate feedback from patients No-show rates
Documentation	Ability to fill out documentation correctly	Feedback on documentation design and instructions	Aggregate quality of the documentation Quality assessment measures

Instructional tapes are expected to play a significant role in the telemedicine training program at UTMB/TDCJ. Tapes provide a high level of flexibility for demonstration and instruction. Tapes can be widely distributed and viewed at the convenience of the person(s) being trained. Tapes can also be coupled with interactive telecommunication sessions for feedback and questions.

Regularly scheduled meetings via multipoint telecommunication among the telemedicine hubs and Hospital Galveston for training and problem solving are anticipated. These meetings are envisioned as a major component in the training program. The meetings will provide an efficient means of direct feedback for training in physical examination skills. The meetings can also provide a venue for discussion and problem solving between physicians and presenters and among presenters at separate sites.

A number of the participants in the focus groups thought there should be training sessions scheduled at sites away from the participant's regular work site. It is too easy for training, even when it is scheduled, to be preempted by patient-care needs when training sessions are conducted on-site.

In developing a training program, it is important to include a continuing education component to maintain and update the skills and knowledge of presenters and physicians. Both the telecommunication equipment and the procedures for conducting telemedicine will change. It is important to develop a continuing education system to keep both the physicians and presenters abreast of these changes.

As with any educational program, evaluation is key for success. This includes evaluation of the trainees, as well as evaluation of the training program. It is necessary to evaluate both the process of delivering education and the impact of training to determine how the telemedicine system functions. A number of different evaluation modalities are needed to assess the competency of the trainees and the effectiveness of the training program. Table 20-1 presents examples of how different knowledge and skills dimensions can be assessed.

The focus group participants suggested developing a certification program for telemedicine presenters and possibly physicians. Telemedicine is a new, emerging field that clearly requires unique skills both on the part of the physician consultant and patient presenter. The development of a certification program facilitates the process of delineating the skills and knowledge required by professionals delivering health via telemedicine. A certification program also facilitates quality assurance. As the UTMB/TDCJ system has one of the largest, if not the largest telemedicine program in the world, it is an ideal setting for developing a training program leading to certification.

CONCLUSION

After conducting thousands of telemedical consultations, it is clear that appropriate protocols and adequate training are key to an efficient and effective telemedicine program. Insights from the experience of the several dozen focus group participants has provided detailed suggestions on what an effective training program for UTMB/TDCJ telemedicine must include and the protocols and information systems necessary for the program. Although the UTMB/TDCJ healthcare system is unique, many of the suggestions are relevant to other telemedicine programs.

Telemedicine: Practicing in the Information Age,
edited by Steven F. Viegas and Kim Dunn.
Lippincott–Raven Publishers, Philadelphia © 1998.

21

Physician Assistant Distance Learning: Project between the University of Texas Medical Branch at Galveston and the University of Texas–Pan American at Edinburg

Richard Roland Rahr

School of Allied Health Sciences, University of Texas Medical Branch at Galveston, Galveston, Texas 77555

HISTORY

The University of Texas Medical Branch (UTMB) at Galveston Physician Assistant Program became involved in the use of interactive television as a major modality of educational delivery after the development of a new satellite training program located 400 miles from Galveston on the Texas–Mexico border in Edinburg, Texas. The new training site linked a health science center campus, UTMB, with an academic campus, the University of Texas–Pan American (UTPA). The new training site was started in the summer of 1994 with the admission of 20 students from the South Texas border area. UTMB, located on Galveston Island and with its beginnings in 1895, is the oldest medical school west of the Mississippi. UTPA is a primarily Hispanic university (80% Hispanic) with an undergraduate enrollment of 12,000 students. The physician assistant program is located within the School of Health Professions with other allied health programs (i.e., occupational therapy, nursing, social work, recreation therapy, medical technology).

Private practice physicians taught basic science courses (i.e., anatomy, physiology, neuroanatomy, pharmacology) during the satellite program's first year, but this was very difficult because of the large time commitment needed. Therefore, interactive television was implemented and used 10 hours per week with both the Galveston and Edinburg classes conducted at the same time. Psychiatry, pharmacology, anatomy, physiology, patient education, interviewing, and neuroanatomy courses were taught on a semester-by-semester basis using UTMB professors. During the program's first year, physician assistant faculty traveled to UTPA each month; however, interactive television made it possible to decrease the number of visits to one per semester. The most valuable sessions were 1-hour interactive meetings per week with the project coordinator, UTMB chair, UTPA chair, and senior instructor from UTPA. These sessions allowed discussion of administrative issues, finances, student issues, and campus politics. A UTMB and UTPA junior class "Chairperson Hour" (department chair meets with students weekly) was added, including interaction between the two classes and seminars on special issues via interactive television.

Establishment of an interactive television course requires support of a Web page (school wide or by instructor) where the instructor can place a syllabus, class handouts, readings, and special medical cases (paperless curricular courses). The basic sciences teachers at UTMB used the Web page to make assignments and to communicate via electronic mail (e-mail) with local and Edinburg students. UTPA has a 24-hour computer center with ultra modem equipment for use by all students on campus. This equipment allowed for CD-ROM course materials to facilitate the anatomy and physiology courses. Students could access these materials from their homes if they had a computer and modem.

THE FIRST 2 YEARS

There was a strong South Texas influence on the development of interactive television at UTMB. UTPA was rapidly growing, with the intent to link rural citizens to major universities and libraries. UTPA was rapidly developing the computer capabilities as well as the interactive television capabilities to compete at the cutting edge of education state of the art. UTPA's development drove UTMB to rapidly accelerate its teleeducation capabilities. The UTMB allied health program expanded rapidly to meet the clinical primary medical need of South Texas. UTPA has the finest computer and interactive television facilities of any state institution; this drove UTMB to meet UTPA's excellence.

Instructor Reaction

Initially, there was a great deal of resistance to teaching via interactive television from the clinical and basic science instructors. Instructors were concerned with being able to keep students' attention at the distant site. Basic scientists were concerned about the ability of offering a comparable or of same quality course over television when cadavers were involved. In the first year, dissection of cadavers was viewed via television. In the second year, cadaver specimens were acquired to do a live session on-site at UTPA.

It became apparent that the reluctance to use interactive television was due in part to the increased complexity of preclass preparation and setup. Instructor resistance continues to be a problem, but teaching faculty resistance is to be expected when a new interactive television teaching modality is introduced. Each basic scientist or clinician has a different set of concerns. These concerns can be overcome; however, it takes a great deal of individual accommodations to make it work.

Student Reaction

Student motivation at rural sites is high when students are working on a degree plan they could not normally obtain without leaving their hometown area. The UTPA students were interested and involved. A major priority, however, is the development of an esthetic environment and large-screen television. Use of an excellent sound system is necessary so that students can hear other student responses when questions are being asked at the host or distant site.

In the pharmacology course, a research study was performed by Dr. Jack Runyan, director of UTPA's program, in which the students' satisfaction and overall grades were measured and compared (unpublished study). There were no statistical differences between the grades or level of student satisfaction. In very difficult basic sciences courses using teachers unskilled in telecommunication, however, the grades and satisfaction differential can be markedly different, with lower satisfaction by students at the distant site.

DEVELOPMENT OF A MODEL TEACHING PROTOTYPE FOR INTERACTIVE TELEVISION

Interactive television teacher needs are very different from traditional classroom teacher needs. One common addition to interactive television is the availability of an Internet connection, allowing each student to access all materials and lectures on a computer (paperless course).

A good interactive teacher should keep distant classes small enough so that he or she can call all students by name. A large name tag for the teacher to see facilitates this process. It is important to ask at least ten questions of the distant-site students during a 3-hour class. This keeps the distant students interested and feeling a part of the class. It is important during a long semester for the teacher to travel to the distant site to conduct at least one of the classes, providing an opportunity for both groups of students to appreciate the value and difficulty of interactive teaching. A class visit also allows distant-site students to get to know the teacher.

Increased visual aids and handouts are needed for distant-site students. Extra videos, graphics, and case examples are appreciated and facilitate learning. One absolutely essential communication tool is the use of a Web site for courses. A Web site allows a paperless curriculum, as well as a chance for the student to interact with faculty (and other students) by e-mail.

The UTMB Nursing School has three networks to communicate. One is for student assignments, a second is for student-to-student interaction, and the third is for faculty-to-student interactions. The future will include multiple sites at one time, further adding complexity to teacher effectiveness while on live television. The best teachers in the modality are the ones who can deal with many variables at one time.

THE FUTURE OF INTERACTIVE TELEVISION IN LONG-DISTANCE EDUCATION

The use of interactive television as a modality for long-distance education will escalate as the quality of teaching improves through the use of additional graphics, prerecorded videos, and live, interactive, off-site presentations of clinical patients. The future of all teachers depends as much on their stage presence as the content of their lectures. In the future, there will be one to two instructional support personnel for each teacher doing the background graphics. Teaching illustrations should be presented so they have the same impact on distant site audiences as at the host site. New teaching delivery systems will develop to facilitate teaming at distant sites, such as case analyses with live patients at home, computer test banks, and interactive student laboratories over interactive television. Flexibility of class time and student preferences for when to learn will also be dramatically enhanced with computer and interactive television innovations.

There is often competition for host-site room scheduling when more than one program transmits classes. There were some scheduling conflicts between allied health and nursing at UTMB for transmission of their courses, which were resolved. There was a time conflict for transmission of the pharmacology course over an early afternoon period. These conflicts are likely to accelerate as the traffic increases on the interactive television network. Universities will have to have multiple rooms to accommodate the 8 a.m. to 5 p.m. preference for teaching time. The buying of more equipment for additional rooms is a better alternative than long-term conflicts.

The new teaching modality will also result in new fears and faculty staffing competition as it changes the culture in education. Interactive television will be feared as a few good teachers replace existing teachers because a larger number of students can be reached at one time; therefore, one teacher reaching larger groups could be more effective and efficient than the existing model, resulting in fewer teachers needed.

Additionally, teachers will become actors and actresses, and the use of humor and other delivery strategies will be just as important as the content of the material taught. The mark of a good teacher is having students learn the material, retain the material, and enjoy the process. The days of the hard, somber, flat-affect teacher will soon be over. The computerized information society is molding student and teacher behaviors: They will never be the same again. The strong need for faculty will not dissipate because distant sites will need teachers who can nurture and facilitate learning. It is possible that the number of teachers will not change as much as the roles they play. There may be senior lead teachers and secondary facilitator teachers.

THE FUTURE OF INTERACTIVE TELEEDUCATION IN ALLIED HEALTH

The future of allied health education will see the establishment of large consortiums of universities with the "university without walls" concept. There will be a conglomerate of universities that offer the same degree by pooling the resources of schools belonging to the "virtual university." The students of the future will take the largest part of their classes at home by the use of interactive television and computer Internet Web-support pages. The curriculum will be downloaded from the Internet and developed at the learner's pace. Times will be set aside to return to the universities to receive testing and professional workshop development. Computerized testing centers will be established throughout the country with security-code clearance for students to prevent cheating. Improved graphics, clinical case conferences, and computer interaction will facilitate learning and communication. Universities will have larger numbers of support staff for computers, television technicians, and instructional graphics artists to facilitate teachers' work. Educators will do more traveling, reading, and humor development than present teachers. Universities will have to think bigger with national and international audiences. Tenure will quickly erode, because faculty will be paid by many universities. There could be a very basic, standardized curriculum for allied health and nursing. Overall, there may be fewer teachers, but all instructors will be more challenged to know the current precepts of not only educational theory but also computer science and the entertainment arts.

PERSONAL COMMENTARY ON INTERACTIVE TELEVISION

The development of interactional television with computer support at UTMB has been very important for my department and the School of Allied Health Sciences. School faculty have some firsthand experience and a broader concept of what the future of allied health education will be. There will be fewer teachers but with increased skills. This will bring increased faculty resistance on the order and magnitude of what the introduction of computers into education brought. Universities will have to become risk takers and develop consortia of degree plans. It will take larger financial outlays for television and computer equipment. There will be less construction of new buildings but more innovative equipment and technology. The competition for excellent students and teachers will be keen. A national identity, not a university identity will be developed. Future emphasis will be on both quantity (multiple sites) and quality of educational delivery if a university is to survive.

BIBLIOGRAPHY

Reichard JP, Youngs MT, Balison AR. *Telemedicine source book, 1998*. New York: Faulkner and Gray Inc., 1997.

Telemedicine: Practicing in the Information Age,
edited by Steven F. Viegas and Kim Dunn.
Lippincott–Raven Publishers, Philadelphia © 1998.

22

Distance Education in Nursing: Strategies, Successes, and Challenges

Jeanette C. Hartshorn

School of Nursing, University of Texas Medical Branch at Galveston, Galveston, Texas 77555

A major component of the University of Texas Medical Branch (UTMB) at Galveston School of Nursing's mission is to meet the healthcare demands within the state through practice and educational programs. To help meet this need, the school has been involved in distance education since the 1980s. This chapter discusses the School of Nursing's distance education programs, identifies the school's conceptual base, and describes the successes and challenges in distance education experienced by the faculty, students, and administration.

Much of Texas is rural, and some areas do not have access to higher education; consequently, the School of Nursing frequently receives requests for specific educational programs in these communities. For example, a rural community may not have a physician or enough physicians to meet the needs of the community. Therefore, within that community, nurses may approach the school with a request to provide a family nurse practitioner program. Potential students for the program are employed in the community and may have family responsibilities that preclude them from traveling several hundred miles to Galveston to participate in weekly classes or from moving to Galveston to attend the program on a full-time basis. From the school's perspective, although the desire to help meet these needs is strong, the reality of sending faculty to a rural community to teach the program on-site raises concerns about cost-effectiveness. As the School of Nursing continued to receive multiple requests of this type, it became evident that the establishment of a distance education program would be an excellent way to meet local needs in a cost-effective way.

The School of Nursing's distance education program was initiated with one outreach campus. As of this writing, there are five, with several others under consideration. Programs offered through distance technology from the UTMB School of Nursing include family nurse practitioner, neonatal nurse practitioner, and baccalaureate completion.

DISTANCE EDUCATION TECHNIQUES

In general, distance education depends at least partially on advanced information technology. Although older, less advanced technologies, such as audiotapes and videotapes, are used, they provide backup and support rather than being the focus of the educational experience. The distance educational experience is designed to overcome the barriers of time and place, to be fully interactive, and to focus on special learning opportunities rather than simulating traditional learning techniques. Current distance education programs at the UTMB School of Nursing use a combination of techniques, including two-way interactive television, computer conferencing, fax, telephone, and mail.

Much of what is known about distance education programs has been learned through experiences in nonclinical programs. Although many nursing programs participate in distance education, few reports are found in the literature about the uniqueness of the curriculum for a professional, practice discipline presented through distance technology. The challenges of presenting a clinical program at a distance site are considerable. Although classes are offered through two-way live interaction or other technology, teaching of clinical skills and providing clinical supervision is more complex.

CONCEPTUAL MODEL

To attempt to meet this unique need, the UTMB School of Nursing established a conceptual model that demonstrates the interaction among variables critical to the success of a distance education program. The partners in the program are the receiving agency (e.g., rural host organization, generally a hospital or university), the sending site (UTMB), and the community. We in the School of Nursing believe that all three partners are critical to the success of the program.

For UTMB, many of the community relationships are supported through our relationship with area health education centers. Individuals who work for or are involved with the centers live and work in the community and are able to assist in developing the linkages essential to the program's successful implementation. Members of the community can be actively involved in the planning process for the educational program. Their support is essential to finding the best and most appropriate sites for clinical placement and providing program planners with adequate information concerning the uniqueness of the individual community.

The cultural influence of a particular community must be taken into account for successful implementation of a program. For example, in one community requesting a distance education program, cultural influences discouraged women from attending evening classes. Although students were interested in attending classes and participating in the program, they had to do so within the constraints of their cultural beliefs. In this case, scheduling meetings and classes for the students in the evening would have led to failure of the program. By working with the community before making class scheduling decisions, however, the planners were able to arrange classes at a time acceptable to that community and the students. This scenario is replayed in each community, albeit with different issues and needs surfacing. For professional, clinical programs, working with the community and gaining support and involvement are essential to program success.

A related benefit from use of the model of partnership at UTMB (i.e., sending university, receiving site, and the community) is that the sending university can develop a relationship with the receiving site designed to assist the host in meeting other goals. For example, one of the receiving sites for the UTMB Family Nurse Practitioner Program wanted to develop its own faculty. Part of our responsibility was to assist them in this process. For other receiving sites, their only goal is to increase the number of providers in the area with a particular credential. No matter which direction, it is imperative that the goals of the receiving and sending organizations be considered in the development of any distance education program.

CHARACTERISTICS OF DISTANCE EDUCATION

One of the most advantageous characteristics of a distance education program is that it allows for greater individuality in the learning process. Within any distance program, individual learning differences can be considered, including presentation of information matched to specific learning styles. For example, with difficult information, students can review the media as many times as needed to assure their grasp of important content. Another important aspect of distance education is that repetition of information can be eliminated. Although most faculty attempt to do this during the lecture process when students do not seem to understand a basic concept that has been presented, it is difficult to move on while repeating past information. With distance learning, the professor can refer students to other programs that provide this basic information and expect them to review and learn this before returning to the current program.

Distance learning can facilitate more quality faculty-student interaction. In a distance format, students approach faculty with specific questions and issues. As their discussions are generally very focused, the quality of the interaction can actually improve. With distance programming, students can access faculty through a variety of different means, including telephone contact, discussions during televised courses, and electronic mail (e-mail). By offering a variety of means to approach faculty, various communication styles are supported. For example, some students are intimidated to call a faculty member whom they consider to be very busy. For them, the e-mail approach may be superior, because they know that their question can be answered at the faculty member's convenience.

Distance education can also provide additional opportunities for flexibility in scheduling and the location of courses. Alternative schedules designed to meet the individual needs of the particular student group can be explored. Although students at the main campus may be accustomed to the regimentation of weekly class meetings, students at distant sites may need an alternative approach, including weekend, evening, and compressed class schedules. UTMB has found that a combination of weekly classes and compressed schedules serve well.

For faculty, a major strength of the distance education experience is that it allows for innovation and strengthening of the educational pedagogy. An important consideration is to determine who the students are and how to meet their individual needs. In a nursing program, often the demographics of the student group provide some insight into their potential needs. For example, nursing students are predominately female and often in their 30s or older. Students who participate at the distant site most commonly have family and work responsibilities in addition to their school demands. Success for these students is dependent on their ability to balance these responsibilities. The challenge to the educational system is to identify a flexible means of presenting course work that allows students to meet all of their obligations. Traditional beliefs about the time students have to devote to their studies must be challenged. Although faculty can expect students at the distance campus to spend the same amount of time on a course as do the students on the main campus, they may not do it in the same blocks of time. For example, they may arrange for vacation time before examinations or papers to give them an opportunity to concentrate on their school work.

POTENTIAL ISSUES AND CHALLENGES

Students in a distance education program must accept responsibility for their learning and thus learn to take an active role in the educational process. At UTMB, we have found that many students have a passive learning style. Some of the traditional learners have been encouraged to be passive and may have difficulty in adjusting their style to this newer, active mode. As they make this transition, students may find themselves floundering and, without the expected rigid structure, may fall behind in their work. Given this situation, it is important to set up routine check points to assist students in staying on track. For passive learners, opportunity for independent work may lead to increased stress and little outcome.

Students should be familiar with the technology and be comfortable with its multiple applications. Their ability to problem solve with the technology will improve their overall learning experience. Students require access to all types of the various technologies needed for success in the educational program. Additionally, the technology must be available at times and places convenient to students. For example, at one distance education site, all students requested personal copies of the videotapes used in the televised class, because they preferred to review the videotapes at home. Although the faculty understood the needs of the students, there were concerns about potential copyright problems and cost of this strategy. As a compromise, videotapes were made available in the library and learning center, which had weekend and evening hours, allowing students access at times convenient to their complex schedules.

The learning program conducted at remote sites includes an emphasis on learning from other students as well as teachers. The support offered from one student to another is critical to the success of the program. Because the students are isolated, in a sense, from the main campus, they should have support from their fellow students. To assist students in developing these linkages with each other, the UTMB School of

Nursing accepts distance education classes in "cohorts." Depending on the program, a cohort may be six to 15 students. These individuals progress through the program at the same pace and participate in the same activities. Students quickly develop a sense of "belonging" and have the opportunity for identification with a peer group. As is true on the main campus, many of these relationships continue after graduation.

In a professional clinical program, such as nursing, role socialization is essential to program success. How students are socialized into a role for postgraduate work is critical to their ability to effectively function in a professional group. Although the struggle with role socialization continues in the traditional educational environment, it presents particular problems at the distant-site campus. The strategies UTMB uses to improve socialization at the remote site include frequent interactions with faculty from the main campus, maintaining exactly the same standards at the remote site as at the main university, and providing consistent clinical support and review. Post-graduation surveys of students from the distance education sites suggest that these strategies are effective, as graduates are employed in positions for which the program prepared them. Several graduates have become active members in professional organizations, suggesting the success of role socialization.

FACULTY ISSUES

The development of multiple distance education sites presents unique challenges to faculty. Some faculty look forward to providing distance education, while others do not. When is it a choice and when is it no longer a choice for faculty to participate? Do faculty have the right to refuse to participate in distance education courses, or is it a component of their current positions? Clearly, faculty who want to participate would be preferred because anyone tends to be more successful when participating in courses of interest. However, at UTMB we are finding that faculty may not be able to have as many choices in this area as we may have wanted. As the number of distance education programs grows, there is an increasing need for involvement of all faculty. As more faculty become involved, the responsibility of administration is to provide them with the support they need to be successful.

Faculty may need graphic design support for production of media for distance education courses. Faculty also need in-service education to assist them in understanding the pedagogy and how to adapt their current style to the type of media being used. Faculty need an opportunity to work with the equipment and learn basic troubleshooting. In addition, faculty should be exposed to new and innovative technological advances that can improve their teaching effectiveness. At UTMB, we are focusing on ways to assist faculty in learning the techniques needed to be successful in broadcasting to multiple sites. This type of broadcasting not only includes development of media but also classroom techniques, such as how to handle interaction from three sites simultaneously.

Faculty need time and support to develop strong relationships with members of the community, particularly clinical instructors and preceptors. Financial resources for faculty travel to distance sites are required so that continual interaction with students and preceptors is possible. Other financial resources to provide education to preceptors is critical. The UTMB School of Nursing, through the primary care nurse practitioner program, has developed a preceptor manual that is supported by a periodic educational program for preceptors. The emphasis in the manual and program is on articulating the expectations of the faculty and students, expectations of students within specific courses, and opportunities for problem solving. This type of standardization of management of students in the clinical courses is essential to the overall success of the program. These activities are essential in demonstrating how students at distance sites are treated in the same way as those on the main campus.

ADMINISTRATIVE ISSUES

One of the major dilemmas for administrators of distance education programs is analysis of the balance between the needs to serve the community, meet healthcare needs of the state, and present programs that are cost effective. Although it can be argued that distance education is a cost-effective strategy, it is much more difficult to argue that these programs represent cost savings. The technology needed to present distance education is expensive, and its continued operation requires a routine outlay of money. State-of-the-art technology may not be available in some areas (e.g., dedicated lines are necessary for real-time video transmission). For a clinical program such as nursing, the number of students must be kept small to provide the type of educational experience required. Thus, it is not always possible to increase the number of students to make the program more cost effective. Distance education programs may represent a technique to increase revenue by opening opportunities to students who would not have been able to attend a higher education program before the distance site's opening.

Multiple legal and ethical issues must be considered in planning the education program. A cornerstone of the distance education program is that it is the same as the program offered on the main campus. Students graduate with a degree from the main university, so they must be assured that they are receiving the same educational experience. Most program accreditors at state and national levels look for evidence of this during their review. For example, some accreditors evaluate the pass rate on national licensure examinations at distance campuses and compare them with the rates at the main campus and results from other comparable schools. Test results such as this can potentially reflect the comparable nature of the experiences on both campuses.

Throughout distance education programs, issues of privacy and confidentiality must be considered. In many clinical programs, there are times dedicated to discussion of patient case studies. In the event these are about real people, faculty and students must consider confidentiality. If patient cases are discussed over two-way interactive television or on the Internet, it is always possible that confidentiality is at risk. At UTMB, we work with the individuals involved in the telemedicine program to provide proactive leadership in this area. The risk that confidentiality may be breached can extend past the actual broadcast time if the broadcast is preserved on videotape or audiotape.

Administrators must be aware of the implications of intellectual property laws from distance technology. Faculty are encouraged to produce new, creative materials to facilitate learning at the distance sites. By doing so, faculty produce materials that are of potential interest to others and must therefore be protected by copyright. Specific policies concerning copyright and "fair use" of program materials, such as syllabi and videotapes and audiotapes, must be developed and implemented. It is imperative that the principles behind these policies include the principles of making access to materials as easy as possible for students and protecting the faculty's work. These are difficult issues that should be considered throughout a program's duration.

A final ethical issue for distance education involves the responsibility of the main university for lifelong learning for those educated at a distant site. For those involved in professional education, lifelong learning is essential. If the university brought education to the distance site because none was available in the area, it is also possible that continuing education will be difficult for the program's graduates. Each university providing distance education should consider this situation as it commits to new educational opportunities for distant campuses.

CONCLUSION

Distance education will play an increasingly important role in the university and community. Much of the groundwork for distance education strategies has been provided in nonprofessional curricula. The current challenge is to determine the best methods for providing professional education at distant campuses.

The UTMB School of Nursing has had a long history of providing educational programs at distance sites. For a successful venture of this type, the cooperation of students, faculty, administrators, and members of the community is essential.

Distance education presents a number of challenges to those who provide the service and those who receive it, but it is one of the best ways to meet the healthcare needs of rural communities in a cost-effective way.

Telemedicine: Practicing in the Information Age,
edited by Steven F. Viegas and Kim Dunn.
Lippincott–Raven Publishers, Philadelphia © 1998.

23

Documenting the Clinical Encounter

Maurice Willis, J. Rick Adams, Meena Husein, and Kim Dunn

Department of Internal Medicine, University of Texas Medical Branch at Galveston, Galveston, Texas 77555; Michigan State University Kalamazoo Center for Medical Studies, Kalamazoo, Michigan 49001; Texas Department of Criminal Justice Outcomes Management and Research, University of Texas Medical Branch at Galveston, Galveston, Texas 77555; and Department of Internal Medicine, Texas Department of Criminal Justice, University of Texas Medical Branch at Galveston, Galveston, Texas 77555

It is becoming increasingly important to accurately document a clinical encounter. With the onset of new regulations by Medicare (IL-372), requirements from insurance companies (particularly managed care), and new HEDIS reporting requirements, clinicians are required to document more in the medical record, and to do so legibly. These requirements demand more time and can result in loss of income and high cost to capture data to meet reporting requirements. Computerization of the clinical encounter provides one answer to this dilemma. The telemedicine clinic is a good testbed for piloting computerized medical record systems for clinician acceptance.

COMPUTERIZATION OF DOCUMENTATION

The mainstay of clinical documentation has always been the handwritten note. Not only is this time consuming, but rarely is it legible, and it often does not contain a complete accounting of the clinical encounter. Physicians and other medical personnel have realized these shortcomings and thus have been interested in a computer medical records system since the 1950s (1). Although computers were available during the 1950s, only large organizations had access to them due to the size and price of technology. In the 1980s, the personal computer was introduced, opening many opportunities for public computer access. Medically related software was produced, but it concentrated principally on the administrative aspects of clinical care, including office scheduling and billing. Little effort was made toward computerizing the documentation portion of the medical record.

Implementation

Computerized medical documentation has not been implemented for several reasons. The hardware required for the task has been one hurdle. Even the smallest laptop forces the clinician to alter his or her normal routine. Technology should be as unobtrusive as possible, so as to ease the burden on the healthcare worker and not interfere with patient interaction. Technological breakthroughs have made this a reality.

Handheld Computers

Handheld computers are becoming a documentation tool in many clinician practices. These computers are not only capable of performing the majority of tasks of a desktop or notebook computer, but are also light enough and small enough to fit into a coat pocket. The first of these capable of documentation was the Newton MessagePad made by Apple Computer, Inc. (Cupertino, CA), in 1993. Handwriting recognition was the mainstay of character input; thus, one had the benefits of handwriting speed and the legibility of typewritten text, all in a portable package. The first few incarnations of this machine, however, were far from ideal. Handwriting recognition was relatively poor, necessitating time-consuming corrections, and the inherent speed of the machine was far from adequate (2).

In 1996, Microsoft Corp. (Redmond, WA) announced the Windows CE operating system and many computer manufacturers began producing handheld computers that could use it. Many manufacturers are making handheld devices for this operating system. In 1997, Apple Computer released the latest version of its Newton MessagePad, the MessagePad 2000. The advances over the original MessagePads were great: Speed was dramatically improved, and handwriting recognition was reported to be 98% accurate. Even so, there seemed to be little mainstream acceptance for the device, and the device is now discontinued. Most wanted something to decrease the time spent documenting and to increase the accuracy and completeness of documentation. To many healthcare workers, writing on a piece of paper was equivalent to writing on a computer screen.

Template System

A solution that many have come to appreciate is template-based documentation. The template system takes advantage of the fact that healthcare workers documenting a clinical encounter use the same phrases from day to day and follow a general standard such as the *SOAP* mnemonic (*s*ubjective, *o*bjective, *a*ssessment *p*lan) as developed by Weed (3). Many began to document encounters using what could be termed *transcription templates*. While dictating notes using the standard method, healthcare workers using the system would state, "Use chest pain template number two, and in blank number one put 47-year-old white male; blank number two should read. . . ." The transcriptionist typing these notes would use a computer file of chest pain template number two to fill in the blanks as directed and would have a completed note in a fraction of the time and with a fraction of the errors of standard dictation. The template system has saved both time and money for many healthcare workers.

Many remain dissatisfied with this template system. Reasons include errors in transcription, time expended reading and correcting transcription, and the turnaround time for dictation to finally become a part of the medical record. Why not have a template-based system on a handheld computer so that the healthcare worker can document his or her encounter at the bedside, have a typewritten document in the medical record at the completion of the encounter, have the bill completed, and bypass the time and expense of other forms of documentation?

Combination System

There are already several incarnations of a system combining templates with handheld computers in use. Each presents the user with a series of selections and fills in the blanks of a clinical template with those choices. For example, a popular program on the market for the Newton MessagePad is PocketCHART (Physix Corp., Houston, TX) (http://www.physix.com) (Fig. 23-1). The template has been predefined (and is user configurable with a separate desktop-based program) to write the sentence according to the user's selections. The front-end client is wirelessly connected to an SQL server (Microsoft). A variety of handheld devices can link to this software. A description of the process for developing templates is included in Chapter 24.

Another popular program for the MessagePad is Transcriptionist (Tactile Systems, Inc., Parker, CO) (http://www.tactile.com/medical.html). Transcriptionist presents a

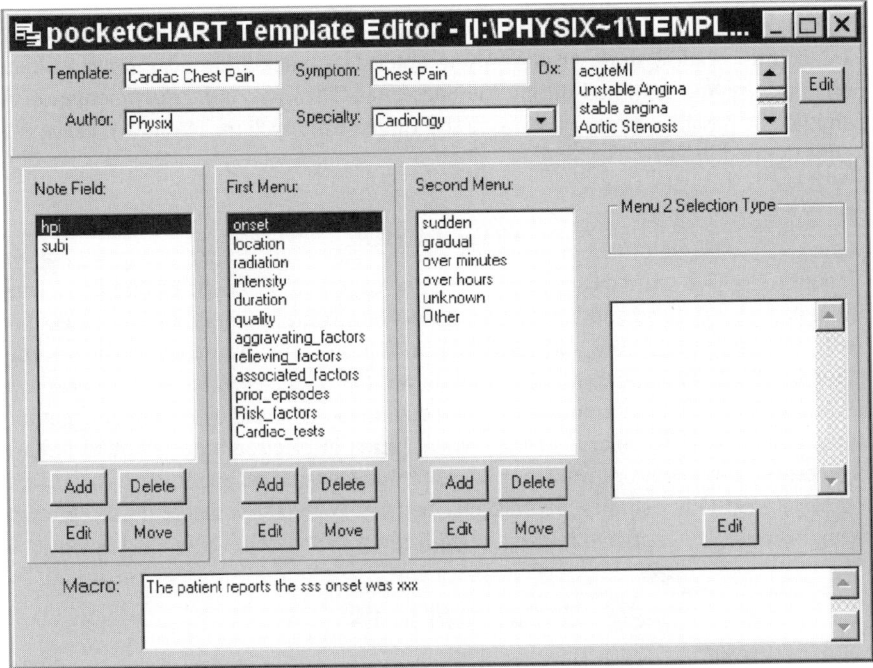

FIG. 23-1. Documentation template in PocketCHART (Physix Corp., Houston, TX).

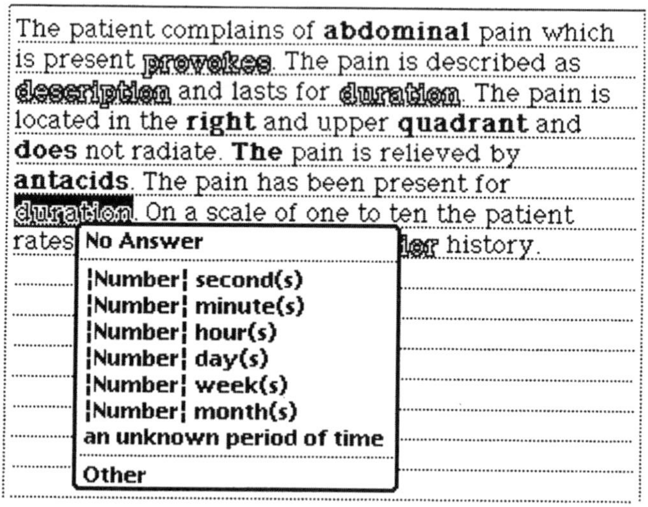

The patient complains of **abdominal** pain which is present provokes. The pain is described as description and lasts for duration. The pain is located in the **right** and upper **quadrant** and **does** not radiate. **The** pain is relieved by **antacids**. The pain has been present for duration. On a scale of one to ten the patient rates ... ler history.

No Answer
¦Number¦ second(s)
¦Number¦ minute(s)
¦Number¦ hour(s)
¦Number¦ day(s)
¦Number¦ week(s)
¦Number¦ month(s)
an unknown period of time
Other

FIG. 23-2. Documentation template in Transcriptionist (Tactile Systems, Inc., Parker, CO).

paragraph with editable blanks that are highlighted. The user taps on the highlighted words to receive a menu of selections. Thus, the sentence, "The symptom lasted for *duration*," would allow the user to select from a menu containing appropriate replacements for the highlighted word *duration* (Fig. 23-2). All the paragraphs, blanks, and menus presented are completely user definable directly on the handheld MessagePad. Both solutions allow the user not only to enter data quickly but also to see all data points that should be asked during the encounter. This makes the documentation as complete as possible, further adding to the value of the system. These two early systems are good prototypes.

CONCLUSION

PocketCHART and Transcriptionist are two excellent prototype examples of what a template-based, handheld solution offers the healthcare worker: portability, ease of use, time savings, legibility, and completeness. These programs are presently evolving in medical documentation and are certainly not the final step. The future holds such advances as voice recognition, audio-based documentation, and other implementations not yet conceived. The merits of the present forms of electronic documentation have been proved for healthcare workers such as physicians, nurses, pharmacists, and social workers (4–9). Other studies are currently under way to assess the benefit to government, university, and private medical organizations (1,4–6,10,11).

REFERENCES

1. Denner D. The computer-based patient record: moving from concept toward reality. *Int J Biomed Comput* 1996;42:9–19.
2. Ebell MH. Hand-held computers for family physicians. *J Fam Pract* 1995;41:385–392.

3. Weed L. Automation of the problem oriented medical record. *NCHSR Research Digest Series DHEW* 1977;(HRA)77-3177.
4. Kilsdonk A. The NUCLEUS integrated electronic patient dossier: breakthrough and concepts of an open solution. *Int J Biomed Comput* 1996;42:79–89.
5. Metsemakers J. Unlocking patients' records in general practice for research, medical education and quality assurance: the registration network family practices. *Int J Biomed Comput* 1996;42:43–50.
6. Rigby M. Practical success of an electronic patient record system in community care: a manifestation of the vision and discussion of the issues. *Int J Biomed Comput* 1996;42:117–122.
7. Buxton C. Diabetes information systems: a key to improving the quality of diabetes care. *Diabet Med* 1996;13:S122–S128.
8. Pabst MK. The impact of computerized documentation on nurses' use of time. *Comput Nurs* 1996; 14:25–30.
9. Zimmerman CR. A computerized system to improve documentation and reporting of pharmacists' clinical interventions, cost savings, and workload activities. *Pharmacotherapy* 1995;15:220–227.
10. Hofdijk J. The proactive medical record. *Int J Biomed Comput* 1996;42:51–58.
11. Gundersen M. Development and evaluation of a computerized admission diagnoses encoding system. *Comput Biomed Res* 1996;29:351–372.

Telemedicine: Practicing in the Information Age,
edited by Steven F. Viegas and Kim Dunn.
Lippincott–Raven Publishers, Philadelphia © 1998.

24

Overview of Template-development Process for Automating the Telemedicine Encounter

C. Sloan Teeple, Kim Dunn, and Michael M. Warren

University of Texas Medical Branch at Galveston, Galveston, Texas 77555; Department of Internal Medicine, Texas Department of Criminal Justice, University of Texas Medical Branch at Galveston, Galveston, Texas 77555; and Departments of Surgery and Urology, University of Texas Medical Branch at Galveston, Galveston, Texas 77555

During an 8-week period between the first and second year of medical school, a first-year medical student developed 32 urology templates for use in a digital assistant device. This chapter uses the development of these 32 templates to provide an overview of how the template-development process can make clinical care maximally efficient and how the template-development process is a useful educational experience for students. The templates can be customized for any automated record system and adapted for telemedicine or nontelemedicine use. The digital assistant device the templates were designed for is outlined in Chapter 23.

DEVELOPMENT PROCESS

The first step in the development process is to obtain an overall picture of the project so the purpose is understood, thus allowing higher productivity. It is important to understand the setting in which the templates will be used, as well as how the system will be used. The next stage requires comprehensive template-development training from the vendor that is selected for use in the telemedicine setting. For the development of the 32 urology templates, Physix (Houston, TX), the maker of PocketCHART, was selected. PocketCHART's template editor is the development tool, and the template engine allows the user to picture how the templates will actually work.

The next stage is time-consuming but is key to assuring that actual template development goes smoothly. It consists of gathering the base of information from the physicians, institution, and textbooks. The following approach was used for the development of the urology templates:

1. Identify the 30 most common diagnoses with their International Classification of Disease-9th Revision (ICD-9) code numbers from hospital billing data (e.g., prostatic hyperplasia #600).

2. Identify the 30 most common chief complaints that relate to the diagnoses from interviews with physicians (e.g., frequency).
3. Determine the key components of the history and physical and laboratory data needed to move from the initial presenting problem to the diagnosis (e.g., degree, onset, retention, stream pattern).
4. Identify the physical examination findings pertinent to the specialty (e.g., digital rectal examination [prostate size]).
5. Identify medication history pertinent to the specialty (e.g., doxazosin mesylate [Cardura]).
6. Identify common laboratory and pathology data pertinent to the specialty (e.g., prostate specific antigen and biopsy of the prostate).
7. Identify common radiologic studies pertinent to the specialty (e.g., transrectal ultrasound of the prostate).
8. Identify common nonspecialty studies such as electrocardiogram, electroencephalogram, or cystometrogram.
9. Determine from institutional guidelines or published data careplans for each diagnosis.
10. Determine pertinent information for follow-up and postoperative visits from review of notes and physician interviews.

Once the base information has been obtained, template development can begin. The first objective is to develop a broad, generic template that is useful for the majority of the types of problems that the subspecialist would see. This allows copying a general template and changing the information pertinent to each individual chief complaint. In urology, for example, most of the physical examination, past medical history, past surgical history, and social history are the same for complaints of hematuria, dysuria, anuria, and pneumaturia. After a revised, general template has been completed, it can be modified to comply with each different chief complaint.

The general template includes common sections from the traditional history and physical examination, but the sections are catered to the specific subspecialty; in this case, urology. The following list of eight note sections comprises the template.

1. HPI = history of present illness
2. PMH = past medical history
3. PSH = past surgical history
4. PObH = past obstetric history
5. FH = family history
6. SH = social history
7. GU = physical examination for urology
8. Careplan = careplans for each diagnosis

The HPI section changes with each chief complaint and only includes information pertinent to the specific problem of the patient at the current office visit. The remaining seven note sections should be generic enough to use with every urologic chief complaint.

The 32 templates can be used for the following chief complaints:

1. Anuria
2. Chills
3. Constipation
4. Curved erection
5. Decreased force of stream
6. Dysuria
7. Foul-smelling urine
8. Frequent urination
9. Hematospermia
10. Hematuria
11. Hesitancy of urination
12. Impotence
13. Incomplete emptying of bladder
14. Incontinence
15. Infertility
16. Malaise
17. Mass
18. Nausea
19. Nocturia
20. Oliguria
21. Generalized pain
22. Penile lesions
23. Pneumaturia
24. Polyuria
25. Priapism
26. Scrotal mass
27. Trauma
28. Undescended testicle
29. Urethral discharge
30. Urgency of urination
31. General feeling of weakness
32. Weight loss

The careplan section is unique in that it is specific to each diagnostic ICD-9 code number. For example, careplan #600 includes the workup for a suspected prostatic hyperplasia. As of this writing, there are eight careplans for these diagnoses:

1. Stress incontinence #625.6
2. Bladder neck obstruction #596.0
3. Prostatic hyperplasia #600
4. Hydrocele #603.9
5. Varicocele #456.4
6. Spermatocele #608.1

7. Torsion of testis #608.2
8. Phimosis #605

The careplan includes information such as recommendations for both general measures and surgical measures, laboratory tests, pathology tests, radiology studies, and a follow-up date and location. Once the generic template is designed, the HPI and careplan are the only sections that need altering to be compatible with each chief complaint.

After the templates have been developed, it is important to ensure that they are useful in the care setting. Therefore, it is important to test them in practice, both via telemedicine and in person. The advantage of template development for telemedicine is that it allows the pertinent data to be collected ahead of time by the remote presenter to make the encounter as efficient as possible.

During the patient interview, either the physician must be able to enter information in a logical order or review the data that have been previously entered. The data-capture process must follow the usual flow of how physicians work. The templates and the data-capture process then are modified based on the use of the templates in the real-world setting.

EDUCATIONAL VALUE FOR STUDENTS

Development of the urology templates proved to be an excellent educational tool for providing insight to the world of clinical medicine. The challenge of designing a program to be used by practicing physicians propels one into the physician's shoes and thus provides an invaluable learning process.

Many aspects of clinical medicine are introduced to the student through the template, such as taking a history and performing a physical examination, documentation procedures, how to approach a chief complaint, clinical protocol, and gaining knowledge about the different fields of medicine in general. Documentation is a vital part of the medical profession and using a personal digital assistant, such as the PocketCHART, teaches the student what information is important for maintaining a high-quality medical record, particularly when it is deployed in a real-time setting such as telemedicine. The vocabulary of a first- or second-year medical student who designs these programs increases to a level consistent with that of a junior student working in the hospital wards.

Patient history and physical examination provide the base of information from which a physician will determine a differential diagnosis and careplan for the patient. History taking and performance of the examination are also the first tools to be mastered by a student doctor. Template development allows a student to form pertinent questions regarding HPI, PMH, PSH, FH, and social history that will be used throughout his or her career. Through interactions with the resident physicians and faculty, a medical student can learn how to approach each different chief complaint by using the information gathered to order laboratory and radiologic tests and to prescribe medication. Recommendations for procedures and surgeries will also be understood through formation of the careplans.

Exposure through template development allows a medical student to be introduced to a particular field of interest so that a decision about a medical career is made a little easier. Template development provides an opportunity to experience firsthand the day-to-day activities in specific specialties. This experience can be achieved through telemedicine clinics, x-ray conferences, grand rounds, and time spent in the clinic.

CONCLUSION

Overall, personal digital assistant devices have a promising future of fulfilling a much-needed role in electronic medical record development as well as medical education. Template development is the first stage, followed by actual use in the clinical setting to weed out all the "bugs." Personal digital assistant devices allow clinical information to be captured at the point of care and assist the practitioner through guidelines recommended by the institution or through up-to-date reference material. The devices hold promise for improving the practice of care in the information age.

Telemedicine: Practicing in the Information Age,
edited by Steven F. Viegas and Kim Dunn.
Lippincott–Raven Publishers, Philadelphia © 1998.

25

Diagnostic and Support Services in the Telemedicine Environment: Pharmacy

Matthew R. Keith

*Managed Health Care Division, College of Pharmacy,
University of Houston, Estelle Pharmacy, Huntsville, Texas 77340*

Participation in the implementation of a telemedicine service is a valuable tool in defining roles and responsibilities as well as informatics needs of several departments within a healthcare organization. The initial engineering of the telemedicine service, if properly planned, identifies many of the shortcomings of existing operating systems and hardware. These findings and experiences, along with the process of planning and implementing telemedicine services, can be used as an outline for pharmacy reengineering. Conceptualizing informatics systems is the most abstract and critical aspect of a successful and optimal reengineering effort. This chapter focuses on conceptualizing the reengineering of pharmacy and related informatics systems.

Informatics has been described as the use of information technology to improve or enhance patient care and healthcare administration. Reengineering is an introspective process of evaluating a business's mission and methods used to meet and improve on defined goals and outcomes. The process requires a fundamental review of roles, responsibilities, efficiency, value, and quality of practice performed. Informatics reengineering cannot be undertaken without prior definition of the service or practice to be supported.

In broad overview, it is first necessary to define the need for reengineering in general and specifically for information systems. The process is initiated by assessing the departmental mission and services to be rendered. Consideration must be given to the need of patients, healthcare providers, and ancillary departments such as billing, inventory, medical records, quality review, and administration. It may be necessary to market the need for information and service reengineering to administrators and clinicians who are unaware of current system limitations and advantages to reengineering. This is particularly true if no similar process has occurred or is occurring elsewhere in the healthcare system.

The remaining processes are equally important but cannot be successful if the initial conceptualization phase is flawed. Various publications discuss implementation of a reengineering plan (see Bibliography). The process includes determining whether the new informatics scheme will include reprogramming in-house, vendor purchases, or a combination of both. On determining the optimal method to proceed, a request for proposal to supply an information software system, hardware system, or both must be prepared. When identifying potential products, a demonstration should be scheduled to allow assessment of product capabilities. A request for bid is then developed based on information provided in response to the request for proposal and interactions during the product demonstrations. The reader is referred to the Bibliography for numerous readings specific to these phases of pharmacy reengineering.

DEFINING A PHARMACY DEPARTMENTAL MISSION AND PRACTICE MODEL

The initial step toward informatics reengineering is defining the institutional mission for pharmacy services and the practice model to be followed. The first phase is to assess the existing mission and responsibilities as compared to legal and regulatory standards, as well as the minimum practice standard for comparable healthcare settings. This includes a review of state and federal legal statutes, organizational standards (e.g., the Joint Commission on Accreditation of Healthcare Organizations, National Commission for Correctional Health Care, American Society of Health-System Pharmacists, American Society of Consultant Pharmacists), and the primary literature identifying practice levels within comparable settings. Responsibilities currently under the pharmacy department are added to the list. The next phase requires an open-minded assessment of the institutional mission, a practice model for the future, and a determination of the role of pharmacy personnel in that mission. Pharmacy personnel should have completed a review of current services and developed a plan for future services and practice responsibilities before establishing working groups with other clinical departments, administration, and finance.

Pharmacy administrators must be cautious to prevent preplanning from limiting their consideration of mission responsibilities offered by others. The changing mission of pharmacy toward a pharmaceutical care model is not well understood by those from other disciplines, however, and it may be necessary for pharmacy personnel to lead the discussion on new responsibilities for pharmacy and integration into the new institutional practice model. It may also be necessary to sell or market the plan for service change to the other clinical departments and administration, as they may be unaware of the contribution these newer services can offer.

Once the greater questions of philosophy in mission, roles, and responsibilities for care are identified, the logistics of service process and structure can be determined. Determining logistics requires the development of a working group with enthusiastic commitment from every department involved. The group should include, at minimum, members from clinical services such as medicine, nursing, and radiology, as well as laboratory, purchasing, administration, and information management (the computer software and hardware people). The group works as a team to define the scope and volume of the planned services. Process issues should be defined in flowchart form to allow visualization of interrelationships.

TABLE 25-1. *Pharmacy clinical service options*

Service category	Service options
Direct patient care	Medication history, patient teaching, referral clinic and physician extender roles in primary care, disease-specific therapeutics management participation on work rounds, pharmacokinetic and parenteral nutrition services, psychopharmacy consultation, telemedicine services
Clinical support	Data support for healthcare management of services, departments, and individuals; medication use evaluation; nonformulary and restricted drug authorization; drug information services; pharmacoeconomic consultations; clinical intervention
Centralized services	Formulary management, disease management guideline development, target drug program administration, institutionwide data support for healthcare management, decision support software development, newsletter

PRIMARY ISSUES FOR PHARMACY

The department of pharmacy should have developed a proposal for a new practice model and case responsibilities, which may require significant justification both in terms of impact on clinical outcomes and finances. This is particularly true as the profession moves toward a greater clinical involvement through pharmaceutical care concepts. Fundamental and detailed issues related to mission, responsibilities, processes, and roles must be defined. There are an unlimited number of approaches to this process; however, as pharmaceutical care is patient focused rather than product focused, it seems reasonable to begin with patient-oriented clinical services and work toward distribution.

Clinical Services

Clinical activities can be subdivided into direct patient care, clinical support, and centralized services. Table 25-1 provides a list of various options for clinical services. The list is not exhaustive but can serve to initiate discussions for future responsibilities. Once service responsibilities are defined, it is necessary to define the information necessary to efficiently support the service. The list of needed information should not be based on what information is currently available in the existing operation or what can be purchased but rather what would be ideal.

Drug Distribution

Before determining a process plan for drug distribution (e.g., purchasing, inventory, delivery, quality review, control, administration, billing), an overall distribution method must be chosen. The most common methods described in the literature include centralized or satellite distribution, point of care, and outsourcing. This should be placed in the context of the setting, such as inpatient, ambulatory, home care, and so on, and whether the setting is managed care, preferred provider, third-party insurance, university-based, for profit, not for profit, or fee for service. Processes must be structured to meet the needs of the patient and design of the healthcare system. The reader is referred to the literature for in-depth review of the distribution services identified.

The type of distribution system chosen influences other aspects of the drug-use process, such as drug administration, inventory and purchasing, order entry, and quality improvement, as well as the support devices used. Robotics systems exist for a wide variety of applications, including unit-dose medication, intravenous preparation, patient medication order packing, point-of-care drug delivery, administration documentation, and others. A number of articles are included in the Bibliography for review of available robotics systems.

INFORMATICS REENGINEERING SUPPORT REQUIREMENTS

Informatics reengineering is a resource-intensive process. The scope of involvement and expense involved must be understood and supported by both administrators and the personnel identified as participants in the working group. Working group membership should include participants from clinical departments (e.g., medicine, nursing, radiology, pharmacy), laboratory, purchasing and inventory, administration, and information systems. Information systems participants may be multiple and include persons with expertise in software, hardware, mainframe, networking, and personal computer applications. Healthcare system dynamics can dictate participation from other areas, such as shipping, transportation, billing, use review, and others. It may also become necessary to involve consultants at some point. Pharmacy administrators must be prepared to provide a point person with ample time dedicated to the reengineering project and provide autonomy in delegation of various tasks to other people. The pharmacy point person also needs appropriate resources (e.g., information access in-house, literature, travel to pertinent scientific meetings, off-site tours) to be successful and efficient. It may also be necessary to hire a person with an information science background or experience with informatics reengineering. Large healthcare providers are more commonly hiring a pharmacist position dedicated to ongoing informatics maintenance in systems that are highly computerized and automated.

CONCEPTUALIZING THE ULTIMATE SYSTEM

It is often difficult for people to conceptualize a system rather than trying to build an information system based on available vendor products. However, reengineering plans should be based on mission, process, and needs rather than being limited to identified product availability. To begin the process, a detailed flow diagram should be developed outlining service flow and logistics to be followed. The information needed to support the people and processes can be determined through discussion in the working group and inserted into the flow diagram. A good starting point can be to develop a list of the current system's strengths and weaknesses within the context of the flow diagram. Each department representative should, in turn, provide his or her perspective for data needs in each area or process reviewed. This provides a list of information needs, per service, which can be used to determine integration needs across departmental boundaries. Finally, wish lists for information access, decision support, and data presentation can be developed. Specific data presentation or layout should be defined by each department and service to help organize data into an efficient tool and prevent data overload or placement of unnecessary demands on the information system.

Once the ideal system is defined, it is possible to begin the assessment process to determine if existing systems can be reprogrammed to meet the requirements of the new plan supplemented with add-on products or if the existing system must be replaced entirely.

BIBLIOGRAPHY

Aldridge GK, MacIsacc D, Gouveia WA. Managing the implementation of a pharmacy information system. *Am J Hosp Pharm* 1993;50:1198–1203.

American Society of Health-System Pharmacists. ASHP guidelines on a standardized method for pharmaceutical care. *Am J Health Syst Pharm* 1996:53:1713–1716.

Borgsdorf LR, Miano JS, Knapp KK. Pharmacist-managed medication review in a managed care system. *Am J Hosp Pharm* 1994;51:772–777.

Boyd AF, Hartzema AG. Computerized monitoring protocols as a pharmaceutical care practice enhancement: a conceptual illustration using diabetes mellitus. *Ann Pharmacother* 1993;27:963–966.

Dasta JF, Greer ML, Speedie SM. Computers in healthcare; overview and bibliography. *Ann Pharmacother* 1992;26:109–117.

Felkey BG, Barker KN. The power of information in an integrated health care system. *Am J Health Syst Pharm* 1995;52:537–540.

Garnick DW, Lawthers AG, Palmer RH, et al. A computerized system for reviewing medical records from physicians' offices. *J Qual Improvement* 1994;20:679–694.

Johnson RE, Hornbrook MC, Nichols GA. Replicating the chronic disease score (CDS) from automated pharmacy data. *J Clin Epidemiol* 1993;47:1191–1199.

Klein EG, Santora JA, Pascale PM, et al. Medication cart-filling time, accuracy, and cost with an automated dispensing system. *Am J Hosp Pharm* 1994;51:1193–1196.

Landis NT. Patient care fills out VA pharmacists' schedule, as automation lifts the dispensing load. *Am J Health Syst Pharm* 1995;52:584–588.

Landis TN. Automated dispensing systems vary by function, location. *Am J Hosp Pharm* 1993;52:2242–2248.

Lee MP. Automation and the future practice of pharmacy—changing the focus of pharmacy. *Pharm Prac Manag Q* 1995;15:23–35.

Magnus GH. Preparing for automated dispensing devices. *Am J Health Syst Pharm* 1995;52:2406–2408.

Miller DA, Zarowitz BJ, Petitta A, et al. Pharmacy technicians and computer technology to support clinical pharmacy services. *Am J Hosp Pharm* 1993;50:929–934.

Neal T. Evaluating and selecting an information system, part 2. *Am J Hosp Pharm* 1993;50:289–293.

Neal T. Justifying an information system. *Am J Hosp Pharm* 1993;50:476–482.

Nold EG. Preparing to implement an information system. *Am J Hosp Pharm* 1993;50:958–964.

Perini VJ, Vermeulen LC Jr. Comparison of automated medication-management systems. *Am J Hosp Pharm* 1994;51:1883–1891.

Pharmacy in integrated health care systems. *Am J Health Syst Pharm* 1996;53(Suppl 1):3–49 [13 articles from various institutions].

Ryan ML, Rinke R, de Leon RF. Selecting a pharmacy computer system for the future. *Pharm Prac Manag Q* 1995;15:1–14.

Saya FG, Shan R. A stepwise approach to the evaluation and selection of a hospital pharmacy information system. *Pharm Prac Manag Q* 1995;15:15–22.

Schafermeyer KW. Basics of managed care claims processing: from claims payment to outcomes management. *J Managed Care Pharm* 1995;1:200–205.

Schneider PJ, Lazarus HL, Puckett WH, Kolar GR, Eckel FM. Outsourcing drug distribution services. *Am J Health Syst Pharm* 1997;54:41–55.

Schwarz HO, Brodowy BA. Implementation and evaluation of an automated dispensing system. *Am J Health Syst Pharm* 1995;52:823–828.

Ukens C. RoboR. Ph. *Drug Topics* 1996;April:60–68.

Zilz DA. The changing health system: implications for pharmaceutical care. *Am Pharm* 1995;(Suppl):6–12.

Telemedicine: Practicing in the Information Age,
edited by Steven F. Viegas and Kim Dunn.
Lippincott–Raven Publishers, Philadelphia © 1998.

26

Diagnostic and Support Services in the Telemedicine Environment: Clinical Laboratory

Daniel F. Cowan, Beverly C. Campbell, and Sue Schneider

Laboratory Information Services, Department of Pathology, University of Texas Medical Branch at Galveston, Galveston, Texas 77555

Telemedicine has been defined as a diverse collection of technologies and clinical applications, the essence of which is the use of electronic signals to transfer information from one site to another (1). This has included real-time still and video images and voice and even microscopic images in telepathology. Full participation by a clinical laboratory in the telemedicine practice environment is a demanding task because of the special circumstances in which a telemedicine system is likely to be established. The existence of a telemedicine system at all implies that units in the system are so geographically dispersed that communication using television technology is feasible, desirable, and cost-effective. The business of the clinical laboratory is providing information, and it seems on a superficial level that links between the telemedicine system and the laboratory system are the critical feature.

There are, however, certain important differences. Most of the goals of a telemedicine system are accomplished by the transmission of video images and sound. Once the data links are established, distance between points is for practical purposes irrelevant. If the clinical laboratory is located in the place where the patients are, the issue is merely the inclusion of results in an accessible database. If the laboratory is at a distance from the patients, however, before the clinical laboratory can begin to contribute its information, tangible objects (i.e., specimens for testing) must be collected and transported to the laboratory. In such instances, geography can be a critical, if not the determining, factor. The need for rapid turnaround time, the perishability of many specimens, and the demands for economy and efficiency in the provision of services mean that frequent and reliable transportation must be available, which usually implies that over a wide geographic area satellite testing centers must be established. Local laboratories that provide a limited menu of immediate testing in a remote facility may be needed. These are not issues in a clinical telemedicine system or even in a telepathology system, but they must be resolved before the clinical laboratory can participate.

Telemedicine systems rely on transmitted pictures and sound, implying high-quality video technology. In contrast, the laboratory information product is supplied as numbers and brief text statements, using digital technology. The telemedicine clinical workstation therefore necessarily includes not only video and voice equipment but also a computer terminal.

Functional integration of the computer record and access to computer functions in the telemedicine workstation are necessary because of the tightly scheduled nature of telemedicine interaction. Scheduling is critical. All persons must be in the right place at the right time, and patient transportation must be arranged.

Ideally, the telemedicine consultant has immediate access to a computer terminal on which the patient's record is displayed, including clinical notes, laboratory and radiology orders and results, and medications. If a system of clinics, hospitals, offices, and prisons are all linked through a common computer system and one organization is responsible for all laboratory services, then the laboratory supports a single, integrated, longitudinal database. This means that for any patient, it makes no difference where he or she was when the laboratory test was done and whether he or she is being seen at a new location: The laboratory information is available to any authorized viewer. Furthermore, the laboratory information will not be limited to the most recent results; the whole record will be accessible. Also, orders for tests to be done now or in the future (e.g., just before the next telemedicine consultation) can be entered by the consultant, assuring that recommended testing is in fact carried out. Display of test status, such as ordered, drawn, in laboratory, or final, prevents duplication of orders entered by someone else.

Providing some discrete identifier, such as a hospital unit history number, is assigned to every patient, that patient's medical record will follow the patient from one clinic to another or from a prison clinic to a free-world clinic. The issues remaining for full and easy implementation are ease of access to the terminal on the user side and provision of laboratory information through a single service organization.

DISTRIBUTED LABORATORY SERVICES

Laboratory services can be organized according to one of two basic structures: the centralized laboratory, in which all testing for a discrete geographic area is done in one place; or the distributed model, in which testing is done in centers at a distance from the home laboratory. The most familiar example of the centralized model is the typical hospital laboratory, in which samples from patients throughout the hospital are collected by laboratory staff and brought to the testing location. The strengths of this model are concentration of resources and efficiency and standardization of testing methodology and result reference ranges.

As a local area begins to sprawl, however, service needs may not be well met by a centralized laboratory. Target turnaround times may be exceeded because too much time is spent moving the specimen from the care site to the laboratory. Under those circumstances, a subset of tests can be done in the clinical care area, with full knowledge that from a strictly business point of view, the arrangement is inefficient and introduces problems of standardization.

The Clinical Laboratory of the University of Texas Medical Branch at Galveston has adopted a distributed model of testing based on the recognition that geography is a determining factor. The service needs of physicians in the system include test turnaround times that cannot be met if specimens have to be transported many miles to a laboratory, where some specimens may deteriorate beyond usefulness if testing is not begun within a few hours of collection.

In this distributed model, one or more satellite testing centers are established, the sites being determined by the concentration of patients to be tested. Often, several facilities are clustered within a few miles of each other. Depending on the distance from the main laboratory in Galveston, a satellite laboratory may be considered as a response to a new service need. A satellite laboratory logically concentrates on tests that require a short turnaround time, typically those needed to establish the nature of a presenting complaint, and refers all specialized, high-cost tests to the central laboratory, which is the referral laboratory for the distributed testing centers. Other factors include the nature of the patient population being served in the local area. Some tests demand rapid turnaround, whereas other more esoteric tests, although important to care, are not related to acuity and can be performed on a planned basis. This pattern of care allows development of a courier service to assure prompt delivery to the central laboratory.

Still another testing scenario would take place in an isolated, distant site, in which a patient presents with an acute problem requiring immediate attention. A test result turnaround time of several hours might be medically unacceptable. If no physician or other medical caregiver is on-site, the patient may be transported to a local hospital emergency room. If a physician is on-site, then it is more appropriate to perform the tests in the care site. This implies a small panel of on-site tests relating to emergent medical conditions.

The problem for a central testing information organization is to assure that a test done at one site is as reliable as the same test done at any other testing site in the system, and that the results are comparable. A major satellite testing center may literally be integrated into the central laboratory through direct computer connections with all testing instruments interfaced with the central computer over a distance of 100 miles or more. All results are entered automatically into the integrated record and, when verified, are instantly broadcast over the communications network to the ordering physician. This arrangement allows central oversight of all quality-control functions and technician work load and similar dissemination of information of interest to laboratory physicians, scientists, and managers. Smaller testing centers, such as the clinic laboratory in an isolated location, are in effect physician office laboratories (POLs). Because of distance and cost, testing instruments are not directly integrated into the laboratory information structure. The results of the tests may be manually entered into the information system either in the clinic or faxed to the central laboratory for manual entry there. In this way, the clinic POL is structurally treated like a reference laboratory for the central laboratory. It is common for even large hospital laboratories, based on cost-benefit considerations, to send esoteric tests to a specialized laboratory and enter the specialty laboratory results into the local record, either manually or over an electronic interface. The POL-generated results are reviewed and entered into the database, in which various quality control procedures can be applied.

IMPORTANCE OF COORDINATED SCHEDULING

Organizing testing and accumulating results provide the basis for the integrated, longitudinal laboratory record. This is the outcome side of the testing event. For testing to take place, it is necessary to organize the flow of samples from the place of origin to the testing laboratory, wherever it is. With the provision of a terminal at the telemedicine consultation workstation, the test can be initiated by the consulting physician's order.

From that point on, events are determined by the location of the patient, not the consultant. A specimen must be collected at the care site. It must then be moved for transportation to the testing site. If that is not in the local facility, then the specimen must be collected by a courier along with any other samples for testing. It is unlikely that a courier serves one location only; it is more likely that he or she has a collection route that extends over many miles. The courier collects from each facility according to a schedule. If the sample is not ready to go when the courier arrives, it is left behind for the next courier run, typically the next day. This means that for telemedicine consultations to be maximally efficient, not only must all parties to the consultation be in the right place at the right time, but sample collection must also be performed with the scheduled courier run in mind, which may have taken place before the consultation. Therefore, the specimen ordered (for example) at 10 a.m. may be done that day, but one ordered at 1 p.m. may wait until the next day. Furthermore, a test requested for completion just before the next scheduled teleconsultation must be collected at the appropriate time. All this implies that the custodians of the patient must have a refined scheduling capability, which may have to be linked not only to the day of the consultation but also the time of the courier pickup and the known pattern of testing in the laboratory. For example, is the test done on the day shift, night shift, or any time of the day? Is it done every day, or (as is not unlikely for low-intensity, chronic diseases of a type that are concentrated in a telemedicine practice) is it done only on particular days of the week?

COMPUTER AS CONSULTANT IN A TELEMEDICINE SYSTEM

Full computer availability, complete with appropriate policy support, an aggressive training program, and physician order entry, has another important benefit. The telemedicine consultant is available episodically. The laboratory computer consultant is available 24 hours a day, 7 days a week. The laboratory's user manual, available on-line, provides information about the availability of tests, patient preparation (if any), the kind of tube for specimens, and the reference range for every test. The manual may also include courier schedules. Using currently available technology, a system of notification of duplicate orders awaits development of a set of rules about how close together repeat testing is sensible, the meaning of out-of-range results, and suggestions as to what to order next. Development and deployment of rule-based expert systems in support of the off-campus, isolated physician or other medical caregiver can be developed as an integral part of telemedicine, the computer-based consultation service. The technology is in place. It awaits only policy direction and a commitment to move ahead.

REFERENCE

1. Perednia DA, Allen A. Telemedicine technology and clinical applications. *JAMA* 1995;273:483–488.

Telemedicine: Practicing in the Information Age,
edited by Steven F. Viegas and Kim Dunn.
Lippincott–Raven Publishers, Philadelphia © 1998.

27

Diagnostic and Support Services in the Telemedicine Environment: Radiology and Clinical Imaging

Oliver Esch

Department of Radiology, University of Texas Medical Branch at Galveston, Galveston, Texas 77555

With the arrival of digital imaging, the basic rules have changed from the simple film or no-film paradigm, which everyone could relate to, to a more complicated scheme of choices and problems. From an information management point of view, the radiologic data-set "filmplate" would be created by radiology, was an original, and could not be shared effectively. Thus, film management in a traditional department focused on keeping films within radiology and getting them back. With a digital data set held in a single or distributed database and accessible through a network, new paradigms needed to be developed with respect to sharing information. Thus, the picture archiving and communication system (PACS) is the basis for distributing information throughout an enterprise, regardless of its size: It can range from an enterprise-wide, high-performance network to a single workstation, connected to the acquisition device by phone.

DEFINITIONS AND STANDARDS

The condition sine qua non for sharing image information is digital data to start with, and the phrase *picture archiving and communication system* describes accurately the components necessary for simultaneous and instant access to image information and diagnostic reports. The term *teleradiology* has been coined for the process of remotely displaying radiologic studies for interpretation, consulation, or both. Although the principles of teleradiology have been explored since 1948, generally accepted standards have been finalized and published only since 1980.

DIGITAL IMAGING AND COMMUNICATION IN MEDICINE 3.0 STANDARD

In collaboration with the National Electronics Manufacturers Association (NEMA), the American College of Radiology (ACR) was instrumental in creating and publishing standards and is currently the only professional organization in the medical field that has released stringent recommendations applicable within and outside of radiology. Based on the ACR-NEMA standards first published in 1983, the Digital Imaging and Communication in Medicine (DICOM) 3.0 standard was published by NEMA in 1992 (1) and presented as a working model at the Annual Meeting of the Radiological Society of North America (RSNA) in November 1993 (2). Unlike its predecessor, DICOM 3.0 was created as a standard for medical informatics and is thus not restricted to imaging. It defines (a) a network environment, that includes the physical network, communication protocols (TCP IP, the Internet protocol), and upper layer protocols for handling of image and related information; (b) service classes for data transfer and processing (i.e., display, distribution, printing); (c) information objects that include images, but also reports, studies, lists, and so on; (d) unique identification of these information objects, thus allowing their complete integration; and (e) a definition of minimum of conformance with the DICOM 3.0 standard.

The standard is long and difficult to read, and little can be found in the current literature to help the reader understand the complex terminology (3). Analogous to a name and a class B IP address that describe the recipient of an electronic mail uniquely worldwide on the Internet (e.g., jdoe@129.109.80.50), DICOM assigns a unique number (e.g., 1.2.840.113619.2.1.27854.2471650931.3.23.858166.339) to the individual image that allows someone to identify server, image modality, patient identification, and all related information in an environment that can be scaled from intradepartmental to principally enterprise, nation, or even worldwide sharing of patient information using widely accepted communication protocols. Thus, DICOM defines an open PACS standard and allows teleradiology to expand from a point-to-point technology using vendor dependant proprietary protocols and hardware to an Internet-like network.

AMERICAN COLLEGE OF RADIOLOGY STANDARD FOR TELERADIOLOGY

The ACR has published a second standard to address the professional issues related to the remote interpretation of radiologic studies in such an environment (4). It defines (a) teleradiology and its major component, diagnostic reporting, for all modalities; (b) recommends adherence to the DICOM 3.0 (and other) standards; (c) describes minimal technical requirements for image digitization and display; and (d) addresses professional issues such as patient database and licensing.

Combined, these standards govern diagnostic radiology in an electronic environment and allow the standardization of digital image formats of different vendors and modalities as well as the conversion of nondigital modalities.

RATIONALE

Digital imaging and its potential impact on processing and distribution of radiologic studies are an issue confronting many physicians and hospitals. Although a few radiology departments around the country, such as the Veterans Administration Medical Center in Baltimore (5), have converted to a filmless or almost filmless operation, most still embrace the methods of conventional acquisition, view box interpretation, and physical film storage to meet their imaging needs. In 1995, less than 1% of imaging practices used an electronic image management system (6).

The rationale for institutional establishment of a PAC-teleradiology system depends greatly on the viewpoint and specialty of the end user. For the clinician, a PACS means timely accessibility of finalized reports and imaging and concurrent access to various types of studies (5,7). At the Mayo Clinic Jacksonville, radiologists are able to deliver digital chest images along with authenticated reports in 45 minutes after exposure (8). Computed tomography (CT), magnetic resonance imaging (MRI), nuclear medicine, and ultrasound examinations are available in 60 to 120 minutes in their practice. The simple addition of teleradiology can eliminate the downtime associated with sending films by courier from small clinics to an off-site radiologist for interpretation. Soft copy preliminary interpretations can be available in 10 to 15 minutes in such a scenario (9).

Increased availability of studies is also a tremendous benefit of PACS. At some institutions, up to 30% of images are not available when requested (10). This is due not only to "lost" films, but also to films legitimately on loan to other consulting physicians. Having the same images available simultaneously to multiple clinicians and radiologists is especially important for integrating diagnostic information by enabling its dissemination.

For the radiologist, a PACS allows more time to spend with referring physicians and focus on patient needs and less time coping with the mechanics of hard-copy distribution (11). By automating image display rather than hanging films by hand, images can be accessed quickly and efficiently. By using a localized high-speed parallel transfer disk as a server and an automated work list for newly acquired images yet to be read, studies can be presented on a monitor for reading in less than 2 seconds for a chest x-ray or 4 seconds for a CT or MRI scan (12,13). Increased productivity of 10% to 15% by radiologists has been documented despite a paradoxically longer reading time per study. This has been attributed in large part to increased access to old images and reports and elimination of interruptions by clinicians and file room staff who are looking for films. The ability to quickly change window and level combinations on screen for multiple images subtracts time formerly spent hanging these images and may result in increased discovery of clinically important findings (5).

Radiologists may also exploit the technology of PACS to fundamentally change the nature of radiologic reporting. By integrating the latest technology in voice processing, a radiologic study can be linked to a digitized recording of the radiologist's interpretation (14). A multimedia document can be created consisting of a selected image or series of images with an animated cursor pointing to the significant findings while the radiologist's spoken interpretation is played (15). Stand-alone, or as part of a PACS, speech recognition technology can significantly increase the availability of diagnostic reports throughout an enterprise (16,17).

With respect to patient care, dissemination of studies and the decrease in lost or misplaced images creates a potential for fewer repeat examinations, resulting in less radiation exposure and patient inconvenience (8). At the Veterans Administration hospital in Baltimore, film retake rates have dropped from 4% to less than 1% after the transition from film to filmless operation (5). At the same time, prompt image availability in a medical intensive care unit setting has been shown to decrease the time between examining images and initiating certain clinical actions such as positioning and placing lines and tubes (18).

The different components of an imaging system pose different challenges and should be carefully adapted to the situation; otherwise the prices will be exorbitantly high. The functionality of an imaging system, however, depends as much on technology as on preexisting image management that did not work very well and resulted in the decision to purchase new technology. This technology alone cannot solve image management problems. It also requires training and adjustment to a new system by the operating staff, who do not necessarily see the necessity for change. All operational errors, old and new, will be added to technological failure that is likely to occur in the introductory phase, and thus the system will be blamed. This is complicated by constant adjustments to the short half-life of both software and hardware. *Half-life* means that within half a year after purchase, your equipment will be half as powerful as new systems, which then will be available at half the price you paid for the old one.

COMPONENTS

The heart of a PAC-teleradiology system is its archive. In an ideal scenario, a patient's complete imaging "jacket" would be instantly available from the archive from any viewing station in the hospital. Images would never become lost and the archival media would not decay or take up space. Consulting physicians could manipulate the images to enhance contrast and other variables to meet their needs. A radiologic report would be simultaneously accessed in the form of a multimedia document with the radiologist's voice and animated pointers to describe findings.

Image server(s) and archive(s) provide access to images and related information to any part of the network and provide connectivity with other networks (and information systems). Speed and safety are as important as the effective use of hardware and manpower on the other side; if you have someone pull optical disks from a shelf, the same person could be pulling films, folders, or slides. Again, server hardware is as important as software, and probably not the place to save. Mass storage is now available at very low cost at all levels. This starts from individual 4- or 9-GB hard drives with tape backups, arrangements of disks (e.g., redundant array of inexpensive disks), cheap CD-ROM writers, and magneto-optical devices, to robotic storage archives in the terabyte range. Though many forms of data storage are available, the excellent long-term stability and storage capacity of optical disks have made them the preferred choice for most digital archives since the early days (7,19). A single optical disk can store up to 10 GB with 20 expected in the near future. Data retention is not affected by magnetic fields, and a 10-year or greater life expectancy can be expected per disk. Data can be written, read, and transferred in excess of 1 MB/second. Various robotic jukeboxes have been designed to allow access to a large library of individual disks. In an effort to further improve on the performance of the archive, data compression techniques are available.

IMAGE PROPERTIES AND DISTRIBUTION

The requirements for distributing image information are high. The smallest component of an image is called a *picture element (pixel)*. The value allowed for any pixel is what determines the range of information (grayscale or color) available and is referred to as a *bit*. To allow for 256 possible values of gray to range between the blackest and whitest extremes requires 8 bits (1 byte). Most manufacturers quote 12 to 16 bits (7). Research suggests that a pixel matrix of 2,048×2,048 may be required for digital chest radiography (19,20), which when viewed at 12 to 16 bits would require approximately 8×10^6 bytes or 8 MB. By comparison, an average CT or MRI study would require 12 to 25 MB of storage (12). A single CT scanner may produce 15 GB in 1 year (21) or more. A fully digital radiology department will easily generate many gigabytes (10) of raw data per day, and exceed several terabytes (10^{12}) in 1 year. Table 27-1 illustrates typical imaging studies, their properties, and transmission times, dependent on network infrastructure.

Fiberoptic transmission of images using the FDDI protocol is the prevalent network backbone at the time of this writing, but the asynchronous transfer mode (ATM) is emerging as the preferred mode in the healthcare environment due to its superior performance at steadily decreasing cost (22). High-speed networks are nec-

TABLE 27-1. *Image properties and transmission rates*

Modality	Image matrix	File size	Modem: 28.8 Kbps	T1: 1.5 Mbps	Ethernet: 10 Mbps	FDDI: 100 Mbps	ATM: 1 Gbs(+)
Magnetic resonance image	$256^2 \times 12$ bits	0.06 MB	25 secs	0.7 sec	0.2 sec	0.05 sec	0.001 sec
Magnetic resonance imaging study	—	4–6 MB	1.5–3 mins	2–3 secs	0.4–0.5 sec	0.1 sec	0.01 sec
Computed tomography scan	$512^2 \times 12$ bits	0.52 MB	3.3 mins	15.0 secs	2.0 secs	0.4 sec	0.01 sec
Computed tomography study	—	7+ MB	30+ mins	50+ secs	10+ secs	3+ secs	0.1 sec
Chest x-ray	2.0×2.5 ×12 bits	10.4 MB	68.0 mins	1.7 mins	33.0 secs	8.0 secs	0.2 sec

ATM, asynchronous transfer mode.

essary to support distribution of image data. For teleradiology, it is advisable to use existing networks on a fee-for-service basis. These range from switched 56-Kb circuits to ATM on fiber backbones. In larger cities, integrated services digital network lines are available for $50 per month for individual users. Hardware requirements are as important as network protocols and should be evaluated carefully for the projected traffic. Certainly, bandwidth on demand offers advantages here; you get what you pay for. The creation of such a network is an institutional or enterprisewide effort and should only be treated as such; thus, it is far beyond the scope of radiology alone.

COMPRESSION

The goal of compression of digital images is to allow fast display and image transmission over networks, and decrease the amount of archive space necessary for long-term storage. Compression usually falls into two categories termed *lossy* and *lossless*. Lossy compression deletes elements of the original data set and attempts to maintain a visual simulacrum at the cost of the ability to postprocess the image. This is euphemistically termed *visually* or *perceptually lossless* (23) and includes the Joint Photographic Expert Group (JPEG) standard (24), also part of DICOM. Although early reports from investigators indicated that final diagnostic interpretation of images by radiologists from anything other than the full data set would be inadvisable, some studies have shown that images with lossy compression ratios of up to 25 to 1 can be used for adequate diagnosis of chest disease (25,26) as well as for CT and ultrasound scans (22), and even for dynamic studies (27). Lossy algorithms are capable of 20 to 1 to 50 to 1 ratios, whereas most lossless algorithms can only compress images up to 3 to 1 (28). Compression for archiving can also be achieved by simply resizing and storing a smaller pixel matrix, though restoration to full size would obviously reveal inconsistencies.

INFORMATION SYSTEMS: INTEGRATION

A seamless integration of imaging and information systems is essential, but not easy to achieve. The Health Level 7 (29) standard provides demographic information, but integration is anything but seamless. To use an imaging system effectively, it cannot be stand-alone. Incorporation or extraction, or both, of patient demographics, scheduling, billing, hospital, follow-up, and other data is a basis for the effective use and maintenance of the imaging system. Good system integration will not be cheap, but will pay off in the long run, especially if it includes a bidirectional interface with related clinical information systems.

SOFT-COPY INTERPRETATION OF DIAGNOSTIC STUDIES

The amount and type of archiving and compression will vary significantly with the needs of the institution and more specifically with each end-user of the PACS.

For instance, is it the goal of the institution to use PACS for soft-copy interpretation or solely for image distribution? Sending and displaying images of orthopedic films demonstrating gross fractures would require less display resolution than a chest x-ray showing the fine interstitial markings of early pulmonary fibrosis (30). In the case of the fracture, a high-compression algorithm and a low-resolution monitor would suffice to convey the relevant clinical information. Obviously, sharper resolution is required for primary diagnosis of difficult cases with subtle findings. Experience and research findings are mixed on whether contemporary technology suffices and is dependent on the relevancy of findings under differing clinical situations. Presently, there is no hardware or software combination sufficient to exactly visually replicate view box examination of plain films. But perhaps this is not necessary. Researchers at the University of California, Los Angeles, have shown that 1,024×1,024 monitors displaying uncompressed computed radiography-acquired chest films are sufficient for primary diagnosis by radiologists of nine findings considered essential to guide patient care in the coronary care unit (30). These findings included the presence or absence of pulmonary venous hypertension, diffuse edema or lung disease, localized infiltrates or atelectasis, pleural effusions, and significant pneumothoraces, as well as estimations of heart size and positions of various lines and tubes. In this setting, the findings of tiny lung nodules, minimal interstitial disease, pneumothoraces of <5%, and tiny effusions were considered inconsequential in terms of daily management and were not studied. In a study designed to magnify the disparity between hard- and soft-copy reading conducted at Johns Hopkins University, emergency department cases with high diagnostic difficulty were chosen and a statistically significant difference was found in interpretation of the findings of fracture, pneumothorax, pneumoperitoneum, lung mass, lung infiltrate, and small bowel obstruction on 1,200×1,600 monitors versus traditional alternators by both radiologists and emergency department physicians and residents (31). Obviously, the final word on whether monitor reading can safely and effectively replace the traditional view box is not out. Clinicians and radiologists alike have conducted numerous studies with mixed results since the introduction of digital imaging for conventional examinations (32–36). Only some studies using lower-resolution monitors and older technology do not support that using PACS yields at least equal, if not superior, results (37–42). With evolving standards and technology, some authors are now emphasizing the advantages of soft-copy interpretation (43–49). Those studies favor high-resolution monitors with equipment meeting the current state of the art, paired with radiologists who have had significant training and experience with the new technology. As with any new imaging advance, a learning curve is traversed before reaching a comfortable level of diagnostic accuracy and an efficient workflow (50).

IMAGE DISTRIBUTION: A MULTI-TIERED APPROACH

Redistributing radiologic studies on diagnostic quality workstations throughout an institution is cost prohibitive. According to specific needs and budgets, every institution should define the needs of its individual components and make decisions based on eco- and ergonomics. No hospital would like to have or could afford giant diagnostic quality monitors (and their maintenance) on all nursing stations, primary care areas, or doctor's offices; whereas for diagnostic interpretation and in specialty care areas, such as intensive care units and operating rooms, this would make sense to everyone. The usual argument about "high-" versus "low-quality images" in the digital age shows a lack of understanding of basic principles: As a film plate, the original data set exists and will not go away; however, it can be distributed much more easily for diagnostic and review purposes as part of an enterprise-wide PACS according to the specific needs of the end user.

A bit more complicated are the distribution of images to those whose need for a full data set is less clear and technically more challenging (e.g., the distribution of regular chest x-rays with no pathologic findings). It may be nice to have this information, but does it make a difference, and if it does, does this difference justify the cost? The solution to this problem is the creation of a second, less expensive tier for image distribution in the form of a cost-reducing filter between the fully sized diagnostic quality images and a smaller version of the same image, closely tied to the diagnostic report. Thus, a compressed and practical version of the original, augmented by a full diagnostic report, can serve the purpose of conveying the necessary information without challenging the system. Practically, that can be done by feeding reduced sized images from the primary PACS server into a second images server that incorporates those radiologic images and other electronic data, such as laboratory and pathology information, and then make this electronic patient record available on a low-cost personal computer (PC) platform. Again, this is far beyond the scope of radiology and requires an organized institutional approach.

In any such system, people not used to working with computers are suddenly forced to do nothing else: This takes some incentive. In the office environment, it took many years to replace typewriters with PCs and a lot of training and technological improvement before general acceptance of the technology in spite of good arguments. Still, the paperless office has not happened (some studies suggest the opposite); and going paperless was one of the most convincing arguments at the time. The same also is true for PACS. It will only prevail in areas in which there is a significant need for solutions that a technology can provide, or where there is no alternative. Operational issues are as important as the right choice of technology, and there are strong interdependencies. But if it does not work, usually the technology will be blamed (and the people who installed it); rarely the people who staff it.

Finally, those parts of the system that are not fully functional because the environment has changed, or the technology has improved, should be upgradable without changing the whole system. A modular approach that leaves key elements in place can ensure this, as well as the strict adherence to prevailing industry standards that are now available. These standards do not solve all problems, but most of them. And their compatibility will result in the free exchange of information in different systems according to the necessity of practical and economical considerations. For images, this development originates and will receive its major directive from radiology for economically improving patient care in a new era.

REFERENCES

1. The National Electrical Manufacturers Association. *Digital imaging and communications in medicine (DICOM)*. NEMA Publications PS 3.1–PS 3.12. Rosslyn, VA: The National Electrical Manufacturers Association, 1992–1995.
2. Ackerman LV, Giltin JN. ACR-NEMA Digital imaging communication standard: demonstration at RSNA '92 InfoRad. *Radiology* 1992;195:394.
3. Bidgood WD, Horil SC, Prior FW, Van Syckle DE. Understanding and using DICOM, the data interchange standard for biomedical imaging. *J Am Med Inform Assoc* 1997;4:199–212.
4. American College of Radiology. *ACR Standard for Teleradiology. Resolution 21*. Reston, VA: American College of Radiology, 1994.
5. Siegel EL, Diaconis JN, Pomerantz S, Allman R, Briscoe B. Making filmless radiology work. *J Digit Imaging* 1995;8:151–155.
6. Reicher MA. Filmless automation: from vision to reality. *Admin Radiol J* 1995;14:24–35.
7. Frost MM, Honeyman JC, Staab EV. Image archival technologies. *Radiographics* 1992;12:339–343.
8. Morin RL, Berquist TH, Rueger W. The Mayo Clinic Jacksonville electronic radiology practice. In: Kilcoyne R, Lear J, Rowberg A, eds. *SCAR 96*. Carlsbad, CA: Symposia Foundation, 1996:146–151.
9. Lawson C. PACS vendor is helping pediatric hospital system realize online advantages. *ADVANCE Administrators Radiol* 1996;63–64.
10. Wiltgen M, Gell G, Graif E, Stubler S, Kainz A, Pitzler R. An integrated picture and communications system—radiology information system in a radiology department. *J Digit Imaging* 1993;6:16–24.
11. Honeyman J, Messinger JM, Frost MM, Staab EV. Evaluation of requirements and planning for picture archiving and communication systems. *Radiographics* 1992;12:141–149.
12. Wong AW, Taira RK, Huang HK. Digital archive center: implementation for a radiology department. *Am J Radiol* 1992;159:1101–1105.
13. Piqueras J, Carreno JC, Ovelleiro M, Lucaya J, Enriquez G, Creixell S. Worklists, preloading and archiving strategies: 3 years of clinical experience in the Barcelona PACS. *Med Inform* 1994;19:123–128.
14. Breant CM, Taira RK, Huang HK. Integration of a voice processor machine in PACS. *Comput Med Imaging Graph* 1993;17:13–19.
15. Kurdziel KA, Hopper KD, Zaidel M, Zukowski MJ. "Robo-Rad": an inexpensive user-friendly multimedia report system for radiology. *Telemed J* 1996;2:123–129.
16. Ramaswamy M, Chaljub G, Esch O, Fanning D, vanSonnenberg E. Impact of continuous speech recognition in MRI reporting. 83rd Annual Meeting of the Radiological Society of North America, November 30–December 5, 1997, Chicago, IL. *Radiology* 1997;205:587.
17. Esch O, Everling S, Farr R, Chaljub G, Kavanagh PV, vanSonnenberg E. Impact of continuous speech recognition on finalization of diagnostic reports in a large academic department. 83rd Annual Meeting of the Radiological Society of North America, December 3, 1997, Chicago, IL. *Radiology* 1997;205:403.
18. De Simone DN, Dundel HL, Arenson RL, et al. Effect of a digital imaging network on physician behavior in an intensive care unit. *Radiology* 1988;169:41–44.
19. Arenson RL, Chakaborty DP, Seshadri SB, Kundel HL. Digital imaging workstation. *Radiology* 1990;176:303–315.
20. Dwyer SJ, Cox GG, Cook LT, McMillan JH, Templeton AW. Experience with high-resolution digital grey scale display systems. *Proc SPIE* 1990;1234:132–139.
21. Grimes S. Modular implementation of PACS: preliminary results of the RiksPACS project. Imaging equipment considerations. *Eur J Radiol* 1992;16:62–63.
22. Huang HK, Wong AW, Zhu X. Performance of asynchronous transfer mode (ATM) local area and wide area networks for medical imaging transmission in clinical environment. *Comput Med Imaging Graph* 1997;21:165–173.
23. Kennedy TE, Bronkalla M, Herro P. Evaluating digital archive system performance: looking beyond the jargon. *J Cardiovasc Manag* 1995;6:33–34.
24. Yamamoto LG. Using JPEG image compression to facilitate telemedicine. *Am J Emerg Med* 1995;13:55–57.
25. Aberle DR, Gleeson F, Sayre JW, et al. The effect of irreversible image compression on diagnostic accuracy in thoracic imaging. *Invest Radiol* 1993;28:398–403.
26. MacMahon H, Doi K, Sanada S, et al. Data compression: effect of diagnostic accuracy in digital chest radiography. *Radiology* 1991;178:175–179.
27. Baker WA, Hearne SE, Spero LA, et al. Lossy (15:1) JPEG compression of digital coronary angiograms does not limit detection of subtle morphological features. *Circulation* 1997;96:1157–1164.

28. Mun SK, Elsayed AM, Tohme WG, Wu YC. Teleradiology/telepathology requirements and implementation. *J Med Syst* 1995;19:153–163.
29. *An application protocol for electronic data exchange in healthcare environments. Version 2.2.* Ann Arbor, MI: Health Level Seven, Inc., 1994.
30. Steckel RJ, Batra P, Johnson S, et al. Comparison of hard and soft-copy digital chest images with different matrix sizes for managing coronary care unit patients. *AJR Am J Roentgenol* 1995;164:837–841.
31. Scott WW Jr, Bluemke DA, Mysko WK, et al. Interpretation of emergency department radiographs by radiologists and emergency medicine physicians: teleradiology workstation vs. radiograph readings. *Radiology* 1995;195:223–229.
32. Goodman LR, Foley WD, Wilson CR, Rimm AA, Lawson TL. Digital and conventional chest images: observer performance with film digital radiography system. *Radiology* 1986;158:27–33.
33. Halpern EJ, Newhouse JH, Amis ES Jr, et al. Evaluation of teleradiology for interpretation of intravenous urograms. *J Digit Imaging* 1992;5:101–106.
34. Wegryn SA, Piraino DW, Richmond BJ, et al. Comparison of digital and conventional musculoskeletal radiography: an observer performance study. *Radiology* 1990;175:225–228.
35. Krupinski EA, Weinstein RS, Rozek SL. Experience-related differences in diagnosis from medical images displayed on monitors. *Telemed J* 1996;2:101–108.
36. Ackerman SJ, Gitlin JN, Gayler RW, Flagle CD, Bryan RN. Receiver operating characteristic analysis of fracture and pneumonia detection: comparison of laser-digitized workstation images and conventional analog radiographs. *Radiology* 1993;186:263–268.
37. Cox GG, Cook LT, McMillan JH, Rosenthal SJ, Dwyer SJ. Chest radiography: comparison of high resolution digital displays with conventional and digital film. *Radiology* 1990;176:771–776.
38. Curtis DJ, Gayler BW, Gitlin JN, Harrington MB. Teleradiology: results of a field trial. *Radiology* 1983;149:415–418.
39. MacMahon H, Metz CE, Doi K, Kim T, Giger ML, Chan HP. Digital chest radiography: effect on diagnostic accuracy of hard copy, conventional video, and reversed gray scale video display formats. *Radiology* 1986;158:21–26.
40. Scott WW Jr, Rosenbaum JE, Ackerman SJ, et al. Subtle orthopedic fractures: teleradiology workstation versus film interpretation. *Radiology* 1993;187:811–815.
41. Slasky BS, Gur D, Good WF, et al. Receiver operating characteristic analysis of chest image interpretation with conventional, laser printed, and high resolution workstation images. *Radiology* 1990;174:775–780.
42. Franken EA Jr, Driscoll CE, Berbaum KS, et al. Teleradiology for a family practice center. *JAMA* 1989;261:3014–3015.
43. Slovis TL, Guzzardo-Dobson PR. The clinical usefulness of teleradiology of neonates: expanded services without expanded services. *Pediatr Radiol* 1991;21:333–335.
44. DiSantis DJ, Scatarige JC, Cramer MS, Kim MH. Feasibility of digital teleradiology for imaging evaluation of patients with acute right upper quadrant abdominal pain. *Radiology* 1990;177:707–708.
45. Elam EA, Rehm K, Hillman BJ, Maloney K, Fajardo LL, McNeill K. Efficacy of digital radiography for the detection of pneumothorax: comparison with conventional chest radiography. *AJR Am J Roentgenol* 1992;158:509–514.
46. Goldberg MA, Rosenthal Di, Chew FS, Blickman JG, Miller SW, Mueller PR. New high-resolution teleradiology system: prospective study of diagnostic accuracy in 685 transmitted clinical cases. *Radiology* 1993;186:429–434.
47. Krupinsky EA, Maloney K, Bessen SC, et al. Receiver operating characteristic evaluation of computer display of adult portable chest radiographs. *Invest Radiol* 1994;29:141–146.
48. Straub WH, Gur D, Good WF, et al. Primary CT diagnosis of abdominal masses in a PACS environment. *Radiology* 1991;178:739–743.
49. Yoshino MT, Carmody R, Fajardo LL, Seeger J, Jones K. Diagnostic performance of teleradiology in cervical spine fracture detection. *Invest Radiol* 1992;27:55–57.
50. Lund PJ, Krupinski EA, Pereles S, Mockbee B. Comparison of conventional and computed radiography: assessment of image quality and reader performance in skeletal extremity trauma. *Academ Radiol* 1997;4:570–576.

Telemedicine: Practicing in the Information Age,
edited by Steven F. Viegas and Kim Dunn.
Lippincott–Raven Publishers, Philadelphia © 1998.

28

Faculty Development Program Overview

*Nancy B. Bell, *Anne Brasier, *Jennifer C. Dudley,
Jean L. Freeman, T. Howard Stone, David J. Solomon,
Daniel H. Freeman, Jr., and Kim Dunn

**Office for Research, University of Texas Medical Branch at Galveston, Galveston, Texas 77555; Departments of Internal Medicine and Preventive Medicine and Community Health, University of Texas Medical Branch at Galveston, Galveston, Texas 77555; Program on Legal and Ethical Issues in Correctional Health, Institute for the Medical Humanities, Department of Preventive Medicine and Community Health, University of Texas Medical Branch at Galveston, Galveston, Texas 77555; Department of Internal Medicine and Office of Educational Development, University of Texas Medical Branch at Galveston, Galveston, Texas 77555; Departments of Preventive Medicine and Community Health and Psychiatry and Behavioral Medicine, University of Texas Medical Branch at Galveston, Galveston, Texas 77555; and Department of Internal Medicine, Texas Department of Criminal Justice, University of Texas Medical Branch at Galveston, Galveston, Texas 77555*

The University of Texas Medical Branch (UTMB) at Galveston has taken a proactive approach to faculty training in proposal development to address research needs in the application and delivery of telemedicine. In this light, UTMB has offered proposal development classes to young clinical investigator faculty so that they can develop the skills necessary to secure external funding and to use telemedicine as a testbed for developing leadership skills in healthcare delivery.

RATIONALE

Clinicians undergo extensive training in disease prevention, patient care, and the curing of patients. Although research findings' importance to improving medical care is a major component of medical school training, the development of skills for most physicians-in-training does not focus on the finer points of how to conduct research or how to apply for funds to perform proposed research. This lack of research training is unfortunate, as clinicians during practice have the opportunity to change or improve the delivery of healthcare outcomes yet lack the resources or training to design a statistically valid research plan that validates their hypotheses. Physicians may even lack the background experience that permits them to state goals, hypotheses, and objectives correctly, thus reducing their chances of receiving funding.

IDENTIFICATION OF POTENTIAL AREAS OF FUNDING

Armed with knowledge about the aspiring physician-investigator, three prime areas in which young faculty could realistically compete for external funding were identified. The first was to study and refine the mechanisms that support the delivery of excellent medical care through telemedicine. To focus on a local concern, the second area was to improve the quality of healthcare for prisoners of the Texas Department of Criminal Justice (TDCJ) through the use of telemedicine. UTMB delivers healthcare services to more than 80,000 prisoners incarcerated in more than 67 units in the northern, eastern, and southern sections of Texas. Any treatment that reduces the expenses associated with (a) long-distance transportation, (b) overnight lodging, (c) security risks, and (d) lowered inmate productivity significantly reduces the state's economic burden of incarceration. The third, related area included the use of informatics to develop mechanisms to improve retrieval of patient records to deliver cost-effective, quality healthcare. As informatics in healthcare improve, the potential for using healthcare data to improve patient outcomes and cost-effectiveness increases. Clinical faculty can take advantage of this new development to do clinical care research.

UNIQUE CHARACTERISTICS OF THE PROGRAM

Proposal development was taught with a multidisciplinary approach to faculty development. Young clinicians from all medical fields on campus that used telemedicine were invited to participate, promoting the interaction of clinicians from different disciplines and specialties. Most patients experience multiple symptoms or problems. UTMB encouraged the participants to consider multidisciplinary approaches to solving patient problems and designing clinical studies. The benefits of hearing other clinicians express concerns that were common to all disciplines was especially beneficial.

To make the course cost-effective, UTMB used faculty and staff from the university. The faculty development mentors met on a regular basis with the clinicians. No one had to leave the campus to attend class or change a clinical schedule to participate on a regular basis. To meet the needs of the clinicians, the group met at 5 p.m. on Thursdays.

The faculty for the development course included (a) a biostatistician, (b) a biomedical database specialist, (c) a lawyer who specialized in correctional health and medical ethics, (d) a proposal development specialist, (e) a post-award specialist, (f) a medical research librarian, (g) a medical educational psychologist, and (h) a telemedicine/TDCJ medical administrator. Each of the faculty contributed in his or her area of expertise and served as a mentor for each clinician's specific needs. A description of the strengths of each of the faculty follows:

1. Biostatistician: The biostatistician contributed to the project by serving as an expert in the analysis of clinical studies. For example, clinicians would share their preliminary data with the biostatistician who, in turn, used that data to

develop a power analysis. This helped the investigator determine the number of samples needed to complete a study with statistically significant test results. The biostatistician also assisted with the selection of the appropriate statistical test for the proposed data. Helping the investigator focus the research design was also a contribution from the biostatistician.

2. Biomedical database specialist: The major contribution of the database specialist was access to the opportunity to improve telemedicine healthcare delivery through the use of information contained in the databases. The biomedical database specialist provides access to patient and hospital records and develops mechanisms to increase the database integrity. The database specialist provides assistance when investigators wish to design a research project that uses database information.
3. Lawyer: UTMB provides managed healthcare for more than 100,000 inmates incarcerated by the TDCJ. It was decided that a legal representative who understood both the constraints on using the inmates for managed healthcare outcomes research and the ethical obligations to patients receiving telemedicine should be a part of the advisory group. The lawyer advised investigators on such issues as health law affecting the practice of telemedicine, correctional law and correctional health law as it applies to the practice of telemedicine, and federal regulations affecting the conduct of telemedicine.
4. Proposal development specialist: Investigators received theory, examples, and hands-on practice through a variety of instructional modules that functioned as vignettes of the grant application from the proposal development specialist. Investigators were taught how to discriminate among and write goals, hypotheses, and specific aims or objectives; how to write summary statements and scientific abstracts; and how to develop research design and proposal formats to make the application easier to review. In addition, considerable time was spent on strategies to prepare a better application. These topics included (a) knowing the reviewers and the review process; (b) how to self-evaluate science for importance, significance, and feasibility; and (c) how to develop collaborations and partners. These activities comprised the bulk of the class meetings.
5. Post-award specialist: A representative of the university's proposal processing and post-award financial operation also attended the classes. When clarification was needed on the rules and regulations regarding the use of human subjects in research, the protocol development for using human subjects in research, and the process by which approvals are given, an on-the-spot authority was essential. Other contributions were in the areas of (a) developing a budget and writing a budget justification, (b) using electronic forms and templates and the future of electronic submission, and (c) obtaining signatures and certifications for application submission.
6. Medical research librarian: A reference librarian trained the faculty participants in the use of electronic information retrieval systems. These systems are used by faculty to enhance the selection of a potential funding agency or solicitation and applying this information to the proposal writing process. Specific databases

explored were SPIN (Sponsored Programs Information Network, a funding opportunity database), CRISP (Computer Retrieval of Information on Scientific Projects), and *MEDLINE*.

7. Medical educational psychologist: The medical educational psychologist was involved with the design of courses that train the users of telemedicine. For example, a successful telemedicine consult is highly dependent on a knowledgeable "presenter" who represents the patient at the client end. UTMB's educational psychologist provided valuable input as to the design of research conducted via telemedicine consults.
8. Telemedicine/TDCJ medical administrator: The medical administrator organized and supported the faculty development program. Speakers and specialists were identified by the medical administrator. The medical administrator also served to break down barriers to the performance of the research for the faculty by providing access to databases or specialty personnel.

CONCLUSION

The support group continues to meet on a weekly basis to develop and refine a faculty development process. The blend of a successful program contains an appropriate support group for the proposal development process, a willing faculty, and an administrative support system that promotes scholarly pursuits while using telemedicine as a testbed for both developing leadership skills to improve system performance and learning to do proposal development for external funding.

Telemedicine: Practicing in the Information Age,
edited by Steven F. Viegas and Kim Dunn.
Lippincott–Raven Publishers, Philadelphia © 1998.

29

Evaluating Patient and Clinician Satisfaction

Russell A. LaForte and David J. Solomon

Department of Internal Medicine, University of Texas Medical Branch at Galveston, Galveston, Texas 77555; and Department of Internal Medicine and Office of Educational Development, University of Texas Medical Branch at Galveston, Galveston, Texas 77555

Telemedicine has numerous participants, each with unique needs and expectations. Patients desire effective, compassionate care that proceeds in as expeditious a manner as possible. Primary care givers desire effective consultation but are also interested in the time spent preparing and presenting a case. Consultants are concerned about the duration of the visit and the quality of presentation. The system collectively is concerned with cost-effectiveness and patient management issues. A complete assessment of telemedicine satisfaction must keep all of these perspectives in mind.

One *MEDLINE* search revealed no articles assessing patient satisfaction with telemedicine. As outlined in Chapter 6, consultants, primary caregivers, and patients participating in telemedicine think that consultations meet their needs at one institution. In this study, the participants were asked to rate on a scale of one to five to what extent their consultation was adequate to meet all of their needs. Patients and consultants averaged a score of four of five, and primary caregivers averaged a score of five. From these 276 consultations, there was only one complaint letter and one official grievance. The study at University of Texas Medical Branch (UTMB) at Galveston is an initial attempt to assess satisfaction and provides a favorable preliminary view of telemedicine.

The first obstacle to increasing patient and provider satisfaction with telemedicine is the identification by all parties of specific concerns. One view of the UTMB study may be that telemedicine is great, but past formal experience with medical care shows that inexact questioning fails to uncover specific problems (1,2). Specific areas of care need to be assessed by each type of participant in telemedicine, most easily, via questionnaires. Examples of each follow.

QUESTIONNAIRES

Patient

The patient questionnaire (Fig. 29-1) should assess what the patient expected to obtain from the visit and whether he or she obtained it. The questionnaire should

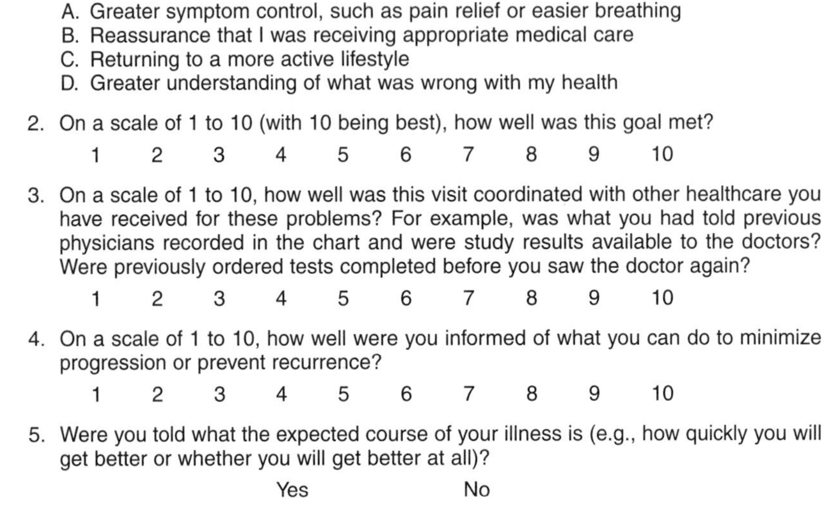

1. Which of the following best characterizes your goals in this doctor visit?
   A. Greater symptom control, such as pain relief or easier breathing
   B. Reassurance that I was receiving appropriate medical care
   C. Returning to a more active lifestyle
   D. Greater understanding of what was wrong with my health
2. On a scale of 1 to 10 (with 10 being best), how well was this goal met?
   1 2 3 4 5 6 7 8 9 10
3. On a scale of 1 to 10, how well was this visit coordinated with other healthcare you have received for these problems? For example, was what you had told previous physicians recorded in the chart and were study results available to the doctors? Were previously ordered tests completed before you saw the doctor again?
   1 2 3 4 5 6 7 8 9 10
4. On a scale of 1 to 10, how well were you informed of what you can do to minimize progression or prevent recurrence?
   1 2 3 4 5 6 7 8 9 10
5. Were you told what the expected course of your illness is (e.g., how quickly you will get better or whether you will get better at all)?
   Yes No

FIG. 29-1. Patient satisfaction questionnaire.

address whether the visit was effectively integrated into the overall medical care plan. As telemedicine is also used to counsel patients, whether the patient believes he or she left the visit with a better understanding of what to expect in the future should also be determined. Whether the patient perceived any limitations of telemedicine during the patient-physician interactions must also be determined. Finally, the patient must compare the time and inconvenience of the visit with standard visits.

Presenter

One critical aspect of effective telemedicine is the accurate, concise presentation of patient information to the consultant. The individual who performs this function, called the *presenter*, must also receive a questionnaire. This questionnaire must assess the ease of information delivery to the consultant. The presenter questionnaire should also address the presenter's level of comfort in presenting the case to the consultant. If not the primary caregiver, the presenter should further evaluate the legibility, quality, and availability of information from the primary care site.

Primary Caregiver

The primary caregiver should be sent a follow-up letter after each visit (Fig. 29-2). Primary caregivers should be asked if they found the consultation helpful in the management of the patient. They should be questioned specifically about the appropriateness and legibility of the written records provided. The timeliness of the supply of those

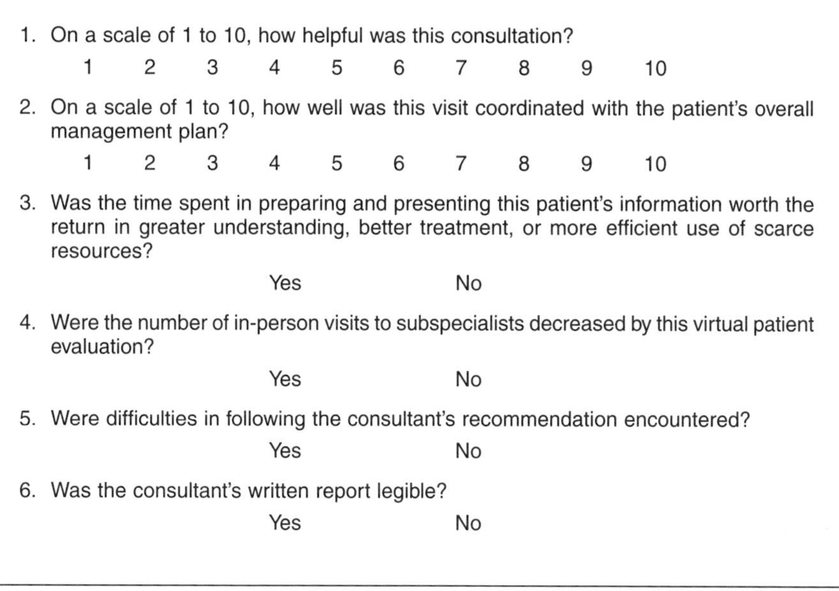
1. On a scale of 1 to 10, how helpful was this consultation?
   1 2 3 4 5 6 7 8 9 10
2. On a scale of 1 to 10, how well was this visit coordinated with the patient's overall management plan?
   1 2 3 4 5 6 7 8 9 10
3. Was the time spent in preparing and presenting this patient's information worth the return in greater understanding, better treatment, or more efficient use of scarce resources?
   Yes No
4. Were the number of in-person visits to subspecialists decreased by this virtual patient evaluation?
   Yes No
5. Were difficulties in following the consultant's recommendation encountered?
   Yes No
6. Was the consultant's written report legible?
   Yes No

FIG. 29-2. Primary caregiver satisfaction questionnaire.

records should also be assessed. The primary caregiver should further note whether the virtual consult decreased the number of in-person consult evaluations received by a given patient. An attempt to determine patient compliance must also be made at this point.

Consultant

The actual telemedicine visit is centered around the consultant. Consultant questionnaires (Fig. 29-3) should determine whether the time spent evaluating the patient was longer, shorter, or similar to that which would be used in an in-person evaluation. Ultimately, these questionnaires should also question whether the consultant was able to fully assess and recommend treatment for the patient, and, if not, whether an on-site evaluation would have allowed a better assessment. Consultants must also be asked whether a visit to their office was saved by telemedicine. If a specific protocol was available, the consultant should record compliance with the stated protocol. The consultant must further identify if the exact reason for consultation was apparent to him or her at the time of evaluation.

CONCLUSION

The ultimate goal is a system that delivers compassionate, competent care in a cost-effective way, including minimization of patient travel and time use. The time from initial consultation until return to an expected functional status should be followed and compared to a standard-care delivery system. Also, the time from patient

1. Was the time spent in evaluation of this patient more or less time-consuming than an in-person evaluation?
   A. Less time-consuming
   B. About equally time-consuming
   C. More time-consuming
2. How complete was your patient assessment compared to assessment of similar patients in your regular practice?
   A. Less complete
   B. About as complete
   C. More complete
3. How complete was the data supplied to you, as compared to the data you are supplied in your regular clinic?
   A. Less complete
   B. About as complete
   C. More complete
4. Was a visit to your office saved by this remote evaluation?
   Yes No
5. Were the results of testing forwarded to you in a timely manner?
   Yes No
6. If a protocol was available to be used, was it followed?
   Yes No N/A (no protocol)

FIG. 29-3. Consultant satisfaction questionnaire.

referral to patient evaluation can be recorded. Whether compassionate, effective care is rendered is certainly subject to interpretation by various participants, but the relative number of complaints, grievances, and lawsuits can be used to compare this aspect of telemedicine to standard in-person care within a given care delivery system.

Telemedicine is a powerful new tool in the management of the practice of medicine. If properly applied, telemedicine maximizes communication via rapid transmission of data and allows for a unique freedom in consultant-patient-caregiver conferencing. To make telemedicine increasingly productive, efficient, humane, and cost-effective, the same problems faced by all physicians in day-to-day practice must be identified and solved.

REFERENCES

1. Delbanco TL. Enriching the doctor-patient relationship by inviting the patient's perspective. *Ann Intern Med* 1992;116:414–418.
2. Bruster S, Jarman B, Bosanquet N, Weston D, Erens R, Delbanco TL. National survey of hospital patients. *BMJ* 1994;309:1542–1546.

Telemedicine: Practicing in the Information Age,
edited by Steven F. Viegas and Kim Dunn.
Lippincott–Raven Publishers, Philadelphia © 1998.

30

Cost Accounting for Telemedicine

Keith Gran

Department of Internal Medicine, University of Texas Medical Branch at Galveston, Galveston, Texas 77555

This chapter addresses the practical application of how to create an income statement, balance sheet, and cash flow statement. A few ratio analyses that can be conducted to determine performance are discussed and details of what should be included in each of these statements according to generally accepted accounting principles are provided. There are other methods of accounting for universities and hospitals (i.e., fund accounting), but they are beyond the scope of this text.

The three statements described in Table 30-1 and Appendices A, B, and C—income, balance sheet, and cash flow statements—allow any size enterprise to determine how a telemedicine program is performing, whether it is the only service offered by the enterprise or a small subsection of the enterprise. The following discussion provides a short explanation for each and shows what items to look for when dealing with a telemedicine consult practice.

INCOME STATEMENT

The income statement is important because it helps predict the amount, timing, and uncertainty of future cash flow. The income statement also is an indicator of how an enterprise has performed for a specific period. The two main sections of the income statement are the revenue and expenses sections.

Revenue Section

The revenue section should include all gross revenue from the telemedicine consult service. Revenue should be broken down by payor, so the reader can determine where revenues are generated. The main payor groups for an academic institution would be managed care, commercial insurance, Medicare, Medicaid, and guarantor. It is important to understand where revenues come from to be able to maximize billings. It would also be useful to track separately the level of billings for each payor, so the enterprise can be sure to maximize its billing for the level of care provided. A

TABLE 30-1. *Three types of financial statements*

Statement type	Major components	Strengths	Weaknesses
Income	Revenues: Inflows or other enhancements or settlement of liabilities. Expenses: Outflows or using up of assets or the incurrence of liabilities. This section includes directly related costs, as well as general costs. Gain: Increase in equity. Loss: Decrease in equity.	Helps predict the amount, timing, and uncertainty of future cash flows. Investors and creditors can use the information to evaluate past performance. Helps determine the risk of not achieving particular cash flows. Uses historical cost, so as not to mislead the statement reader.	Important that bad debt is calculated accurately. Net income can have items included that are not cash, such as depreciation, that will affect net income. Only reflects activity for a certain period, so there is a need to compare previous performance.
Balance sheet	Assets: Probable future economic benefits obtained or controlled by a particular entity as a result of past transactions or events. Liabilities: Probable future sacrifices of economic benefits arising from present obligations of a particular entity to transfer assets or provide services to other entities in the future as a result of past transactions or events. Equity: Residual interest in the assets of an entity that remains after deducting its liabilities. In a business enterprise, the equity is the ownership interest.	Provides tool for determining the net worth of the enterprise. Provides ability to track capital expenditures. Provides ability to analyze debt. Investors and creditors can use to evaluate liquidity of the enterprise.	Majority of capital expenditure is based on historical cost, so it does not reflect market value. Allowance for doubtful accounts is an estimate and should be calculated carefully.
Cash flow	Operating activities: The case effects of transactions that enter into the determination of net income. The excess of cash receipts over cash payments. Investing activities: Those items considered investing activities (e.g., equipment purchase). Financing activities: Any activity that helps fund the enterprise or relieves the debt of the enterprise.	Helps user evaluate the liquidity, solvency, and financial flexibility of the enterprise. Enables the reader to determine if the enterprise will be able to meet future obligations. Most important statement for a start-up enterprise.	Does not represent profit but available cash.

telemedicine consult service will probably be billing at lower levels. As the collection rates have decreased since 1994 due to managed care reimbursement, it is important to make note of the collections in the footnotes to the income statement so there will not be any misunderstanding. It is also important that bad debt expense is calculated accurately and reflected in the expense section of the income statement. Any other funding related to telemedicine could be indicated in this section of the income statement. For instance, federal or state grants that are specific for telemedicine can be included as other funding, but only that part that is used to pay expenses related to telemedicine.

Expenses Section

The costs of the telemedicine service should be calculated separately based on the time spent providing the service. For instance, the portion of time a physician and his or her support staff spend on the actual service should be counted. The rest of the time administrating the enterprise should be counted in operating expenses. By doing this, the break-even point for the enterprise may be determined. If all expenses directly related to the service are added to the fixed costs, such as equipment and setup cost of the enterprise, revenue that must be generated to break even may be calculated.

Net Income

Once all expenses are determined, the income statement is complete. Revenues less expenses equal net income. Net income is what is used to determine how the enterprise performed during a specific period. At the end of each year, net income would close to the retained earnings account in the equity section of the balance sheet, thereby moving net income to the balance sheet.

BALANCE SHEET STATEMENT

The balance sheet provides information about the nature and amounts of investments in enterprise resources, obligations to enterprise creditors, and the owners' equity in net enterprise resources at a point in time. The balance sheet contributes to financial reporting by providing a basis for (a) computing rates of return, (b) evaluating the capital structure of the enterprise, and (c) assessing the liquidity and financial flexibility of the enterprise.

Balance sheet accounts are classified so that similar items are grouped together to arrive at significant subtotals. The three general classes of items included in the balance sheet are assets, liabilities, and stockholders' equity.

Assets

The asset section of a balance sheet is broken into two parts, current and those items that are not current. In the current section for a telemedicine consult service, cash and accounts receivable would be the main categories. The accounts receivable would include all receivables, collectable or not, with an estimate of doubtful accounts subtracted from it. This would provide a net receivable amount.

The noncurrent section would include the setup cost of the consult service along with the equipment needed to operate the service and would be expensed over the useful life of the equipment. Equipment would only be included if the equipment was purchased. If the equipment was leased, it would be a rental expense in the income statement.

Liability

The liability section also is broken down into current and noncurrent items. The current would include those items that are due or payable within 1 year or the operating cycle, whichever is shorter. Such items would be accounts payable, salary payable, and that portion of debt due within the 1-year period. If the equipment were financed for 10 years, the first year of debt would be in current and the 9 remaining years would be in long term. For a telemedicine consult service, debt on the purchase of equipment would probably be the major noncurrent liability, unless the purchase of property takes place to conduct the service.

Stockholders' Equity

The stockholders' equity section of the balance sheet contains ownership interest in the telemedicine consult service. It is the interest in the assets that remains after deducting the liabilities. If the consult service were a corporation, the stockholders' equity section would include stock ownership and any excess that is paid above the par value of that stock. The stockholders' equity section would also include the retained earnings, which is an accumulation of net income and losses from all the previous years, along with any paying of dividends or repurchase of stock.

CASH FLOW STATEMENT

The last statement is the statement of cash flow. This statement is important in that it allows the reader to determine if the enterprise can meet its future obligations from cash flow. The primary purpose of the cash flow statement is to provide relevant information about the cash receipts and cash payments of an enterprise during a period. To achieve this, the cash flow statement reports (a) the cash effects of an enterprise's operations during a period, (b) its investing transactions, (c) its financing transactions, and (d) the net increase or decrease in cash during the period.

Operating Activities

Operating activities include the cash effects of transactions that enter into the determination of net income. Cash provided by operations (the excess of cash receipts over cash payments) is usually determined by converting net income on an accrual basis to a cash basis. This conversion is accomplished by adding to or deducting from net income those items in the income statement not affecting cash, such as depreciation expense on the telemedicine equipment and the gain or loss on selling any equipment. Changes in balance sheet accounts should also have an effect on cash, such as an increase or decrease in accounts receivable or accounts payable, comparing the beginning of the year to the end of the year. Once all these items are reconciled to net income, the net cash flow provided by operating activities is known.

Investing Activities

Cash flow from investing activities would include very few items, such as the sales price or purchase price of the telemedicine equipment. This provides cash flow from investing activities.

Financing Activities

Cash flow from financing activities is derived by reconciling all financing activities, such as payment of dividends or the issuance of stock. Many cash flow statements would not have this section if there were not any financing transactions.

Net Increase or Decrease

Once the three sections have been completed and reconciled to net income, the net increase or decrease in cash will be known. This number will always differ from net income, unless there is zero change from one year to the next or the consulting service is already on a cash basis of accounting.

RATIO ANALYSIS

Ratio analysis helps determine how an enterprise is performing. Data on other similar enterprises will help determine where yours falls on the scale. The following describes a few of the ratios that help in analyzing financial statements:

1. Liquidity ratios help determine the firm's ability to meet its current debts.
   - Current ratio (current assets/current liabilities): the ratio of total current assets to total current liabilities.
   - Acid-test ratio (cash + marketable securities + net receivables)/current liabilities: the same as the current ratio except it leaves off inventories and prepaid items. For a telemedicine consult business, it will not vary much from the current ratio.
2. Activity ratios measure how effectively the enterprise is using the assets.
   - Receivables turnover (net revenues/average net receivables): The ratio is computed by dividing net revenues by average receivables outstanding during the year. This information provides some indication of the quality of the

receivables and an idea of how successful the firm is in collecting its outstanding receivables. The faster the turnover, the more credence the current ratio and acid-test ratio have in financial analysis.

3. Profitability ratios indicate how well the enterprise has operated during the year. These ratios answer questions such as the following: Was the net income adequate? What rate of return does it represent? Generally, the ratios are either computed on the basis of revenues or on an investment base such as total assets. Profitability is frequently used as the ultimate test of management effectiveness.
   - Profit margin on sales (net income/net revenue): indicates what financial cushion is available in the case of higher costs or lower revenues in the future.
   - Rate of return on assets (net income/average total assets): a combination of the asset turnover ratio and the profit margin on sales ratio. Asset turnover is calculated as net revenue divided by average total assets, and the profit margin on sales is calculated as net income divided by net revenue. As net revenue is in the numerator in the first formula and the denominator in the second formula, when multiplied together they cancel and net income divided by average total assets is left. A high rate of return is desired.
4. Coverage ratios are computed to help predict the enterprise's long-term solvency. Coverage ratios indicate the risk involved in investing in the enterprise. The more debt added to the capital structure, the more uncertain the return. There is only one coverage ratio discussed here, debt to total assets.
   - Debt to total assets (debt/total assets): provides creditors with some idea of the enterprise's ability to withstand losses without impairing the interests of creditors. From the creditor standpoint, a low ratio is desirable.

Because a ratio can be computed precisely, it is easy to attach a high degree of reliability to it. The reader of financial statements must understand the basic limitations of ratio analysis when evaluating the enterprise. The ratios are only as good as the data on which they are based.

OTHER INFORMATION

Finally, many important factors about an enterprise are not reflected in financial statements. Events involving industry changes, management changes, technological developments, and government actions are often critical to the success of an enterprise.

At the end of each financial statement, any notes that will enable the statement reader to understand more clearly what took place should be included. Financial statements should be prepared in such a way that someone without a financial background can understand them. The last thing desired is to mislead a reader of financial statements. To avoid misleading information, the accounting industry uses historical cost, which is a more conservative approach when presenting financial information. Always err on the conservative side.

BIBLIOGRAPHY

Fischer PM, Taylor WJ, Leer JA. *Advanced accounting*, 5th ed. Cincinnati: South-Western Publishing Co., 1993.

Homgren CT, Foster G. *Cost accounting, a managerial emphasis*, 7th ed. Englewood Cliffs, NJ: Prentice-Hall, 1991.

Kieso DE, Weygandt JJ. *Intermediate accounting*, 7th ed. New York: Wiley, 1992.

Niswonger CR, Fess PE, Weygandt JJ. *Acounting principles*, 12th ed. Cincinnati: South-Western Publishing Co., 1977.

The Stanley H. Kaplan CPA Review. Practice and theory seminar. Dallas, TX, October, 1994.

The University of Texas at Arlington CPA review material. Arlington, TX, 1994.

Appendix A

XYZ Company Income Statement for the Year Ended December 31, 19XX

Telemedicine consult revenue				
Managed care charges	xxxxx			
Commercial insurance charges	xxxxx			
Medicare charges	xxxxx			
Medicaid charges	xxxxx			
Guarantor charges	xxxxx			
Federal grants	xxxxx			
State grants	xxxxx			
Other charges	xxxxx			
Total telemedicine revenue			xxxxx	
Cost of goods sold (services rendered)				
Salaries				
Physicians	xxxxx			
Nurses	xxxxx			
Nurse practitioners	xxxxx			
Physician assistants	xxxxx			
Other support staff	xxxxx			
Total salaries related to consult service		xxxxx		
Telecommunications expense		xxxxx		
Bad debt expense		xxxxx		
Supplies		xxxxx		
Total cost of goods sold			xxxxx	
Gross profit on telemedicine consults				xxxxx
Operating expenses				
Administrative and other salaries		xxxxx		
Travel		xxxxx		
Advertising		xxxxx		
Freight and postage		xxxxx		
Depreciation of telemedicine equipment		xxxxx		
Depreciation of office equipment		xxxxx		
Telephone		xxxxx		
Insurance		xxxxx		

Utilities	xxxxx	
Office supplies	xxxxx	
Miscellaneous expenses	xxxxx	
Total operating expenses		xxxxx
Net income before taxes		xxxxx
Income tax		xxxxx
Net income after taxes		xxxxx

Appendix B

XYZ Company Balance Sheet, for the Year Ended December 31, 19XX

Current assets			
Cash		xxxxx	
Marketable securities		xxxxx	
Accounts receivable	xxxxx		
Less allowance for doubtful accounts	xxxxx	xxxxx	
Note receivable		xxxxx	
Supplies on hand		xxxxx	
Prepaid expenses		xxxxx	
Total current assets			xxxxx
Long-term investments			
Property, plant, and equipment			
Land: at cost		xxxxx	
Buildings: at cost	xxxxx		
Less accumulated depreciation	xxxxx	xxxxx	
Telemedicine equipment	xxxxx		
Less accumulated depreciation	xxxxx	xxxxx	
Total property, plant, and equipment			xxxxx
Total assets			xxxxx
Liabilities and stockholders' equity			
Current liabilities			
Notes payable		xxxxx	
Accounts payable		xxxxx	
Accrued interest		xxxxx	
Income tax payable		xxxxx	
Accrued wages		xxxxx	
Other current liabilities		xxxxx	
Total current liabilities			xxxxx
Long-term debt			xxxxx

Total liabilities			xxxxx
Stockholders' equity			
Common stock	xxxxx		
Additional paid in capital	xxxxx	xxxxx	
Retained earnings		xxxxx	
Total stockholders' equity			xxxxx
Total liabilities and stockholders' equity			xxxxx

Appendix C

XYZ Company Statement of Cash Flow for the Year Ended December 31, 19XX: Increase (Decrease) in Cash

Cash flow from operating activities		
Net income		XXXXX
Adjustments to reconcile net income to net	XXXXX	
Cash provided by operating activities	XXXXX	
Depreciation expense	XXXXX	
Gain or loss on sale of telemedicine equipment	XXXXX	
Increase or decrease in accounts receivable	XXXXX	
Increase or decrease in accounts payable	XXXXX	XXXXX
Net cash provided by operating activities		XXXXX
Cash flow from investing activities	XXXXX	
Sale of assets	XXXXX	
Purchase of telemedicine equipment	XXXXX	
Net cash used by investing activities		XXXXX
Cash flow from financing activities		
Payment of cash dividends	XXXXX	
Issuance of common stock	XXXXX	
Net cash provided by financing activities		XXXXX
Net increase or decrease in cash		XXXXX
Cash at the beginning of the year		XXXXX
Cash at the end of the year		XXXXX

Telemedicine: Practicing in the Information Age,
edited by Steven F. Viegas and Kim Dunn.
Lippincott–Raven Publishers, Philadelphia © 1998.

31

Cost Analysis of Telemedicine Consultations

Mary Moore

College of Communications, Arkansas State University,
State University, Arkansas 72467

Telemedicine is implemented for three main reasons: (a) to improve access to healthcare, (b) to improve the quality of care, and (c) to reduce the cost of care.* It is generally accepted that telemedicine improves access to care and early studies established that when telemedicine is provided, more people seek care (1).

In this chapter, the topic of cost analysis is approached by examining definitions and the history of cost studies in telemedicine, considering major variables in the cost analysis of telemedicine, examining cost analysis attempts for numerous specific applications, discussing various approaches to determining the cost of a telemedicine consultation, and summarizing the issues.

Telehealth is defined in this chapter as the use of telecommunications for the delivery of healthcare services across distances. These services may include patient consultations, education, administrative services, or collaborative research. This chapter concentrates primarily on telemedicine. Telemedicine is a subset of telehealth. Telemedicine uses telecommunication to provide medical care and healthcare, expedite research, and improve the diagnosis and treatment of illness (2). The primary focus of this chapter is on the use of interactive video to provide telemedicine consultations.

Costs can include dollar costs, personnel costs, time, or other resources. Cost-benefit and cost-effectiveness analysis are defined as follows:

> [They] are the quantitative examination of alternative ways to accomplish public goals as to their benefits, or effectiveness, to be gained and the costs to be incurred—for the purpose of identifying the preferred alternative.
>
> In cost-benefit analysis, benefits are primarily expressed in monetary, dollar, values. In cost-effectiveness analysis, benefits are primarily left in non-monetary units. (3, p.166)

Finally, cost feasibility is defined as follows:

> [C]osts relative to some figure set as a criterion for decision-making. For example, if we calculated the costs of various telemedical applications relative to related amounts

*A fourth reason for the implementation of telemedicine in underserved or rural areas may be to reduce professional isolation, which may also involve elements common to the other three reasons.

of prospective reimbursement, we would have criteria relevant to whether we might wish to engage in those applications. (4, p. 49)

Cost-feasibility study summaries, characterized by their speculative nature, occur more frequently in the telemedicine literature than do formal cost-benefit or cost-effectiveness reports, which have been rare.

COST STUDIES IN THE LITERATURE

An often-repeated myth at telemedicine conferences has been that there are no cost studies on telemedicine. The common consensus has been that, currently there is no uniform third-party reimbursement for telemedicine in the United States, because there are no cost studies. Sometimes the statement appears in print without qualification. Grigsby wrote, "[t]here are no published data on the cost effectiveness of telemedicine" (5, p. 21). Burdick echoed, "[a]lthough there are no published data on the cost-effectiveness of telemedicine . . . ," attributing the statement to Grigsby (6, p. 313). More often, the statement is qualified when it appears in print. In these cases, authors may state that there are no cost-analysis studies published in peer reviewed journals or that there are no rigorous studies using current technology and evaluative techniques (7–12). The more these individuals qualify the statement, the more likely it becomes that the statement is defensible. Indeed, it does appear that, though the results of cost studies are reported with some frequency, there are no true business plans, income statements, balance sheets, or cash flow statements yet published in telemedicine.

However, valuable cost analysis research already in existence goes unrecognized. Even studies conducted by the U.S. Government neglect to cite research work completed under U.S. Government contracts. When a sample of telemedicine project directors were interviewed in 1992, almost all indicated they had compiled cost-analysis information (13). Only a few published the information. Fewer still published the information in the journal literature indexed by *Index Medicus*. As of this writing, a literature search of the *MEDLINE* database combining the keywords *cost* and *telemedicine* yields 87 articles. Of the 35 articles in the *MEDLINE* database with *telemedicine-economics* as a major heading, 29 were written in the past 3 years. A literature search of the *Telemedicine Information Exchange*, however, yielded 474 articles, including more than 50 new citations appearing in the immediately preceding 3 months.

This chapter does not claim to be a comprehensive review of telemedicine cost analysis. I clearly recognize, however, that there is an untapped wealth of relevant information never indexed by *MEDLINE*.

Early Cost-analysis Studies

Conrath (1) found that cost issues were at the core of telemedicine development and use in the early 1900s.

> Many examples of the early use of specific communications technologies can be cited. Einthovan (1906), the inventor and developer of the electrocardiogram, transmitted EKGs and phonocardiograms via the telephone in the early 1900s, even before his galvanometer was generally accepted and available. This was done because the cost of telephone transmission was less than that of supplying each hospital with an additional galvanometer. (1, p. 24) (For more information on Einthovan, see ref. 14.)

Attempts to specifically analyze costs of telemedicine began occurring in the literature in the 1970s. Muller and colleagues (15) and Cunningham and colleagues (16) wrote of an inner city project in New York that had the objectives of minimizing costs by using nurses instead of physicians and not making unnecessary referrals.

The Sioux Lookout Zone telemedicine project in remote northern Ontario covered an area almost as large as California (1). Three nursing stations were outfitted with interactive, slow-scan television equipment. The authors concluded that telemedicine was not cost justifiable. Increased access had apparently resulted in an increased usage of healthcare. The decreased cost of transfers for emergency care could not balance the increase in total use.

Mark and colleagues (17) reported on a nursing home telemedicine project in Boston in 1976. In this project, the telemedicine technology used was a tone and voice paging system, portable electrocardiogram machines, and telephone-coupled transmitters for analysis of pacemakers. Although the study used a very different definition of *telemedicine* than that used in current studies (usually "interactive video" now), the cost study methodology and analysis used in the report may be valuable to current researchers. Some results were similar to those of the Sioux Lookout Zone Project. The telemedicine study group used more ambulatory care and significantly less hospitalization than the control population.

The WAMI project (18) examined the cost effectiveness of an ATS-6 satellite-based telemedicine project serving *W*ashington, *A*laska, *M*ontana, and *I*daho. The University of Washington in Seattle had the only medical school in the region. Between 1977 and 1979, researchers conducted cost experiments for two examples of consultations: normal consultations and emergency consultations. The consultations for patients in Fairbanks were to be performed by physicians in Seattle. Costs for various options for each example were compared. Pros and cons for each option of each example were also identified. Items that were difficult to cost were also enumerated. In both cases, the telemedicine services were found to be as cost-effective as travel for either the patients or the healthcare providers.

Several early articles (1,15,18–21) reported cost-effectiveness analyses of different types of information-delivering technologies, sometimes with conflicting results. It is sometimes concluded by those reading the reports that comparisons of types of technologies show no significant difference in diagnostic accuracy and therefore the cheapest technology (telephone) is the most effective (1,19). Because several authors have written about the same experiment, this report may appear to have general acceptance and was quoted at conferences as recently as 1995. Before accepting the authors' conclusions, it is necessary to examine the methods used in the original study and their applicability to dissimilar settings, as well as changes due to emerging technologies.

Summary of Early Telemedicine Literature

Early studies reached different conclusions about whether telemedicine costs could be justified because the variables differed in size from project to project. In some projects, the cost of equipment was higher than in others. In some projects, the only alternatives for healthcare provision were at greater distances. In some projects, local nonphysician healthcare providers could substitute for physicians when they were linked to distant physicians who could supervise care. Finally, telemedicine services in some projects were considerably used more than in other projects.

Several early experiments concluded that, due to the high cost of new technologies, such as satellite transmission and full-motion, interactive television, telemedicine could not be cost justified for general use (1,15,16,19,22). The early studies are quite valuable to current researchers, however, in the methodologies used for the cost studies. If relative costs of equipment today were inserted into the equations, different results might occur.

Summary of More Recent Studies

After the initial attempts at cost analysis, there is a gap in the literature, generally corresponding with the gap in U.S. federal funding for telemedicine projects. The next attempts to document cost analysis of telemedicine programs began in the late 1980s. After 1992, projects again began reporting cost studies in the literature (23,24).

Although more than a decade had passed between studies, the same cost variables emerged as issues in cost-analysis studies. The primary variables examined were equipment and technology, transportation, personnel, transportation, and time. Lower costs of local healthcare and revenue generation were sometimes included in the studies. Variables that are more difficult to quantify and less likely to be studied are savings due to faster treatment, avoided tests and procedures, and shorter lengths of stay. Avoided morbidity and mortality costs are sometimes reported but rarely calculated in telemedicine cost studies.

Equipment and Technology

There is a trend toward decreasing costs of equipment and increasing capabilities in telemedicine. If projects were deemed to be cost-effective using 1990 equipment, it is likely that they would be even more cost effective today. Many reports only summarize equipment studies. It is necessary to obtain the initial cost study to determine how equipment costs were estimated. Project reports must be read carefully to determine if the equipment used is relevant to the type of equipment being considered in new project implementation. Often, it is not. An ideal cost study, however, would identify equipment costs, so that the new cost for comparable equipment could be readily substituted.

Network costs have also begun to decline, especially for nonprofit applications in rural areas of the United States. The U.S. Telecommunications Act of 1996 helped assure that rates would become more reasonable for telemedicine applications. In reading reports, one must consider the possibility that the telecommunication rates could have changed since the publication of the article. One must also consider whether the research study was calculated using dedicated lines or with discounts allowed for the use of measured lines and services. Regardless of whether the study is academically rigorous, local network rates must be compared before making assumptions about replicability of the study locally.

Personnel

Cost calculations should include the number of individuals employed to provide the telemedicine services, including those performing technical, scheduling, coordinating, and healthcare provisions and those providing training and evaluative activities. Savings may be realized when healthcare providers are able to increase productivity through grouped, scheduled telemedicine clinics or when the role of nonphysician providers is expanded through telemedicine.

Several early telemedicine trials examined whether nonphysician healthcare providers could provide adequate healthcare when supervised by physicians at a distance and concluded that this type of service was feasible (1,15–17,22).

In early 1996, a trial by a managed healthcare provider in Minnesota reexamined whether nurses supervised through telemedicine could replace on-call physicians in rural emergency rooms at night and on weekends (25). The cost-benefit analysis has not yet been fully disclosed to the public but resulted in additional sites being added in 1997.

Transportation

Elements to consider in evaluating the costs of avoided transportation include who is traveling (e.g., patient, physician, patient's family) and whether the travel is planned or emergency. Potential savings from telemedicine include travel costs and unproductive travel time that are avoided.

One must still consider who is the recipient of transportation savings. If circuit-rider healthcare providers are replaced by telemedicine, the savings accrue to the sponsoring organization. This may be the health sciences center or hospital, the government, the managed care provider, or the individual healthcare provider in private practice.

Patient transportation is fairly easy to calculate if the consultation results in an avoided emergency transfer. If the cost of the transfer would be borne by a third party, the savings would accrue to that party. In some countries (e.g., Norway), in correctional healthcare in the United States, and in military medicine, travel for even nonemergency, routine healthcare is reimbursed or provided. In these cases, the savings would accrue to the government. In other countries, such as the United States and China, costs for travel for routine healthcare is generally borne by the patient, and in these cases the patient would benefit from reduced travel. Examples of projects in which transportation savings have been substantial are

- Texas Tech University MEDNET (now HealthNet) in West Texas (23)
- Texas Telemedicine Project centered in Austin (24)
- Hughes Electronics Company's and the government of Mexico's project connecting a hospital in Chiapas with one in Mexico City (26)
- The Eastern Montana Telemedicine Network (27)

Time

Time savings can include lost opportunity costs to healthcare providers and to patients. Time may be lost to travel or in unproductive time waiting for care. Time may also be lost when consultations are inefficient.*

Preston (25) and Bergmo (28) both addressed lost opportunity costs for healthcare providers. Each study proved cost justification for the respective projects. Halvorsen and Kristiansen (29) also considered patient travel time and leisure time in their cost study of telemedicine. Their conclusion was that leisure time must be valued as much as productive time for a telemedicine program to be cost-effective. At Northwest Covenant Medical Center in New Jersey the emergency department used telemedicine to increase physician productivity (30). Telemedicine services also resulted in patients' stays in the emergency department being cut by approximately one-third. The cost equivalency of the reduced stay was not calculated, but patient satisfaction was enhanced. In 1994, Methodist Hospital of Indiana internally funded its ultrasound telemedicine program, which was designed to be self-sustaining (26). Faster treatment time and more timely care, although reported, were not included in the cost analysis.

Gonzalez's (31) prison healthcare project is reported in Correctional Healthcare. In his cost study, he reported measuring the mean of various types of telemedicine consultations for prisoners. For example, internal medicine telemedicine consultations in his project required a mean of 18 minutes; a neurologic consultation required a mean of 16 minutes. The mean for all consultations was 15 minutes. In the first 6 months of the project, the cost per telemedicine consult resulted in 25% savings over the cost of the conventional correctional care alternative. Due to increased usage in the second 6 months of the project, the savings increased to 29%. The cost savings were attributed primarily to avoided transportation cost and secondarily to increased efficiency in length of the consultation.

Lower Cost of Local Care

At least three studies have looked at the comparative costs of care for similar conditions at urban and rural hospitals (32–34). All concluded that the cost of care at

*The critical point at which shortened consultations lead to decreased quality of care rather than increased efficiency remains to be examined.

rural hospitals was less expensive. In the Culler (32) study, cost savings ranged from $1,560 to $6,306 for knee-replacement surgery in comparable patients. If care is less expensive in rural areas, it follows that healthcare money could be saved if transfers and referrals to urban hospitals were avoided.

The Louisiana State Health Care Authority TELEMEDicine Project was initiated in the fall of 1994. The project was based on the information that rural hospital charges were $600 per day, versus $1,200 per day at urban hospitals (26). At a telemedicine project in Georgia, similar statistics were presented.

> Telemedicine has demonstrated that it can decentralize the provision of care. Since medical expertise is brought to the patients, the patient is kept at lower cost facilities. For example, the average day private bed cost of care in one representative rural hospital in Georgia is $1,100.00. If that patient is transferred to the Medical College of Georgia Hospital, the private bed daily rate escalates to $1,850.00. (35)

The Medical College of Georgia found that more than 80% of patients seen via telemedicine did not require transfer to secondary or tertiary care centers. In addition to that savings, telemedicine allowed savings in transportation, increased productivity, and decreased hospitalization days from treating a patient at an earlier stage (36). The Medical College of Georgia went on to report that if rural hospitals were to retain telemedicine patients, the increase of a single patient per day to the rural hospital census would represent a net cash flow of $150,000 per year for the hospital. Finally, at one small, 20-bed hospital in Sioux Falls, South Dakota, a 7-week telemedicine demonstration resulted in a 10% increase in patient days for the hospital (37).

Revenue Generation

The most obvious example of revenue generation develops when physicians and healthcare organizations are able to accrue additional income from telemedicine consultations. Most of these examples come from teleradiology, telepathology, special situations with approved third-party reimbursement,* and managed care organizations. Additional revenue can be generated by expanding services, as certain services can be supervised via telemedicine. Preston (25) found that revenues of $39,000 annually accrued when a local hospital was able to reinstate obstetric services due to telemedicine consultations with remote specialists. Other revenue can be generated by reselling bandwidth to other professionals to consult with patients or clients at a distance or to use for other purposes such as educational conferences or administrative meetings.

As some benefits are difficult to quantify, they may go unreported in cost-benefit studies. Texas Tech MEDNET reported how the availability of telemedicine services resulted in increased levels of confidence in a rural hospital by the local community and subsequent cost benefits (24). According to the hospital administrator, the availability of telemedicine services led to increased patronage of and increased revenues for the rural hospital, allowing it to remain open, when once it had been threatened

---

*One example would be Medicaid reimbursement for telepsychiatry in Montana.

with closure. This is only one example of increased revenue generation that may not be quantifiable.

The sentiment was echoed in a case study of the Louisiana State Health Authority.

> The effectiveness of the system is being judged by physician usage rates rather than fixed equipment costs. Costs per clinical encounter appear high. However, the "aura of excellence" perceived by patients and the increased reputation of those connected with the system are considered significant payback. (26, p. 15)

SPECIFIC TELEMEDICINE APPLICATIONS IN WHICH COSTS HAVE BEEN JUSTIFIED

Teleradiology

Swartz (38) provided insight into how to prepare a cost-benefit analysis for teleradiology, including a comparison of methods for computing net present value. The costs in both the film-based system and the digital imaging alternatives were identified as capital costs, maintenance costs, consumable costs (such as film and chemicals), personnel costs, training and support costs, and space costs. The benefits were more difficult to quantify, but may include reduction in the number of retakes and lost films, faster access to images, better service to physicians and patients, better clinical outcomes, shorter hospital stays, enhanced competitive position, support for other users of images, and expanded patient base from the support of outreach facilities. Swartz summarized:

> It is unlikely that a hospital can eliminate film. More often the use of film is reduced by 50% to 85%. If the film budget is $800,000 annually it could save $400,000. This savings is compared to the cost of the network, but may underestimate the value of the imaging network. There will be additional savings from reduction in space needed for film storage, reduced need for retakes, etc. (38, p. 32)

When cost analysis of this type is applied to teleradiology services, there may be a need to add additional variables to the equation, such as travel costs. In 1995, a cost analysis was conducted for a teleradiology service in Norway connecting the University Hospital of Tromso to a local hospital that had no radiologist. Teleradiology allowed a 39% savings over the traditional method, which used a circuit-rider radiologist (28).

A report of a 1993 study (29) also in Norway, found that teleradiology could not be cost justified unless leisure-time savings were valued as highly as lost production. This study included direct medical costs, travel costs, and lost production costs. Three options were examined: all examinations conducted at the host site; teleradiology equipment installed at the remote site and read at the remote site; and a small x-ray unit installed at the remote site with other examinations conducted at the remote site.

Bergmo (28) attributed the difference in conclusions to the low patient work load (approximately 2,000 versus Bergmo's reported 8,000 total patients per year) in the study by Halvorsen and Kristiansen (29) and that there was no preexisting radiology equipment in either site in his study, as there was in the study by Halvorsen and Kristiansen.

Correctional Healthcare

Since the 1970s, correctional telemedicine has been documented to be significantly less expensive than conventional care: Figures in the literature determine telemedicine to be at least 25% to 30% less expensive.

In 1973, a prison medical service was instituted in Dade County, Florida (39). A cost study compared the use of physicians providing on-site services, nurse practitioners providing the first line of medical care on-site (supported by physicians if necessary), and telemedicine services provided by nurse practitioners at the prison site to remote physicians. The telemedicine service was approximately 30% less expensive than on-site physician services.

The University of Texas Medical Branch (UTMB) at Galveston conducted 3,200 consultations to correctional facilities from 1994 to 1996, with the volume expected to double in the future. The reported operating costs were $300,000 per year. According to Kim Dunn of the project (personal communication, April 1997), this amount was almost equal to the expenditures on transportation for healthcare alone (40).

Texas Tech University's correctional healthcare telemedicine services are described in Time. Conservative cost estimates for the first year of service indicated that the service would be at least 29% less expensive than conventional alternatives for care (31).

Inmate patients at the Arapahoe County Detention Facility are seen 25 miles away at Denver Health and Hospitals through telemedicine. The majority, 95%, of the cases could be seen and treated through telemedicine. Although cost savings on care could not be calculated, the savings for transportation were projected to be $136,800 annually (41).

Home Care

A pilot study by HELP Innovations, Inc. was conducted in Lawrence, Kansas, at a retirement home and at three patient homes using audio and video transmitted via the local cable television company. The report concluded:

> While formal cost-benefit analysis was not part of this pilot program, preliminary information suggests that patients could receive care in their homes using tele–home health care techniques at less than half the cost of on-site home health nursing. (42, p. 94)

A home-care telemedicine system providing data, voice, and video transmission for monitoring reported the cost of a telemedicine visit to be $30, contrasted with a home healthcare visit cost of $74, a nursing home cost per day of $100, and hospital inpatient costs of $820 per day (26).

Military Care

Although cost studies are difficult to locate on telemedicine in the U.S. military, it has been estimated that the government is spending approximately between $445 million and a half-billion dollars on telemedicine. The bulk of this is spent on military applications. At the 1997 American Telemedicine Association Meeting, Harold Koenig, surgeon general of the U.S. Navy, identified the cost of medical evacuation off navy carriers as being between $1,500 and $4,000 for fuel alone (43). Evacuation from Diego Garcia in the Indian Ocean was reported to cost $40,000 per trip. Koenig reported that the most important cost, however, was the loss of services of the individual airlifted. Russ Zajtchuk, commanding general of U.S. Army Medical Research and Material Command, reported that the army had models that proved cost savings, evacuations savings, and faster returns to service from telemedicine (44).

COST OF A CONSULTATION

One study generated protest when it placed the average cost of a telemedicine consultation as high as $1,184 (45). The figure was arrived at by calculating costs for equipment and networks and dividing by the total number of consultations reported over 1 year.

In 1996, Doolittle (46) compared the costs for types of oncology services over a 1-year period. The average cost of telemedicine consultation was $812 versus $897 for a clinic visit using personnel transported by airplane. The average cost per traditional on-site urban visit was $149. The study did not account for rural patients' costs of traveling to the urban site. If the telemedicine service were used to capacity, the estimated cost per teleoncology visit would be $271.

Gonzalez (31) calculated the mean cost of a correctional telemedicine consultation to be $104.75 in 1995 and $98.89 in 1996, versus the cost of a conventional consultation at $139.57. Included in the conventional care costs were transportation costs of approximately $50.11 per consultation. This cost was the lowest reported for correctional healthcare transportation.

Another correctional healthcare service provided information on the costs of providing services and the number of services provided (40). Even if one added the extremely high figure of $100,000 per year for equipment, the cost would still be relatively reasonable, at $125 per consult. The director of the project indicated that high use was the main reason that consultation costs were so low (40).

The HealthTech Services Corporation report on home healthcare costs, cited in Home Care, estimated only $30 per patient telemedicine visit when the Home Assisted Nursing Care Network was used (26). The system included data, voice, and video services.

Finally, Bergmo (28), in his analysis of teleradiology, identified the lowest figure for a consultation. In his study, the cost of a teleradiology consultation worked out to be $15.94 United States equivalent using 1994 exchange rates versus $26.27 United States equivalent for a visiting radiologist. In Bergmo's study, there was high use of services (28).

In summary, the literature reports costs for a telemedicine consultation ranging from $16 per consultation to almost $1,200. The lowest cost is reported by a teleradiology project in Norway (28). About the same time the Norway study was conducted, the

U.S. Government reported the mean figure of $1,184 per consultation for interactive telemedicine consultations at hub sites (45). The difference can be attributed primarily to usage, network costs, travel costs, and perhaps equipment costs. The number of consultations in Norway was higher, the network charges were lower, and travel costs were included. The U.S. study considered only costs in its estimation of mean cost of a consultation. Savings are not factored into the U.S. equations.

CONCLUSION

This review of telemedicine cost studies indicates that it is easier to cost justify telemedicine when telemedicine is examined on an application-specific basis. In this regard, an emerging pattern is being seen, indicating that telemedicine can be cost justified in certain circumstances. The major variables that determine whether telemedicine can be cost justified include the cost of the equipment (which continues to decline over time); networking costs (which are also declining); travel costs and who bears the costs; the number of consultations performed; and whether physicians or other health professionals conduct the consultations. Finally, cost studies that exclude potential savings and revenue generation must be considered incomplete. See Table 31-1 for a summary of cost studies and conclusions.

TABLE 31-1. *Summary of cost studies and conclusions*

Cost element	Author of report (reference)	Date	Name, location of project or program	Conclusions
Equipment and technology	Einthoven (14)	1906	EKG	Reported on invention and use of EKGs and phonocardiograms via telephone. Transmission of EKGs via telephone was more cost-effective than supplying each hospital with galvanometer.
	Dohner and colleagues (18)	1975	WAMI, (*W*ashington, *A*laska, *M*ontana, *I*daho)	Project linking academic medical center in Seattle, Washington, with remote sites. Linked through ATS-6 satellite using interactive video. Telemedicine was as cost-effective as travel for consultation. Lower cost technologies for telemedicine found to be more cost-effective, but full-motion, interactive video was required to reduce the sense of professional isolation for remote practitioners.
	Conrath and colleagues (1) and Dunn and colleagues (19)	1977	Sioux Lookout Zone, Ontario	Compared costs of various technologies for diagnosis and treatment. Lower cost technologies were found to provide the most cost-effective approach for diagnosis and treatment.
	Grundy and colleagues (20)	1977	Pennsylvania	Interactive television service provided between the critical care unit of a small hospital and a large medical center. Telemedicine, though expensive, was found to be superior to the telephone for consultation.
	Muller and colleagues (15)	1977	New York	Pediatric primary care project linked nurse practitioners to physicians through interactive cable television. Use of 1,750 hours per year was required to reach cost-effectiveness (two-thirds the cost of traditional care). Telephone use could not substitute for television in diagnostic consultations.
Local care costs	Hartman and Moore (22)	1992	Texas Tech University MEDNET (later HealthNet) West Texas	Linked academic medical centers in West Texas to two remote rural sites using full-motion, interactive video, T1 networks. Average savings of $1,500 per patient treated by telemedicine was determined to be due to lower costs of care at rural hospitals and reduced costs for emergency transfer.
	U.S. Council on Competitiveness (26)	1994	Louisiana State Health Authority	Cost-feasibility study for telemedicine was based on rural hospital charges of $600 per day versus $1,200 per day for urban hospitals.

	Sanders and colleagues (35)	1996	Medical College of Georgia School of Medicine	Telemedicine allowed 80% of patients to be retained at rural hospitals. Cost of rural care in a private room was $750 less per day than at an urban center.
Personnel	Mark and colleagues (17)	1976	Boston	Care provided by nurse using paging systems, portable EKG, and facsimile service to reach distant physician. Cost savings of $365,000 per 500 patients.
	Muller and colleagues (15)	1977	New York	Telemedicine cost-effective with five satellite clinics and use of 1,750 hours per year. Cost would be two-thirds cost of direct care.
	Cunningham and colleagues (16)	1978	New York	Pediatric nurses could function with televised supervision rather than on-site supervision 40% of the time (same study as Muller [15]).
	Goodall (23)	1996	Allina, Minnesota	A trial of nurses supervised through telemedicine was determined to be cost-effective, resulting in additional telemedicine sites added in 1997.
Supplies	Swartz (38)	1996	—	Examined cost-feasibility issues in teleradiology. Estimated that teleradiology could reduce the use of radiology films by 50% to 85%.
Time	Preston (25)	1993	Texas Telemedicine, Central Texas	This study of interactive video service between a rural renal dialysis clinic and a physician in Austin, Texas, introduced the concept of "windshield time." The project was cost justified in 2.2 years of operation primarily due to salary savings from both physician travel time avoided and increased efficiency in treatment time.
	Methodist Hospital (26)	1994	Indiana	Faster treatment time and more timely care were reported but were not included in the cost analysis.
	Gonzalez (31)	1996	Texas Tech University HealthNet, West Texas Prisons	Cost savings of telemedicine over traditional transport for prison healthcare resulted in 25% to 29% savings, primarily due to avoided transportation and to increased efficiency in length of consultation.
	Halvorsen and Kristiansen (29)	1996	Norway	Teleradiology services between a large medical center and a remote clinic were found to be cost justified only if lost leisure time was valued as high as lost work production time.
Transportation	Conrath and colleagues (1) and Dunn and colleagues (19)	1978–1980, reported 1983	Sioux Lookout Zone, Ontario	Telemedicine not cost justifiable because increased access resulted in increased usage of services. Decreased transportation costs resulted, however.

Continued

TABLE 31-1. *Continued*

Cost element	Author of report (reference)	Date	Name, location of project or program	Conclusions
	Hartman and Moore (24)	1992	West Texas	Average savings of $1,500 per patient treated by telemedicine was determined to be due to lower costs of care at rural hospitals and reduced costs for emergency transfer.
	Preston (25)	1993	Texas Telemedicine, Central Texas	Savings in travel costs estimated to be between 50% and 95%.
	Allen (41)	1995	Arapahoe County Detention Center	Transportation savings estimated at $136,800 annually.
	Bergmo (28)	1996	Norway	The economic analysis of teleradiology services between a local hospital and a university was compared with the cost of using a traveling radiologist. The study determined that a workload of at least 1,576 patients per year must be reached for the service to be cost justified. The most sensitive variable was found to be the cost of emergency transport of patients.
	Reid (27)	1996	Eastern Montana	Patients saved almost $280 per consult in transportation costs, resulting in $65,00 in annual nonemergency transports. Additional $232,000 in administrative and educational travel costs avoided.
	U.S. Council on Competitiveness (26)	1996	Chiapas to Mexico City	Reduction in the percentage of patients transferred ranged between 34% and 59%; savings reported from $6,300 to $11,200 monthly.
Revenues generated	Hartman and Moore (24)	1992	West Texas	Rural hospital administrator reported that telemedicine leads to increased patronage of and increased revenues for the rural hospital, allowing it to remain open. Specific cost figures not reported.
	Preston (25)	1993	Texas Telemedicine, Central Texas	Revenues generated of $39,000 due to reinstituting infant deliveries and retaining local patients.
	Adams and Grigsby (36)	1995	Medical College of Georgia School of Medicine	Estimated that 80% of patients seen through telemedicine could be retained locally, and the increase of a single patient per day to the rural hospital would represent a net cash flow of $150,000 per year for the hospital.
	Travers and Molseed (37)	1995	Sioux Falls, South Dakota	A 7-week telemedicine demonstration resulted in a 10% increase in patient days.
	Reid (27)	1996	Eastern Montana	98.9% of patients seen by telemedicine were treated locally (instead of some percentage being transferred for care).

EKG, electrocardiogram.

REFERENCES

1. Conrath D, Dunn E, Higgins C. *Evaluating telecommunications technology in medicine*. Dedham, MA: Artech House, 1983.
2. International Space University. Summer Session. *Global Access Telehealth and Education System final report*. Barcelona, Spain: International Space University, 1994.
3. Heyel C, ed. *Encyclopedia of management*. 3rd ed. New York: Van Nostrand Reinhold Company, 1982.
4. Williams F. Sustainability challenges of telemedicine applications. In: Furino A, William F, eds. *Telehealth for Texas: UT Health Science Centers' programs: prospects and potential and special topics in telehealth*. Austin, TX: IC^2 Institutes, University of Texas at Austin, 1995.
5. Grigsby J. Current status of domestic telemedicine. *J Med Syst* 1995;19:19–27.
6. Burdick AK. Response to a telemedicine inquiry from the Florida House of Representatives and text of Model Act to Regulate the Practice of Telemedicine. *Telemed J* 1995;1:309–319.
7. Elford R. Telemedicine—cost effectiveness review. In: *Second International Conference on the Medical Aspects of Telemedicine and Second Annual Mayo Telemedicine Symposium. April 6–9, 1995* [Abstract book]. Rochester, MN: Mayo Clinic, 1995:16.
8. Field MJ, ed. *Telemedicine: a guide to assessing telecommunications in health care*. Washington, DC: National Academy Press, 1996.
9. Kircher M. Rural telemedicine may fail to fill pot-of-gold hopes. *Telemed Telehealth Networks* 1997; 3:28–33.
10. Perendia DA, Allen A. Telemedicine technology and clinical applications. *JAMA* 1995;273:483–488.
11. Emery S. Evolving technology thwarts aim of cost analysis. *Telemed Telehealth Networks* 1997;3: 20–21, 23, 25.
12. Bashshur RL. Telemedicine effects: cost, quality and access. *J Med Syst* 1995;19:81–91.
13. Moore M. Elements of success in telemedicine projects: report of a research grant from AT&T, 1993. http://naftalab.bus.utexas.edu/nafta7/tmpage.html
14. Einthoven W. Het telecardiogram. *Ned Tijdschr Geneeskd* 1906;50:1517–1547.
15. Muller C, Marshall CL, Krasner M, Cunningham N, Wallerstein E, Thomstad B. Cost factors in urban telemedicine. *Med Care* 1977;15:251–259.
16. Cunningham N, Marshall C, Glazer E. Telemedicine in pediatric primary care. *JAMA* 1978;240: 2749–2751.
17. Mark RG, Willemain TR, Malcolm T, Master RJ, Clarkson T. *Nursing home telemedicine project. Vol. 1. Boston City Hospital. Boston, Massachusetts*. Springfield, VA: National Technical Information Service, 1976.
18. Dohner CW, Cullen TJ, Zinser EA. *ATS-6 evaluation: the final report of the communications satellite demonstrations in the WAMI Decentralized Medical Education Program at the Universitv of Washington. Prepared for Lister Hill National Center of Biomedical Communications*. Seattle: University of Washington, 1975.
19. Dunn EV, Conrath DW, Bloor WG. An evaluation of four telecommunication systems for delivery of primary health care. *Health Serv Res* 1977;12:19–29.
20. Grundy BL, Crawford P, Jones PK, Kiley ML, Reisman A, Pau Y. Telemedicine in critical care: an experiment in health care delivery. *JACEP* 1977;6:439–444.
21. Conrath DW, Dunn EV, Bloor WG, Tranquada B. A clinical evaluation of four alternative telemedicine systems. *Behav Sci* 1977;22:12–21.
22. Fuchs M. Provider attitudes toward STARPAHC: a telemedicine project on the Papago reservation. *Med Care* 1979;17:59–68.
23. Hartman JT, Moore M. *Using telecommunications to improve rural health care: the Texas Tech MEDNET Demonstration Project*. Prepared for the US Office of Rural Health Policy, US Department of Health and Human Services. Lubbock, TX: Texas Tech University, 1992.
24. Preston J. *Texas Telemedicine Project report*. Austin, TX: TICS, 1993.
25. Goodall W. Allina Health System promotes telemedicine in rural Minnesota. *TeleConference* 1996; 15:21–23.
26. US Council on Competitiveness. *Highway to health: transforming U.S. healthcare in the information age*. Council on Competitiveness, 1996.
27. Reid J. Eastern Montana project offers lesson in telemedical economics. *Telemed Telehealth Networks* 1996;2:13–14, 41.
28. Bergmo TS. An economic analysis of teleradiology versus a visiting radiology service. *J Telemed Telecare* 1996;2:136–142.

29. Halvorsen PA, Kristiansen IS. Radiology services for remote communities: cost minimization study of telemedicine. *BMJ* 1996;312:1333–1336.
30. Leighty J. New Jersey health center tests viability of interactive consults. *Telemed Telehealth Networks* 1996;2:15–16.
31. Gonzalez WE. Telemedicine in a managed care system. Visions of the Southwest Conference: technology changing the face of education and health care. Presentation at Texas Tech University, Lubbock, Texas, March 1996.
32. Culler SD, Holmes AM, Gutierrez B. Expected hospital costs of knee replacement for rural residents by location of service. *Med Care* 1995;33:1188–1206.
33. Cromwell J, Mitchell J, Calore K, Iezzoni L. Sources of hospital cost variation by urban-rural location. *Med Care* 1987;25:801.
34. Hendricks A, Cromwell J. Are rural referral centers as costly as urban hospitals? *Health Serv Res* 1989;24:289.
35. Sanders JH, Salter PH, Stachura ME. *The unique application of telemedicine to the managed health care system.* January 18, 1996. Submitted to the *American Journal of Managed Care*. HII 96. The Emerging Health Information Infrastructure. Enabling the Vision, April 14–16, 1996. Washington: Georgetown University.
36. Adams LN, Grigsby RK. Georgia State Telemedicine Program: initiation, design and plans. *Telemed J* 1995;1:227–235.
37. Travers H, Molseed R. Patient and physician acceptance of interactive video telemedicine systems linkage in a rural hospital setting. Presented at the Second International Conference on the Medical Aspects of Telemedicine and Second Annual Mayo Telemedicine Symposium. Rochester, Minnesota, April 1995.
38. Schwatz D. Techtalk: teleradiology, mini-PACS, PACS and the digital medical image system. *Telemed Today* 1996;4:32–35.
39. Hastings G, Sasmor L, Sanders J. Primary nurse practitioners and telemedicine in prison care: an evaluation. In: Zoog S, Yarnall S, eds. *The changing health care team: improving effectiveness in patient care*. Seattle: Medical Communications and Services Association, 1976:54–59.
40. University fills Texas-sized need with cost-effective care. *Telemed Telehealth Networks* 1996;2:28–29.
41. Allen A. Prison telemedicine in Colorado. *Telemed Today* 1995;3:26–27.
42. Allen A, Roman L, Cox R, Cardwell B. Home health visits using a cable television network: user satisfaction. *J Telemed Telecare* 1996;2[Suppl 1]:92–94.
43. Koenig HM. Department of Defense Telemedicine Initiatives. Presented at the American Telemedicine Association Conference. Atlanta, April 4, 1997.
44. Zajtchuk R. Military Telemedicine. Presented at the American Telemedicine Association Conference. Atlanta, April 5, 1997.
45. Hassol A. Surprises from the rural telemedicine survey. *Telemed Today* 1996;4:5, 41.
46. Doolittle G. *Tracking and comparing costs associated with two telemedicine practices: oncology and psychiatry*. Atlanta: American Telemedicine Association, 1997.

Telemedicine: Practicing in the Information Age,
edited by Steven F. Viegas and Kim Dunn.
Lippincott–Raven Publishers, Philadelphia © 1998.

32

Neurology

Karen A. Rasmusson

Department of Neurology, University of Texas
Medical Branch at Galveston, Galveston, Texas 77555

Neurology is a specialty that lends itself well to telemedicine. At least 90% of a neurologic diagnosis is made from a careful history, which can be elicited very well via telemedicine.

There are a few patients who do not lend themselves well to evaluation via telemedicine. Patients who cannot speak well, including patients with aphasias and dysarthrias and in whom the neurologic examination plays a much more important role in diagnosis may need on-site evaluation. Even in these individuals, however, an assessment, including demonstration of physical findings by an on-site examiner, can help the neurologist decide if travel to the medical center is warranted.

Telemedicine in neurology can be used in the emergency room setting, in instances of problems thought to be less severe and not life threatening and in acute situations to determine if emergency transport is needed.

NEUROLOGIC HISTORY

The neurologic history, with its history of present illness, past medical history, social history, family history, and pertinent review of systems data, can be obtained via telemedicine. The history proceeds just as in a face-to-face encounter.

After introducing myself, I usually visit for a few moments with the patient to acquaint him or her with the process and to enable the patient to relax and become accustomed to seeing the physician and himself or herself on television screens. The process is a novelty to most patients, and it is necessary to take the small amount of extra time to allow the patient to switch his or her focus to the medical problem.

I do not select my patients before seeing them via telemedicine. At the time of the encounter, I want available the consult from the primary care physician, a list of the patient's current medications, and the patient's vital signs and weight (if possible). Any pertinent studies, clinic notes, or correspondence necessary to complete the consultation can be quickly faxed to me during the encounter.

Rapport with the patient is extremely important in a telemedicine encounter, just as it is in person. Distraction in the telemedicine room or area should be minimized to allow the patient and physician to concentrate on each other. In the optimal situation, telemedicine results in a more focused encounter. (People today are accustomed to focusing on the television screen.)

NEUROLOGIC EXAMINATION

Much information relating to the neurologic examination can be gathered before starting the formal examination portion of the encounter. Careful observation of the patient as he or she sits at the examination table provides useful information about upper and lower extremity function (motor, sensory, coordination). Facial symmetry; speech; eye movement; and spontaneous movement of the head, neck, and extremities are assessable by careful observation.

Under the direction of the physician, the patient can perform maneuvers needed for the physician to assess cerebellar function and station and gait. Close-up views can be used to view rapid alternating movements. The physician should observe for evidence of focal atrophy or fasciculations. A peripheral ophthalmoscope can be used for the funduscopic examination.

A third party is needed to perform the examination of the deep tendon reflexes and the motor and sensory examinations. If the same person assists with the telemedicine encounters during each clinic, it is a good investment to take the time to meet with this individual to train him or her in these portions of the examination so that you feel comfortable with the findings that he or she presents to you. Even so, if the reported findings do not fit the hypothesis I have formed during the interview, then I need to follow up the patient with a face-to-face encounter.

Other examination maneuvers can also be indicated. These include auscultation of the carotid arteries (or other areas of the head or body), which can be accomplished with the use of a peripheral stethoscope. Examination of the back with inspection can be nicely done via camera. Although cervical, thoracic, or lumbar muscle spasm may be suspected by observation, these muscles should be palpated by the on-site assistant. Although active range of motion can be performed at the direction of the physician, passive range of motion requires an on-site assistant. Straight leg raising and assessing for Tinel's sign are other examples of maneuvers that require assistance at the distant site.

DOCUMENTATION

Documentation of the encounter can be accomplished in many ways, just as in a regular office visit. If one's handwriting is legible, notes can be handwritten and immediately faxed to the referral source for review of the assessment and implementation of the recommendations as appropriate. Voice recognition computerized dictation offers another option for immediate transmission of written documentation of the consult. When a copy of the complete written consult cannot be made immediately available to the site, a summary of the assessment and recommendations can be transmitted by fax or electronic mail at the time of the encounter, with a full consult to follow.

PATIENT SATISFACTION

Just as patient satisfaction is important to a practice in a clinic setting, it is important to measure it in a telemedicine encounter. Similar tools can be used to monitor patient satisfaction and identify potential problem areas for improvement. Expressions of satisfaction and dissatisfaction with distant presenters and equipment should likewise be conveyed to appropriate individuals.

CONCLUSION

In summary, a neurology consult delivered via telemedicine can be just as effective as a face-to-face encounter. Care should be used to ensure good patient rapport, a good working relationship with the distant presenter, and effective communication of the results of the consult with the distant site.

Telemedicine: Practicing in the Information Age,
edited by Steven F. Viegas and Kim Dunn.
Lippincott–Raven Publishers, Philadelphia © 1998.

33

Dermatology

Mark H. Lowitt

Department of Dermatology, University of Maryland School of Medicine, Baltimore, Maryland 21201

When I am asked about the range of telemedicine applications, even my most technophobic, nonmedical acquaintances nod vigorously when they hear about teledermatology. The visual nature of the field strikes even the most skeptical as a natural use of the technology. The relative scarcity of dermatologists in rural areas, coupled with a low level of dermatologic comfort on the part of many primary care providers makes teledermatology even more attractive. Having said this, however, it is still appropriate to take one step back and begin to examine the aspects of dermatology that are best or least suitable for telemedicine examination. Inquiry into the specific needs for teledermatology, and how they differ from those of other telemedicine specialties, is also appropriate.

WHICH PATIENTS CAN BE SEEN VIA TELEMEDICINE AND WHICH CANNOT?

All dermatology patients can potentially be evaluated with telemedicine. For store and forward applications, patients with clinically apparent skin lesions are most appropriate. For interactive video examination (IATV), even those with no clinical lesions but a history to give (e.g., generalized itch) can be effectively evaluated and treated.

It is important to examine the relative advantages and disadvantages of teledermatology for different subsets of patients. Both new and follow-up patients can be effectively treated with telemedicine examination. In a study using IATV, Lowitt and colleagues found no differences in patient satisfaction between these two groups (1). The level of diagnostic agreement between video and in-person physicians was no different for new than for follow-up examinations. Similarly, no differences in satisfaction, physician diagnostic confidence, or diagnostic agreement were detected between patients of different racial groups or gender. Age, however, proved to be an important factor in patient satisfaction with telemedicine examinations. The data suggest that older individuals are less inclined to readily accept the technology than younger patients (1).

Specific diagnoses or diagnostic categories for teledermatology application have been examined. From a practical standpoint, some conditions, such as subcutaneous nodules, lend themselves less well to strict visual inspection with telemedicine. Solutions for how to handle some conditions are evolving, such as training escorts or presenters in lesion palpation and verbal description. More high-tech solutions, such as virtual palpitation, are in development and may eventually help to overcome obstacles to teledermatology. In a study comparing diagnostic agreement between in-person examinations and still images, no disease category stood out as particularly easy or particularly difficult for teledermatologic diagnosis (2).

Other elements of the standard dermatologic interview that may not be optimally provided by telemedicine examination include certain diagnostic tests, such as potassium hydroxide preparation, Tzanck smear, and skin biopsy, all of which require different degrees of procedural skill. With appropriate training, remote presenters may be able to perform some of these services, and a video microscope for viewing of potassium hydroxide smears or skin biopsies can be made available. Certain treatments, such as cryotherapy with liquid nitrogen, traditionally requires the presence of a physician; however, with training and visual supervision, in some cases the remote presenter may be able to serve as the hands of the dermatologist.

HOW DO YOU WANT THE REMOTE PRESENTER TO PRESENT TO YOU?

To answer this question, it must be first determined who the remote presenter is. In telemedicine's early years, the referring physician frequently served as the patient presenter. As programs matured, the primary care physicians (PCPs) realized that after a certain point this time commitment became untenable. Additionally, both PCPs and dermatologists recognized that in traditional in-person medicine, the referring physician does not accompany the patient to the dermatologist's office to be physically present for the dermatology examination.

Physician's assistants, nurses, certified medical assistants, and certified nursing assistants all can be involved as patient presenters. Because the presenter frequently must accompany a disrobed patient, patient-related skills are important. Clerical or administrative personnel may not possess the appropriate training to manage the delicate situations that can arise during cutaneous examination. Although the question has been raised as to whether a presenter need be present at all, experienced telemedicine programs have recognized the critical role the presenter plays in facilitating communication between the patient and the (video) physician.

Before connecting with the physician, the presenter can prepare the patient for the examination, explaining what to expect. Once the examination is in progress, however, it is best if the patient be allowed to talk with the dermatologist directly, as would occur in an in-person office examination. The presenter can help to redirect or identify miscommunications between the physician and patient, position the patient for examination, manipulate any peripheral camera devices (see Chapter 16), and assist in transmission of patient chart information.

WHAT DATA DO YOU WANT AVAILABLE WHEN?

Generally, no information is necessary before the time of the patient's examination. At the time of the actual visit, and when necessary after the visit, the following should be available: (a) the most recent dermatology note (hard copy or computerized); (b) all previous available notes; (c) all current and previous laboratory work; (d) all biopsy reports; (e) patient's demographics; (f) list of current medications; (g) list of drug allergies; (h) any available old photos or images; and (i) the referring provider's phone number, fax number, address, and electronic mail address to facilitate easy and open communication. Having all the information in a single location (either by chart or by computerized medical record) and accessible from the examination room is ideal.

DESCRIBE YOUR CURRENT CLINICAL DOCUMENTATION PROCESS

Dermatology outpatient clinic notes tend to be brief and problem focused. Photographic images (either on 35-mm film or with a still digital camera for computerized archiving) are obtained when appropriate.

HOW WOULD YOU LIKE YOUR TELEMEDICINE ROOM ARRANGED?

Because full cutaneous examination is difficult to achieve with a single mounted camera (in a standard small examination room, the distance between the camera and the patient is too short to allow a full body scan), a peripheral handheld camera is almost always required. If a computerized medical record is used, design of the physician's room should ideally allow access to this record without having to move away from the imaging monitor or the camera.

WHAT EQUIPMENT DO YOU NEED TESTED BEFORE THE CLINIC VISIT?

Everything! Each day, before a patient enters the telemedicine room, full video and audio contact must be assured. The project's credibility will suffer immeasurably if patients regularly witness the inevitable start-up dilemmas.

REFERENCES

1. Lowitt MH, Kessler II, Kauffman CL, Hooper PJ, Siegel E, Burnett JW. Teledermatology and in-person examinations: a comparison of patient and physician perceptions and diagnostic agreement *Arch Dermatol* 1998;134:471–476.
2. Kvedar JC, Edwards RA, Menn ER, et al. The substitution of digital images for dermatologic physical examination. *Arch Dermatol* 1997;133:161–167.

Telemedicine: Practicing in the Information Age,
edited by Steven F. Viegas and Kim Dunn.
Lippincott–Raven Publishers, Philadelphia © 1998.

34

Telemedicine in Correctional Psychiatry

Laura K. Slaughter and Alan R. Felthous

Department of Psychiatry and Behavioral Sciences, University of Texas Medical Branch at Galveston, Galveston, Texas 77555

Virtually any psychiatric patient who is medically stable can be seen via telemedicine. If the patient is unstable (e.g., if he or she is suspected to be postoverdosed or in a state of delirium), he or she should be seen in an emergency room setting. However, psychiatric consultation can occur via telephone or television link once emergency interventions are under way.

A few reviews of telepsychiatry have addressed the issue of psychotic patients being seen in consultation, and the concern has been whether the television format can be incorporated into the psychotic thought processes (1–3). In the available literature, this does not seem to be the case. Even patients who have ideas of reference of receiving messages from their televisions were able to differentiate the reality of the consultation from their delusions (1–3).

A study of group therapy via two-way television by Wittison and colleagues (4) suggested that patients with antisocial traits may not cooperate as well and, in fact, in a group therapy setting, used the equipment to increase resistance (4) and whispered to each other without the therapist being able to hear (4,5). Further studies of appropriate on-site supervision and support can help develop a structure to avoid cooperation difficulties.

REMOTE PRESENTATION

Whenever possible, the consulting healthcare provider should make contact with the psychiatrist by telephone or other medium before the consultation to discuss any special concerns and to arrange any assessment procedures that would be helpful before the consultation. Prior contact permits any special arrangements or procedures to be made in advance, thereby allowing consultation time to be used in an efficient manner. The consultant should receive a formal request with a direct question as well as pertinent medical records before the consultation.

At the time of consultation, all parties present should be introduced and their respective roles in the care of the patient explained. The patient should be informed of the format of the consultation in advance and the limits of confidentiality should be thoroughly explained, with an opportunity for any questions or concerns to be voiced and addressed (3).

DATA ORGANIZATION FOR SEEING THE PATIENT

A request for consultation should provide the basic information necessary to allow the consultant to focus his or her interview and evaluation appropriately (3). This should include, but not be limited to, identifying information (e.g., age, sex), chief complaint, recent history (including current treatment), significant medical history, past psychiatric history, social history (including substance use), educational history, and the current question posed by the provider. A standardized form highlighting each of these areas, possibly available for computer entry, is appropriate and would allow for ease of information retrieval.

A thorough medical assessment is a necessary part of any psychiatric evaluation. It is important that a complete physical and neurologic examination be documented on the medical record within 6 months before the consultation and more recently if complaints of a physical nature are present. Likewise, basic laboratory studies can be indicated to rule out treatable conditions, such as hypothyroidism, that can produce psychiatric symptoms.

Information that may be more specific for the correctional setting would be a description of the patient's current setting, for example a psychiatric unit versus a high-security prison, and a description of services available and medications approved for use in the individual's particular setting. Specific information enables the consultant to formulate a practical treatment plan by using services that are currently available.

When the patient is being seen, it is important to know current medications and other therapy and compliance. If any data is available, such as nursing reports and symptom checklists, these should be reviewed as well. If any psychological testing or other evaluation is available, these should be made available to the consultant.

After seeing the patient, the results of any further procedures, such as laboratory tests, psychological tests, imaging studies, and so on, should be forwarded to the consultant. Periodic feedback on treatment efficacy, side effects, changes in treatment, and compliance issues should also be made available so that appropriate revisions of the treatment plan can be made.

A computerized patient record would be ideal for telemedicine. The complete record would be accessible to each provider without delay. A flexible design model has been described that allows for a variety of presentations of stored data (6). Based on the needs of individual providers, the data can be modified, displayed, and communicated to meet specialized parameters. To take advantage of the convenience of telemedicine, it is important to make the medical record as accessible as possible to the consultant. The use of a computerized medical record would allow off-site consultants to easily view the data in its entirety.

CURRENT CLINICAL DOCUMENTATION PROCESS

Consultants at Skyview Unit, the correctional psychiatric hospital in Rusk, Texas, provide telepsychiatric services to providers at McConnell, a regular unit in the Institutional Division of the Texas Department of Criminal Justice (TDCJ). Providers obtain the patient's written informed consent with a consent form developed specifically for telepsychiatry. The providers complete a telepsychiatric information form, a two-page document containing requisite categories of information for the consultant, and this, together with other documents (including medical record reports), is made available to the consultant in advance of the telepsychiatric session. Finally, following the session, the consultant completes a consultation or progress note on a form designed for this purpose. All of these documents are kept on file at Skyview, the hub facility, for further consultations as needed. The completed progress note is then faxed to the primary providers for placement in the patient's medical record.

TELEMEDICINE ROOM ARRANGEMENT

The telemedicine room should use any safety precautions recommended for a particular patient. Whenever possible, the room should be chosen to minimize any distracting sounds or interruptions during the consultations. The seating should be arranged to permit viewing of the entire body and to allow viewing of the presenter and the patient together for assessment of their interactions. The furnishings should be relatively comfortable, allowing for a relaxed atmosphere during the interview.

The equipment should be positioned to ensure a clear view while not becoming distracting to the patient. Dwyer (2) described a setting in which the camera was located directly below each monitor, creating the appearance of eye contact. This setting helps reduce the variation from face-to-face contact and fosters a more comfortable interaction.

NECESSARY EQUIPMENT

All equipment should be tested before the clinic consultation, including sound and visual transmission. If multiple parties are present at the consultation, arrangement of cameras may be necessary to enable viewing of the entire team. Because a clear view of the patient is often important to allow for assessment of a nonverbal nature, a split screen showing both the patient and the consulting parties is helpful and should be set up in advance to prevent wasted clinical time.

CONSULTATION FEEDBACK

At the end of the consultation, a period should be agreed on in which the recommendations can be implemented and their effectiveness evaluated. The time allowed varies depending on the presenting problem and the complexity of the recommended course. Once the treatment plan is initiated, the consultant should be informed of the patient's status, including response to the current interventions, and a follow-up consultation should be arranged as necessary.

CLINIC CONSULTATION EVALUATED

All parties involved in the consultation should complete an assessment survey to enable effective provision of services. In a study of teleconferencing, brief semistructured interviews were used to determine the expectations and criteria for successful consultations (7). Similar questionnaires were used in another study and covered aspects of comfort with the interview, the relationship established, and the helpfulness of the consultation (1). In addition, studies to determine the financial and time saving benefits of telepsychiatry are desperately needed to design cost-effective services for the correctional setting.

REFERENCES

1. Dongier M, Tempier R, Lalinec-Michaud M, Meunier D. Telepsychiatry: psychiatric consultation through two-way television. A controlled study. *Can J Psychiatry* 1986;31:32–34.
2. Dwyer T. Telepsychiatry: psychiatric consultation by interactive television. *Am J Psychiatry* 1973; 130:865–869.
3. Kavanagh S, Yellowless P. Telemedicine-clinical applications in mental health. *Aust Fam Physician* 1995;24:1242–1245.
4. Wittson CL, Affleck DC, Johnson V. Two-way television in group therapy. *Ment Hosp* 1961;2: 22–23.
5. Baer L, Cukor P, Coyle J. Telepsychiatry: application of telemedicine to psychiatry. In: Bashshur R, Shannon G, eds. *Telemedicine theory and practice*. Springfield, IL: Charles C. Thomas Publishers, 1997:265–288.
6. Adelhard K, Eckel R, Holzel D, Tretter W. Design elements of a telemedical medical record. Proceedings of the AMIA Annual Fall Symposium. 1996:473–477.
7. Harrison R, Clayton W, Wallace P. Can telemedicine be used to improve communication between primary and secondary care? *BMJ* 1996;313:1377–1380.

Telemedicine: Practicing in the Information Age,
edited by Steven F. Viegas and Kim Dunn.
Lippincott–Raven Publishers, Philadelphia © 1998.

35

Gastroenterology

Emil P. Miskovsky, Vonda G. Reeves-Darby, and Karl E. Anderson

Department of Medicine, University of Texas Medical Branch at Galveston, Galveston, Texas 77555; Department of Internal Medicine, University of Texas Medical Branch at Galveston, Galveston, Texas 77555; and Department of Preventive Medicine and Community Health, University of Texas Medical Branch at Galveston, Galveston, Texas 77555

The practice of gastroenterology (GE) depends on highly accurate clinical history information; a directed physical examination; and focused laboratory, radiographic, and endoscopic investigations. As clinical history in GE is paramount, a principle taught for decades by Johns Hopkins University Emeritus Professor Dr. Tom Hendrix and Professor Ted Bayless, telemedicine can serve to augment traditional mechanisms of diagnosis and management. Telemedicine methods can lead to a definitive diagnosis in certain cases (e.g., acute hepatitis B, gastroesophageal reflux) and may suggest required procedures leading to a diagnosis in others (e.g., flexible sigmoidoscopy with biopsy for the diagnosis of ulcerative colitis). The telemedicine technique enables accurate evaluations of medical management (i.e., effectiveness of antireflux or inflammatory bowel disease therapy) and decreases travel and inconvenience for the patient, thereby increasing the accuracy of follow-up. This chapter reviews the role and techniques of telemedicine in the practice of outpatient consultative GE.

IDEAL PRESENTER

The ideal presenter should have the capabilities of taking accurate vital signs (including orthostatic indices), facility with the operations of the video equipment, knowledge of the medical capabilities of the presenter's facility (e.g., laboratories, radiology), and access to emergency care (e.g., intravenous fluids, antibiotics, oral rehydration therapy, other medications). Furthermore, the presenter should speak a common language with the presentee, including medical terminology, and, if the patient speaks a different primary language than either of the professionals, an interpreter should be available. Ideally, the presenter should have clinical care experience (i.e., registered nurse, doctor of medicine, or doctor of osteopathy degrees). The reason for the consultation should be clear to the presenter and the necessary data (i.e., laboratory tests, test results, radiology) should be readily available to the presenter.

PRESENTATIONS IDEAL FOR GASTROENTEROLOGY TELEMEDICINE CONSULTATION

The following is a list of complaints that are well suited for telemedicine GE consults:

- Dysphagia
- Odynophagia
- Atypical chest pain
- Heartburn
- Nausea and vomiting
- Chronic abdominal pain
- Hiccups
- "Gas"
- Food-borne gastroenteritis
- Abnormal liver enzymes
- Elevated amylase, lipase
- Acute diarrhea (with or without human immunodeficiency virus infection)
- Chronic diarrhea
- Fecal incontinence
- Mild to moderate hematochezia
- Ascites
- Jaundice
- Constipation

Pre- and postprocedure evaluations are managed well via telemedicine. In general, once a diagnosis is made and therapy instituted, one can monitor response accurately via telemedicine. This is especially true for chronic disorders, such as ulcerative colitis, chronic hepatitis, or gastroesophageal reflux disease.

The following are presentations that are unsuitable for telemedicine:

- The pregnant patient with abdominal complaints
- Abdominal mass
- Acute pancreatitis
- Acute onset ascites
- Hepatomegaly
- Acute abdominal pain
- Toxic-appearing patient
- Hematemesis, melena, or symptomatic gastrointestinal bleeding
- Acute esophageal obstruction

The presentations in the preceding list are better suited to an immediate referral or emergency room visit. In general, the symptom and its context dictate the applicability for telemedicine referral. Those complaints that are straightforward and not emergent can be handled well by telemedicine. Moderately complex, nonemergent complaints should be evaluated by direct referral. Highly complex and emergent issues should be evaluated immediately and via the route that is in the patient's best interest. In most settings, this would mean emergent evaluation by a physician.

IDEAL CLINIC VISIT

A standardized approach to data acquisition, medical record availability, and information transfer is preferred. The caring professional should provide a concise statement of the referring issue. All patients have routine vital signs performed; a list of present medications, doses, and duration of therapy; a past medical problem list; and a medication allergy history. Results of any laboratory data, radiographic studies, or consultations are shared via fax before the telemedicine patient encounter. It is routine to ask for medical records on-site, just as if we were seeing the patient for an outpatient clinic visit. Access to a computer for unforeseen laboratory results is helpful.

The room should be arranged such that the presenter can focus video equipment on the patient and display x-rays if necessary. A mobile camera functions best, but there are not frequent needs to examine x-rays and so on, and, in many instances, a nonmobile camera functions well. Fax machine capability is important. Initially, the patient should be positioned sitting and facing the camera. He or she may need to lie down for a focused physical examination by the presenter.

The presenter should be capable of rudimentary percussion, auscultation, and palpation of the abdomen. Important information includes the frequency and character of bowel sounds, the presence of abdominal tenderness, and the assessment of hernias.

The University of Texas Medical Branch at Galveston documentation process is via a chart kept at both the presenter's and the consultant's site. In an electronic medical record situation, this information could be kept in a single place and made available to all caring professionals via computer. Additionally, it is useful to maintain an on-site telemedicine practice log identifying the date, name of the patient and history number, consulting issues, and a brief description of the plans for the patient.

THE FUTURE

The future of GE telemedicine technology includes the opportunity for interface with radiology in terms of teleradiology-teleendoscopy analysis of complex problems. Virtual endoscopy is possible through telemedicine and may offer an effective means to evaluate patients located in desolate areas. In general, more experience with telemedicine and data outlining its efficacy and ability to deliver quality healthcare are needed before these programs can proceed. There is great potential for telemedicine development in the area of GE consultation.

Telemedicine: Practicing in the Information Age,
edited by Steven F. Viegas and Kim Dunn.
Lippincott–Raven Publishers, Philadelphia © 1998.

36

Hypertension

Fernando Elijovich and Cheryl L. Laffer

Department of Internal Medicine, University of Texas Medical Branch at Galveston, Galveston, Texas 77555

BACKGROUND

Hypertension is a major public health problem in the United States, affecting 50 million people and contributing to cardiovascular morbidity and mortality via its major complications, stroke and heart attack (1,2). The number of individuals labeled as having the disease has increased concomitantly with the progressive reduction in the arbitrary blood pressure cutoffs used to define normal versus abnormal blood pressure. This reduction is the byproduct of the demonstration of therapeutic benefit in milder and milder forms of hypertension from large trials conducted since the 1980s (3–5).

The need to include individuals with the mildest elevations of blood pressure in the population to be treated makes it imperative that blood pressure recordings be obtained in baseline conditions with all the methodologic precautions described in the *Fifth Report of the Joint National Committee on Detection, Evaluation, and Treatment of High Blood Pressure* (2). Otherwise, the natural variability of blood pressure and its response to stressors could lead to misdiagnosis and overtreatment of millions of individuals. Furthermore, accuracy of blood pressure recordings is important for management of established hypertensive patients. In these patients, improper techniques of blood pressure recording can lead to unnecessary adjustments in pharmacologic therapy, with consequent untoward impacts on cost, side effects, and patient compliance.

It is now unequivocal that reduction of high blood pressure leads to reduction of cardiovascular morbidity and mortality (2). Although major progress has been enacted in diagnosis and detection of hypertension since the 1970s, results of therapeutic efforts are still dismal even in the United States, one of the most developed countries in the Western world. Hence, the most recent data indicate that only half of the hypertensive patients who are aware of their disease are under treatment, and, of those, only half achieve normal blood pressure despite receiving treatment (1).

The explanation for these results is probably multipronged. Some factors relate predominantly to the patients (e.g., understanding of disease process, behavioral problems, issues of compliance with management of chronic illness, social and employment effects of diagnostic labeling). Others have to do with the healthcare delivery system (e.g., lack of universal health insurance, other issues of access, technologically oriented care with few resources allocated to patient education). Finally, socioeconomic factors (e.g., affordability of medical visits and medications, cost of time taken from work to take care of medical problems) affect both the patients and the providers of care.

ROLES FOR TELEMEDICINE

The preceding review of the background makes it immediately apparent that telemedicine can accomplish several goals in the management of essential hypertension.

Education of Providers

Physicians, physician assistants, nurse practitioners, nurses, and nurse-assistant personnel (i.e., those who will probably become the most common remote providers for a teleconsultation in hypertension) can undergo initial training and periodic recertification in the correct techniques of blood pressure recording via remote communication. This is particularly important for geographic settings removed from major medical centers, where healthcare providers seldom have an opportunity to update their skills. Helping a massive number of remote providers achieve and maintain the skills for recording unstressed blood pressures has the utmost importance and can only lead to a decrease in unnecessary use of medications or excessive dosages. It can also diminish the number of referrals to major medical centers for treatment of apparently uncontrolled hypertension. The process of provider education via telemedicine can be enacted with mock patients for initial formal training, but the nature of the interaction itself (with telewitnessing by the consultant of the activities of the remote provider) allows for continuous monitoring and reinforcement of appropriate techniques during the course of actual ongoing medical care.

Patient Education

In the current climate of healthcare in the United States, patient education is detrimentally affected by the pressures on provider productivity. Patients per unit time has become a major indicator of performance for health maintenance organizations, managed care organizations, and so on. The physician, in his or her office or in the clinic at the medical center, begins his or her activity by carrying out the scout work (i.e., the gathering of the information acquired during a previous workup, the taking of a history, and the performance of a physical examination). Later, he or she spends a significant portion of the visit documenting all activities with proper record keeping, the importance of which has increased due to liability and financial issues. Finally, the physician plans further workup (which implies paperwork) or recommends pharmacologic therapy (which implies prescription writing). More often than not, these activities preclude a final, extensive, patient-physician interaction devoted to education on the multiple nonpharmacologic aspects of management of chronic illness. In the case of essential hypertension, this is particularly relevant, since several lifestyle modification maneuvers (e.g., weight loss and reduction of salt intake) are known to be powerful antihypertensive agents (6). Teleconsultation offers a unique opportunity for improvement in patient education. The remote provider, by prepreparing the information required for the visit (using predesigned protocols and instruments), allows the consultant to make decisions regarding workup and pharmacologic therapy in a fraction of the time required in a traditional office consultation. Therefore, the consultant has the opportunity and the time necessary to devote to the crucial issues of patient education. In addition to the direct impact on the patient, this activity has a multiplier effect via additional education of the remote providers, as the ability of the senior specialist to counsel on the management of chronic illnesses is passed on during the actual delivery of care to the patient.

Improved Affordability for Recipients and Givers of Care

The time savings are obtained by delegating a series of activities usually carried out by the physician to a provider with less training and years of schooling but equally capable of performing the tasks. In financial terms, time savings translates into a decrease in the cost of the teleconsultation when compared with routine office care. This should be reflected in third-party reimbursement patterns. Although compensation per unit time for the consultant must be preserved, there is a decreased gross payment per patient encounter. This makes the intervention more affordable to patients and to insurance carriers. The latter should pass on this benefit in the form of improved fee-for-service reimbursement rates. In the case of capitated care, a more efficient use of the time confers an obvious financial advantage to consultants.

Optimal Frequency of Interactions

A decrease in the cost of medical care to all participants results in increased flexibility for scheduling of televisits at optimal intervals. It is common in the management of chronic illnesses to resort to less than optimal interactions (e.g., phone contact for follow-up, discussion of workup, or modification of therapy) to minimize the financial burden on the patient. It follows that less expensive care permits more frequent care. In the field of hypertension, this is particularly important because it has been shown that infrequent visits are a deterrent to patient compliance and are associated with higher recurrence of previously corrected unhealthy behavior (7). A classic example of the beneficial effect of frequent follow-up visits is the spontaneous improvement of hypertension observed in volunteers participating in drug efficacy trials (8).

Decreased Time Taken from Work

Chronic illnesses have a major societal impact via lost productivity due to both days of actual disability and days devoted to medical care (9). In nonurban areas, this is compounded by the additional time required for travel to and from the medical office or center, usually with loss of an entire day of work. Teleconsultation for follow-up of hypertension offers the possibility of actually conducting medical care at the worksite, allowing for minimal disruption of worker productivity. Furthermore, there is previous experience from worksite programs conducted in situ (i.e., with medical providers visiting the business or factory) that demonstrates a favorable impact on patient adherence to therapy and on treatment outcomes (10).

Decreased Effect of Labeling

Diagnosis of hypertension is associated with the phenomenon of labeling (i.e., a distorted perception of "stigmata" with untoward psychological effects, diminished self-esteem, and increased absenteeism) (11). Worksite teleconsultation, which can be scheduled "in mass" (i.e., delivery of care to the entire affected population of a business or factory), offers the additional advantage of "destigmatizing" hypertension in patients' minds, placing this health problem in the proper perspective of a prevalent problem that is shared by many, that can be controlled, and that permits a normal life with controlled risk.

TELECONSULTATION PROTOCOLS

Patient Population

Because the protocols described here are for teleinteraction from office to office (between consultant and remote primary provider), they are meant for the population of hypertensives that would normally be followed in a physician's office. Hypertensive emergencies and acute complications that require admission are beyond the scope of this discussion, although this does not preclude the devising of future protocols for teleconsultation from office to remote emergency rooms or intensive care units.

How Does the Interaction Take Place?

Teleconsultation in hypertension requires four discrete steps. First, the remote provider conveys the information gathered on the patient by means of previously agreed-on instruments. The patient is not yet present, to prevent exposing him or her to the medical lingo and speculation about his or her problems that are a necessary part of provider-provider interaction but are not useful and can be anxiety-generating for the patient. The patient participates in the second step, for direct interaction with the consultant (i.e., further gathering of information, witnessing of elements of physical examination) and, most important, for engagement in the process. The third step occurs again in the absence of the patient and is for the consultant and remote provider to discuss issues of diagnosis, workup, and therapeutic plan. The fourth step is with participation of the patient again for discussion of all elements of the plan. The educational efforts on lifestyle modification also take place during this final step.

What Should the Organization, Availability, and Storage of the Data Be?

There are three major situations that a teleconsultation in hypertension can address: a first visit, a follow-up on an established patient, and review of workup without formal patient interaction. For a first visit, the remote provider gathers information using a protocol that does not follow the format of the usual medical history. A problem-oriented approach, tailored to the major aspects of hypertension, addresses the following issues:

1. Should secondary forms of hypertension be investigated? This requires gathering the historical data (e.g., age at onset, presence or absence of family history, episodes of accelerated hypertension, refractoriness of blood pressure, presence of atherosclerotic vascular disease, episodic hypertensive crisis with tachycardia, headaches, sweating, and piloerection), physical examination data (vascular bruits), and previous workup data (e.g., serum potassium off diuretics, imaging of kidneys, proteinuria), which usually lead to the suspicion of concealed secondary forms of hypertension, such as renovascular disease, pheochromocytoma, or hyperaldosteronism.
2. What is the established target organ damage? This requires evaluation of elements of the history (e.g., angina, history of myocardial infarction or stroke, intermittent claudication), past available workup about renal function (e.g., serum creatinine or clearance, random or 24-hour proteinuria), left ventricular size and function (e.g., electrocardiogram, echocardiogram), and established vascular disease (e.g., noninvasive cardiologic workup for ischemia, cardiac catheterization, Doppler assessment of disease in femoral or carotid vessels, abdominal sonograms for evaluation of the aorta).
3. What are the concomitant risk factors for cardiovascular disease? Data on obesity (e.g., body weight and body mass index, history of weight gain), diabetes, lipids, smoking habits (including quitting attempts), and calorie expenditure (i.e., sedentary versus active lifestyle) are gathered for the planning of educational and therapeutic maneuvers.

For a follow-up visit, the remote provider gathers information following a subjective (data), objective (data), assessment, and plan format, with special consideration given to all interim blood pressure recordings (home or otherwise) by the patient, the success or failure at modifying dietary or lifestyle patterns (for further educational intervention), and the tolerance to pharmacologic agents (for adjustment of therapy). Finally, review of workup without formal patient interaction can take place in specially scheduled sessions or before or after teleconsultation sessions. These are intended to expedite adjustments to previous decision making, which may be needed after results of major medical testing become available.

The data gathering instruments for all the type of interactions are predesigned as either forms or computer files (using database software). The forms are to facilitate the tasks of the remote provider, serving as guidelines for systematic, thorough, and complete obtaining of the information. The computer files are to be used for electronic transfer of the information via telephone lines, when the data is to be stored and eventually pooled for statistical analysis (for monitoring of the results of the teleconsultation program, other healthcare delivery research project, or similar endeavors).

Paper-based record-keeping instruments, as well as printed test results, electrocardiogram tracings, and so on, can be made available to the consultant in advance of the actual teleconsultation, if prereview of data is deemed to allow for diminished time allocation to the actual interaction, to shift its focus toward the tasks of patient engagement and education, or to enhance provider-provider joint decision making.

Telemedicine Examination Room and Equipment

As opposed to the needs of other specialties, the hypertension teleconsultation takes place in a traditional office setting. The consultant space and equipment requirements are limited to a desk and the necessary equipment for electronic transmission of information via video, telephone lines, or fax technology. The remote provider requires the usual equipment of an examining room with the caveat that the examining table must allow for the recording of blood pressures in unstressed conditions, including posture devices (arm and back supports) and sound (quiet room). Calibrated or mercury sphygmomanometers, stethoscope, ophthalmoscope, an electrocardiogram machine, and an x-ray viewbox are the required pieces of equipment to conduct a full examination and review the baseline, bedside workup.

Feedback

The best objective assessment of the efficacy of telemedicine intervention for the management of hypertension is the blood pressure curve over time in individual patients. A large-scale, comparative analysis of the results of treatment of essential hypertension via telemedicine versus the clinic must be carried out to validate this intervention. Such a study, conducted in essential hypertensive patients matched for demographic characteristics and disease severity, may prove that telemedicine is as efficacious as (if not more than) the traditional clinic intervention.

Subjective feedback is also important to be able to tailor the intervention to the needs (e.g., educational, emotional) of the remote providers and patients. Particularly important is the devising of instruments that rate the degree of satisfaction of all participants with the interaction. Issues to be addressed include but are not limited to (a) remote providers' perception regarding the benefits of continued education, (b) patients' satisfaction with the remote interaction with a consultant, and (c) perceived barriers to communication (by all providers and patients) due to the impersonal aspects of the intervening technology.

CONCLUSION

The use of telemedicine for the management of hypertension is not only the use of a new tool (derived from technological advances in electronic communications) to accomplish the same ends as usual care in a physician's office or clinic. Use of videocommunications changes radically the allocation of tasks, the time distribution, the geography, and the finances of the interaction. All these changes have potential, positive spin-offs from unresolved issues in the management of hypertension. Improved patient and provider education, diminished cost and impact on societal productivity, closer follow-up, improved compliance, and reduced misuse of resources should result in improved outcome. Thus, telemedicine has a definite role in the management of hypertension and will hopefully improve this prevalent health problem's treatment results, which are still suboptimal in the United States.

REFERENCES

1. Burt VL, Whelton P, Roccella EJ, et al. Prevalence of hypertension in the US adult population: results from the Third National Health and Nutrition Examination Survey, 1988–1991. *Hypertension* 1995;25:305–313.
2. Joint National Committee on Detection, Evaluation, and Treatment of High Blood Pressure. The Fifth Report of the Joint National Committee on Detection, Evaluation, and Treatment of High Blood Pressure (JNC V). *Arch Intern Med* 1993;153:154–183.
3. Hypertension Detection and Follow-up Program Cooperative Group. The effect of treatment on mortality in mild hypertension: results of the Hypertension Detection and Follow-up Program. *N Engl J Med* 1982;307:976–980.
4. SHEP Cooperative Research Group. Prevention of stroke by antihypertensive drug treatment in older persons with isolated systolic hypertension: final results of the systolic hypertension in the elderly program (SHEP). *JAMA* 1991;265:3255–3264.
5. Neaton JD, Grimm RH, Prineas RJ, et al. Treatment of mild hypertension study: final results. *JAMA* 1993;270:713–724.
6. Wassertheil-Smoller S, Oberman A, Blaufox MD, Davis B, Langford H. The trial of antihypertensive interventions and management (TAIM) study: final results with regard to blood pressure, cardiovascular risks, and quality of life. *Am J Hypertens* 1992;5:37–44.
7. Working Group on Health Education and High Blood Pressure Control, National High Blood Pressure Education Program. *The physician's guide: improving adherence among hypertensive patients.* Bethesda, MD: U.S. Department of Health and Human Services, National Heart, Lung and Blood Institute, 1987.
8. Carney SL, Gillies AH, Smith AJ, Floate LF. Effect of trial therapy on subsequent therapy. A review of patients with hypertension who have completed a pharmacological intervention study. *Med J Aust* 1986;144:315–316.
9. Harris L and Associates, Inc. The public and high blood pressure: a survey. Washington, DC: Government Printing Office, 1973 [DHEW Publication no. (NIH) 74-536].
10. Baer L, Parchment Y, Kneeshaw M. Hypertension in health care providers: effectiveness of worksite treatment programs in a state mental health agency. *Am J Public Health* 1981;71:1261–1263.
11. Haynes RB, Sackett DL, Taylor DW, Gibson ES, Johnson AL. Increased absenteeism from work after detection and labeling of hypertensive patients. *N Engl J Med* 1978;299:741–744.

Telemedicine: Practicing in the Information Age,
edited by Steven F. Viegas and Kim Dunn.
Lippincott–Raven Publishers, Philadelphia © 1998.

37

Rheumatology

Bruce A. Baethge and Jeffrey R. Lisse

Department of Internal Medicine, University of Texas Medical Branch at Galveston, Galveston, Texas 77555

Telemedicine is an interactive medium that allows a physician or his or her designee to interview and visually examine patients at great distances from the medical center (1,2). There are limitations to the telemedicine encounter that become apparent as one participates in patient interviews. These limitations can be minimized by prior experience and a working relationship between the healthcare provider accompanying the patient (advocate) and his or her counterpart on the other end of the electronic screen (receiver). It is our goal to optimize the rheumatologic telemedicine experience by training skilled advocates and by developing protocols that best serve this advance in technology. This chapter discusses our recommendations for training advocates to assist in the management of rheumatologic patients, reports our experience with a small successful pilot study (3), and outlines our plans for further implementation of telemedicine in rheumatologic care.

THE RHEUMATOLOGY TELEMEDICINE ENCOUNTER

The rheumatologic patient can be a particular challenge in any clinical setting. As most of rheumatologic problem solving is based on the recognition of clinical syndromes, some prior training of the advocate is appropriate. The advocate assisting in the evaluation of rheumatology patients must be comfortable with the methods used by rheumatologists for diagnosis and treatment. Only by becoming acquainted with the syndromes likely to be encountered is the advocate going to be able to know what to look for to identify these diseases. An example to illustrate the need for prior advocate training is psoriatic arthritis, the inflammatory joint disease associated with the common skin disorder. Most clinicians recognize psoriasis and also notice when a patient has a hot inflamed joint. The relationship between these two clinical findings is often unappreciated and the diagnosis of psoriatic arthritis is therefore missed—something easily avoided by prior training. It is prudent to hold frequent training sessions with the advocate and receiver to discuss potential cases and pitfalls in diagnosis and treatment of systemic rheumatic disorders. A preceptorship may be necessary until the advocate becomes acquainted with the intricacies of rheumatologic syndromes.

The receiver needs, clearly, to be someone schooled in rheumatology. This most likely is a rheumatologist or a rheumatology fellow in training. Other candidates may include a nurse practitioner or physician assistant trained in rheumatologic diagnosis and treatments.

Unless the advocate and receiver are particularly adept at the art of maintaining and operating electronic equipment, the current state-of-the-art telemedicine equipment is best operated with the aid of a technical engineer. His or her task is to make certain that the flow of information between the two sites is smooth and complete, including that transmitted by fax, video, special equipment, and sound. The need for special devices is relatively low in rheumatology, making this task easier than one would anticipate in other specialties such as cardiology or otolaryngology (4).

The patient population in rheumatology is most easily divided into two simple groups, new and follow-up or "old" patients. The two groups have different challenges and therefore should be dealt with separately. All of our experience has been with Texas Department of Criminal Justice (TDCJ) patients, but this information can be readily generalized to other patients interviewed with telemedicine (5,6).

NEW PATIENT VISIT

New rheumatology patients are particularly challenging in any setting. A detailed clinical history, review of systems, and family history all can aid in diagnosis. Obtaining these can be done by the receiver, but eventually it is more cost-effective and appropriate for this information to be gathered beforehand by the advocate, along with other pertinent history, such as medications and allergies. This shortens the interview and increases efficiency of the telemedicine encounter. Information can be sent by fax, presented live, or mailed beforehand in anticipation of the encounter.

There is a great deal of historical information that can be directly asked by the specialist or receiver. The history can be elicited directly from the patient, including the nature of the pain, history and duration of morning stiffness, prior episodes of joint swelling, and a rheumatologic review of symptoms. This includes questions about skin rashes and photosensitivity; eye, oral, or genital ulcerations; bloody diarrhea; and other organ systems that may be affected. Duration and progression of joint symptoms is another important feature. Did the symptoms begin in all of the joints at the same time? Was it migratory? Was the onset insidious or acute? Were there any precipitating factors? All of these can be important questions. Advocates improve their diagnostic skills by listening to the questions of the specialist. It is highly advisable that the same advocate work with the same rheumatologist or specialist to develop the communication skills and trust necessary for optimal care of the patient. Once the advocate is knowledgeable in rheumatologic history taking, this information can be obtained before the telemedicine encounter. The receiver or specialist may need to ask only directed questions to further clarify the history.

The physical examination offers the next challenge to a successful telemedicine encounter. The single sense that is most lacking in telemedicine is touch during the joint examination. Touch is an integral part of the rheumatologic physical examination and must be done by proxy, through the fingers of the advocate to the receiver. This action is performed by sound and sight. The advocate palpates or manipulates the joints in question and relays what he or she feels to the receiver by describing these findings, and the receiver simultaneously observes the maneuver on his or her video screen. This allows the receiver to verify that the advocate is indeed palpating or manipulating the correct joint in the correct manner. He or she must rely on the experience of the advocate to describe correctly what he or she is feeling during the examination. This information can be critical. For example, soft tissue swelling denotes synovitis or fluid, which in turn suggests inflammation, while bony enlargement is more indicative of degenerative changes, or "wear and tear." Many patients have arthralgias, detected by complaints of joint aches with a completely normal articular physical examination.

Advocates for rheumatology telemedicine encounters must be trained in proper joint examination technique. Once the advocate has been trained to perform joint examinations, he or she can be relied on to convey the physical findings detected by palpating the joints. The advocate must be able to identify the number and pattern of abnormal joints involved. This skill differentiates arthritis from soft tissue rheumatism. The advocate should be able to identify the degree of tenderness and swelling, as well as the nature of that swelling in all abnormal joints. Bony or hard swelling can denote degenerative joint disease or osteoarthritis, as well as crystal deposition disease such as gout. Soft tissue swelling is more indicative of inflammatory disorders, such as rheumatoid arthritis. The presence of fluid in the joint may also be detected. The major limitation of telemedicine in rheumatology is the skill of the advocate in performing the joint examination. Only a well-trained observer can fully evaluate the subtleties of the joint examination, so that all the necessary information can be conveyed to the receiver to assure correct diagnosis. This acquired skill can be taught and reinforced by direct televised observation of the physical examination by the specialist.

A preliminary diagnosis can be made through the telemedicine encounter, and further testing to verify the diagnosis can be initiated. It is tempting for the advocate and referring physician to order multiple tests when a patient presents with joint complaints. Advocates should avoid the temptation to overuse the laboratory by ordering unnecessary tests. Laboratory data should be gathered on rheumatology patients for three basic reasons. The first is to support the diagnostic suppositions formed during the history and physical examination. This includes tests, such as antinuclear antibodies, rheumatoid factors, and more specific serologies such as anti–double stranded DNA antibodies. These tests can often be falsely positive. It is important to order tests only when indicated by the history and physical examination. The second is to ascertain end organ involvement in rheumatic diseases, such as renal damage in patients with systemic lupus erythematosus or scleroderma. The third reason is to monitor drug therapy and guard against potential toxicity. This is especially important in follow-up patients. The interactions of the specialist or receiver and advocates ensure the appropriate laboratory testing of rheumatologic patients. This can lead to cost reduction and reduction of unnecessary services.

Once a presumptive diagnosis is made, therapy can be initiated. The exchange of information can form a vital link in the therapeutic chain between consultant, patient, and primary caregiver. Telemedicine is a unique situation in which all three participants in care are face to face. The usual sources of communication, including verbal, written, and second-hand information conveyed through the patient, are unnecessary in the telemedicine environment. Face-to-face interaction can serve to increase patient compliance and correct therapeutics in the hands of the advocate or primary care provider. There is also the opportunity to have questions answered immediately and have the patient question both practitioners concerning his or her care. Such an interchange is not possible in the traditional patient care setting.

FOLLOW-UP VISIT

Most patients with chronic rheumatic diseases require frequent follow-up to monitor medical therapy and toxicity. Patients with rheumatoid arthritis are a common example of this. Current care of the severe rheumatoid patient necessitates using immunosuppressive and other dangerous drugs. Telemedicine offers an effective way to follow patients who are at a great distance from the rheumatologist directing care. An experienced advocate can perform an appropriate examination and evaluate remission or progression of disease. Not having to travel great distances increases patient comfort and assures that appropriate laboratory monitoring is done for safety. Contact with the specialist and the patient can reinforce therapy. There may also be therapeutic benefit to the telemedicine encounter, which should at least equal the benefits of telephone follow up that has been shown to be effective in rheumatologic care (7).

RHEUMATOLOGY TELEMEDICINE PILOT STUDY

In 1996, a 60-day study of rheumatology telemedicine consultations was performed at the University of Texas Medical Branch (UTMB)/TDCJ hospital (3). Ten patients were randomly selected from the Rheumatology Consultation Clinic to participate in the study. The purpose of the study was to test the satisfaction of the physicians and patients with the telemedicine encounter.

The system used for the study was Compression Labs Incorporated's (CLI, San Jose, CA) Radiance System. The patient and consultation stations consisted of a single-monitor workstation. Each patient station had four cameras: a single-chip room camera and a three-chip patient camera with a 16:1 zoom lens, a document stand, and a scope camera that interfaced with the medical peripherals operated by the on-site member. Medical peripherals permitted the use and transmission of findings by a digital stethoscope, otoscope, and ophthalmoscope for physical examination.

The resulting images and annotation were stored as part of the individual patient's encounter within the AccessMed database.

Each visit lasted 15 to 30 minutes with a rheumatologist in the studio and with a referring physician and patient on-site at one of the prison patient consultation stations. After each session, treatment plans were faxed and carried out by the local medical staff.

The patients were later seen in the rheumatology clinic, and the telemedicine diagnosis was confirmed by direct examination. The patients, participating physicians, and consulting rheumatologists were surveyed regarding the encounter. All reported satisfaction with the telemedicine experience and provision of services. The telemedicine consultations were considered equal to the on-site diagnosis and treatment plans. No formal cost analysis was performed on this small pilot study, but it was estimated that telemedicine consultation resulted in a 30% increase in the number of patients that were seen when compared to the same in-house clinic time period. The pilot was considered a success and resulted in formation of further studies that are now in progress at UTMB.

UTMB has a regular program of telemedicine follow-up for patients with rheumatoid arthritis and a program for consultations on patients with other connective tissue diseases. Several questions must be answered before widespread use of telemedicine in rheumatology can be advocated.

- Is it possible to provide the same quality of care relying on physical examinations performed by advocates?
- Is the patient-physician relationship that is so important to successful rheumatologic care harmed by use of the electronic medium?
- Can the same level of care be provided at a reduction in cost?

UTMB hopes to be able to answer some of these concerns in the near future.

CONCLUSION

Telemedicine offers the potential to revolutionize the care of patients with chronic diseases such as rheumatoid arthritis (5). Underserved populations for whom the distance to medical care or security barriers make face-to-face contact with medical practitioners difficult or impossible are especially likely to benefit from this new technology (2,8). Barriers to this new technology include patient and physician satisfaction, legal issues, and reimbursement issues (9,10) that are not within the scope of this chapter. The rapid advances in technology will continue, and one can expect that the ability to perform remote-site examinations will be further enhanced. The rapidly aging population and the way healthcare delivery is changing in a managed-care environment will be other factors that will have profound implications on the use of telemedicine in the future (11,12). We in the UTMB/TDCJ system believe that telemedicine will be a potentially useful tool in the care of the chronically ill patient with systemic rheumatic disease.

REFERENCES

1. Crump WJ, Pfeil T. A telemedicine primer. An introduction to the technology and an overview of the literature. *Arch Fam Med* 1995;4:796–803.
2. Norton SA, Burdick AE, Phillips CM, Berman B. Teledermatology and underserved populations. *Arch Dermatol* 1997;133:197–200.
3. Chase JL, Lisse JR, Brecht RM. Rheumatology in the twenty-first century: telemedicine leading the way. *Arthritis Rheum* 1995;38:R39.
4. Crump WJ, Driscoll B. An application of telemedicine technology for otorhinolaryngology diagnosis. *Laryngoscope* 1996;106:595–598.
5. London JW, Morton DE, Marinucci D, Catalano R, Comis RL. The implementation of telemedicine within a community cancer network. *J Am Med Inform Assoc* 1997;4:18–24.
6. Zelickson BD, Homan L. Teledermatology in the nursing home. *Arch Dermatol* 1997;133:171–174.
7. Pal B. Telemedicine. Pilot study of telephone follow up in rheumatology has just been completed. *BMJ* 1997;314:520–521.
8. Zarate CA Jr, Weinstock L, Cukor P, et al. Applicability of telemedicine for assessing patients with schizophrenia: acceptance and reliability. *J Clin Psychiatry* 1997;58:22–25.
9. LaMay CL. Telemedicine and competitive change in health care. *Spine* 1997;22:88–97.
10. William ME, Remmes WD, Thompson BG. Nine reasons why healthcare delivery using advanced communications technology should be reimbursed [See comments]. *J Am Geriatr Soc* 1996;44:1472–1475.
11. William ME. Geriatric medicine on the information superhighway: opportunity or road kill? *J Am Geriatr Soc* 1995;43:184–186.
12. Wynn-Jones J, Lews L, Groves-Phillips S. Telemedicine: if it is the answer, then what are the questions? [Editorial: See comments] *Br J Hosp Med* 1996;55:45.

Telemedicine: Practicing in the Information Age,
edited by Steven F. Viegas and Kim Dunn.
Lippincott–Raven Publishers, Philadelphia © 1998.

38

Geriatrics

David A. Chiriboga, *Kenneth J. Ottenbacher,
and *Richard Roland Rahr

*Department of Health Promotion and Gerontology, School of Allied Health Sciences, University of Texas Medical Branch at Galveston, Galveston, Texas 77555; and *School of Allied Health Sciences, University of Texas Medical Branch at Galveston, Galveston, Texas 77555*

There is little information available concerning how a clinical protocol for geriatric telemedicine may differ from those developed for specific specialties and other age groups. The reason is that the application of telemedicine to care of the older patient is still in its early stages. This chapter briefly discusses the implications of current clinical knowledge for the development of geriatric protocols and considers several issues in geriatric telemedicine, using its possible application to long-term care as a case in point.

PROTOCOLS AND GERIATRIC TELEMEDICINE

There is an ever-growing number of geriatric demonstration projects dealing with telemedicine. For example, several pilot studies are considering how telemedicine may be incorporated into home health services, and how in-home telemedicine units may benefit older patients during the period immediately following discharge from an acute care facility. In all cases, the underlying premise is that the use of nursing homes and hospitals or medical visits can be reduced.

The University of Texas Medical Branch (UTMB) at Galveston, although it has not focused specifically on geriatrics in its prison-based telemedicine health maintenance organization (HMO), provides care to the older inmate population. At the regional medical facility located at Huntsville, Texas, for example, older inmates are housed not only within the main units but also in units designed for the frail elderly and in extended-care and skilled-care units. All of these inmates are seen on a consultative basis via telemedicine.

Although the telemedicine protocols for older patients, as used in the UTMB correctional HMO, are generally the same as protocols for younger inmates, there are guidelines, gleaned from the literature on geriatrics (e.g., Kane and colleagues

[1]), that help to inform. In general, the older patient, especially if age 75 years and older,

- is more likely to be frail, dependent in one or more activities of daily life, and not easily transferred or moved; hence a reduction in medically related visits to emergency rooms or hospitals is highly desirable.
- is more likely to be taking multiple medications (polypharmacy). Medical necessity of prescribed and over-the-counter medications should be reviewed periodically, as well as side effects, synergistic effects, and dosages.
- presents with a greater likelihood of comorbidities.
- is more likely to have chronic health problems.
- is more likely to present with undifferentiated or atypical symptoms.
- is more likely to have experienced declines in perceptual and sensory abilities (e.g., hearing, vision, sense of smell) that make communication and comprehension more difficult. Glare is of particular concern.
- may have unexpected sociocultural characteristics that can affect comprehension or compliance (e.g., minimal education; different views on health, compliance, and propriety).

The preceding guidelines help illuminate some of the differences the health professional should consider when caring for an older patient. At the same time, it should be noted that the provision of care in any defined specialty area is likely to be similar to the care requirements of younger patients. Thus, the clinical protocols developed in the other subspecialty chapters of this book would generally pertain to this chapter as well.

TELEMEDICINE IN LONG-TERM CARE

To illustrate the potential for telemedicine and facilitate protocol development, long-term care is used as a case example. Sixty percent of the almost 13 million individuals requiring long-term services are 65 years of age and older (2). Although the trend is to provide these people with home health services rather than institutional care, in 1995 approximately 1.5 million Americans age 65 years and older were living in nursing homes (3). This figure translates to 41.3 residents per 1,000 older Americans.

Perhaps of greater social and economic significance is that a disproportionate share of public and private funds allocated for long-term care services are expended for nursing-home care. For example, 24.8% of the Health Care Financing Administration's Medicaid expenditures for fiscal year 1994 were for nursing-home vendors, as compared to 26.1% for inpatient hospitals and 6.7% for physicians.

Because expenditures for nursing-home care not only are substantial but growing, the delivery and management of long-term care has gained national attention. A number of specific concerns have been identified. To highlight just one example, a relatively new focus of attention is on the costs and crises surrounding hospitalization of these residents, as well as a general lack of knowledge about the problem (e.g., see

Creditor [4] and Barker and colleagues [5]). Estimated hospital admission rates per 1,000 nursing home residents range from 265 to 471 (5,6). Many of these admissions could potentially be prevented with minimal additional attention to patient needs (5,7), an outcome that would be facilitated through judicious use of telemedicine.

HEALTHCARE IN THE LONG-TERM CARE SETTING

Although the nursing home industry is subject to heavy regulations, the care actually provided to residents is often minimal. As Kane (2) noted, doctors generally play only a minor and transient role, with most of the formal burden of care falling on nurses and nurse's aides. The context of caring is evolving, however, due in part to changes arising from managed care and from new state and federal regulations. In part, this evolution also reflects a better understanding of patient needs. Technological innovations, such as the use of electronic medical records and care plans, are also beginning to have an effect (e.g., see Weiler and colleagues [8]).

A particular role of telemedicine may be in facilitating how long-term care facilities deal with unusual or unexpected health events. It is generally recognized that the elderly may present with atypical symptomatology, leading to delayed detection and misdiagnosis (e.g., see Kane and colleagues [1]). Fevers and infections, for example, often prompt hospitalization, especially during poorly staffed shifts (9). Hospitalization, in turn, can have its own untoward effects (1,4). In general, reduction of hospitalization and emergency room visits could be expected to result in both reduced costs and improved patient well-being.

COST BENEFITS OF TELEMEDICINE IN NURSING HOMES

Telemedicine and related technology have been proposed as one method to both improve the quality of nursing-home care and reduce costs. In discussing long-term healthcare in general, Willams (10, p. 184) suggested that "what is really needed is a broader approach that maximizes the interactive nature of communication to provide coordinated interdisciplinary care, expanded access to expertise, enhanced person-to-person communication, decreased cost, broadened education opportunities, and improved data integration." These objectives can be facilitated by telemedicine.

With regard to the use and development of telemedicine in geriatrics, a central barrier may be the lack of organizational structures compatible with its use (11). Other potential barriers to full use within nursing homes include the following: (a) the current lack of a systematic protocol for applying telemedicine technology and training in long-term care facilities; (b) cost factors, although these are rapidly decreasing; (c) reimbursement factors, although legislation in California, Texas, and other states is laying the groundwork for payment of healthcare delivery via telemedicine; (d) lack of adequate outcome data, a problem common to all telemedicine applications; and (e) the rapidity of technological change, which can deter or delay planners hesitant about committing their organization to a telemedicine effort.

The idea of integrating telemedicine into the nursing-home care delivery system thus raises a number of concerns. Based on our pilot work at UTMB, it would seem that in implementing a telemedicine unit into long-term care, the planner should consider

- involving nursing home administration and staff at all stages of planning and implementation. Unless telemedicine is viewed as helpful not only to the patient but to the care provider, the effort may fail to obtain full cooperation.
- the portability of the telemedicine unit. To maximally accommodate to the mobility restrictions of patients, units should be portable.
- that training must be oriented to the least trained user and must be repeatable, because nursing homes typically experience a high staff turnaround.
- that training should also include off-site health professional staff.
- that development of protocols for specific presenting conditions, as well as the general case, is important.
- that staff should be encouraged to use the telemedicine equipment as part of their everyday work effort. Otherwise, it is likely to be neglected during unexpected points of uncertainty or crisis.

Although protocols for geriatric telemedicine are minimally developed, most existing subspecialty protocols should be readily adapted if the preceding points are taken into account.

REFERENCES

1. Kane RL, Ouslander JG, Abrass IB. *Essentials of clinical geriatrics*, 3rd ed. New York: McGraw-Hill, 1994.
2. Kane RL. Improving the quality of long-term care. *JAMA* 1995;273:1376–1380.
3. Strahan GW. An overview of nursing homes and their current residents: data from the 1995 National Nursing Home Survey. *Adv Data Vital Health Statistics* no.80, 1997.
4. Creditor MC. Hazards of hospitalization of the elderly. *Ann Intern Med* 1993;118:219–223.
5. Barker WH, Zimmer JG, Hall WJ, Ruff BC, Freundlich CB, Eggert GM. Rates, patterns, causes, and costs of hospitalization of nursing home residents: a population-based study. *Am J Public Health* 1994;84:1615–1620.
6. Mor V, Intrator O, Fries B, et al. Changes in hospitalization associated with introducing the Resident Assessment Instrument. *J Am Geriatr Soc* 1997;45:1002–1010.
7. Kayser-Jones JS, Weiner CL, Barbaccia JC. Factors contributing to the hospitalization of nursing home residents. *Gerontologist* 1989;29:502–510.
8. Weiler PG, Thorpe L, Walters R, Chiriboga D. An automated medical record system for a skilled nursing facility. *J Med Syst* 1987;2:367–380.
9. Yoshikawa TT, Norman DC. Approach to fever and infection in the nursing home. *J Am Geriatr Soc* 1996;44:74–82.
10. Williams ME. Geriatric medicine on the information superhighway: opportunity or road kill? *J Am Geriatr Soc* 1995;43:184–186.
11. Williams ME, Ricketts TC, Thompson BG. Telemedicine and geriatrics: back to the future. *J Am Geriatr Soc* 1995;43:1047–1051.

Telemedicine: Practicing in the Information Age,
edited by Steven F. Viegas and Kim Dunn.
Lippincott–Raven Publishers, Philadelphia © 1998.

39

General Internal Medicine

Russell A. LaForte, Nancy Hughes,
and Stephen J.B. Sibbitt

*Department of Internal Medicine, University of Texas
Medical Branch at Galveston, Galveston, Texas 77555*

Audiovisual computer-assisted teleconferencing is a powerful advance in consultative medicine, and as internal medicine experience with this technology increases, more effective use of scarce resources should result. In the Texas Department of Criminal Justice (TDCJ), referrals to general internal medicine have been evaluated using telemedicine at a site remote to patients' actual location for 3 years. These principles apply to any live telehealth clinical encounter.

PROVIDER-DRIVEN TELEMEDICINE

Telemedicine in the TDCJ has been and will continue to be provider driven. Access to telemedicine by inmates is completely gated through an on-site provider. *On-site* refers to the patient's actual location, and *on-site provider* is the medical personnel providing care to that patient at that site. Although patient-driven telemedicine consultation may be present in the future, we think a system based on this approach is untenable with existing technology and is clearly not the best approach with an incarcerated population.

The on-site care provider is the person responsible for the appropriate selection of patients for consultation. The appropriateness of a consult depends on this provider's educational background. Also, certain problems are more easily and effectively evaluated by telemedicine than other problems. Of particular importance at the University of Texas Medical Branch (UTMB) at Galveston is the follow-up of patients recently discharged from the TDCJ hospital. Because a complete medical record is available to the remote-site physician (i.e., the consultant) in these cases, the patients can be readily seen. Attempts to arrange follow-up visits with the actual discharging physician are important. Of the most common discharge diagnoses at UTMB, most can be seen readily by telemedicine in follow-up (Table 39-1).

TABLE 39-1. *Reasons for visits to internal specialists*

1. Essential hypertension*
2. Diabetes mellitus*
3. Other forms of chronic ischemic heart disease*
4. Acute upper respiratory infections
5. General medical examination
6. Osteoarthrosis and allied disorders
7. General symptoms
8. Chronic airway obstruction*
9. Asthma*
10. Bronchitis*
11. Neurotic disorders*
12. Angina pectoris*
13. Chronic sinusitis*
14. Acute pharyngitis
15. Cardiac dysrhythmias*
16. Other disorders of soft tissue
17. Symptoms involving respiratory system*
18. Heart failure*
19. Peripheral enthesopathies
20. Other and unspecified arthropathies
21. Diseases of the esophagus
22. Other noninfectious gastroenteritis
23. Other disorders of urethra and urinary tract
24. Allergic rhinitis*
25. Hypertensive heart disease*

*Diagnoses readily seen by telemedicine initial visit.
From National Ambulatory Medical Care Survey, National Center for Health Statistics, 1985.

EVALUATION AND DIAGNOSIS

Initial evaluation for the most common diagnoses, however, can prove more difficult in a telemedicine setting. For example, the follow-up evaluation of cirrhosis with ascites could be acceptable without assessing shifting dullness or a fluid wave, as inferences about the ascites and its treatment could be made by assessing the weight, abdominal girth, and appearance of edema in the lower extremities. Such an evaluation would be unacceptable for an initial presentation. The need and ability to examine the appropriate body system should always be addressed before requesting a telemedicine evaluation.

Evaluation of new patients by telemedicine is, of course, frequently and safely performed. Of the 25 most common reasons for ambulatory visits to general internists (see Table 39-1) more than half are appropriate for general telemedicine consultation in the TDCJ. Evaluating a patient for most problems in hypertension, diabetes, heart disease, chronic lung disease, allergies, and psychiatric disorders is possible with existing technologies. As telemedicine continues to improve technologically, better resolution permitting more accurate assessment of the joints and upper respiratory areas is envisioned. Should accurate palpation become possible, the assessment of the abdomen, rectum, and urinary tract would be feasible. Stethoscopes and other analog equipment should be checked on a regular basis by the consulting site to assure high-fidelity transmission.

One important aspect of a telemedicine evaluation is the presentation of data from the patient site. This presentation is best done by the person requesting consultation because such a presentation helps clarify the reason for consultation, which may otherwise remain obscure. Should the consulting physician, nurse, or physician's assistant not be available, other health professionals should present the case after familiarizing themselves with the case and before attempting to present the data. Bedside presentation with the patient who is able and willing to participate usually works well. All patients should have copies of their TDCJ problem list and accurate medication sheet faxed to the remote provider. Compliance lists should be readily obtainable on request. Vital signs and weight should be provided. Laboratory tests ordered on a previous telemedicine visit should be provided, along with any test the on-site provider deems relevant. Patients with hypertension should have a recent chemistry panel with serum calcium, potassium, and renal function. Patients with diabetes should have recent glycosylated hemoglobins and urinalyses. Pulmonary patients should have chest x-ray reports and, if requested, the actual film available for review. Cardiac patients should have an electrocardiogram and chest films with reports. Liver patients should have recent liver function tests, complete blood counts, prothrombin times, and electrolytes. Arthritis patients should have appropriate x-rays.

PATIENT MONITORING

Patient monitoring after the visit can be difficult. The consulting health professional should notify the telemedicine consultant of any decision to deviate from the outlined plan. The consultant should also be made aware of patient decisions not to pursue the recommended course. Laboratory tests ordered should be forwarded to the requesting physician as they become available to the on-site provider. In lieu of an actual follow-up visit, a consultant should be able to request results of treatment evaluation and should be notified by fax on the appropriate clinic day of the on-site provider's patient assessment and satisfaction with the consultation. This procedure would be time saving to both sites.

ON-SITE ARRANGEMENT AND PERSONNEL

Optimum on-site arrangement and personnel are critical. A trained nurse and physician's assistant, if not a physician, should be present on-site. There should be a clear central area where the patient can be comfortably placed and the provider can stand to present. All rooms should contain the necessary materials to perform a complete physical examination on-site if needed. Rooms should also contain a person trained in the use of the remote site equipment. Fax machines are essential to the documentation process.

DOCUMENTATION

Clinic documentation should proceed in an efficient manner. The medical chart should be updated at the time of the visit with a detailed clinic note written by the consultant. This note should reflect the source of all data obtained during the visit because on-site, as well as remote, data gathering is possible. This note should have all data faxed to the remote site attached. Laboratory results should be forwarded to the remote provider as they are obtained.

FEEDBACK

Useful feedback in a complex, busy system is difficult. In a tightly managed care environment, the primary responsible physician should decide the usefulness of a consultation on a case-by-case, as opposed to visit-by-visit, basis. The provider (consultant) should assess the appropriateness of the case for telemedicine. A brief questionnaire should be given to both the providing and referring physicians. The provider's questionnaire should address the appropriateness of the consult for telemedicine, as he or she is the doctor with the closest view of the process in a given case. He or she will know if an effective patient evaluation was possible, if remote treatment was possible, and so on. This data should then be collected on a semiannual basis and sent to the referring physician.

Similarly, referring personnel should complete a questionnaire regarding the usefulness of each consultation. They could evaluate whether therapy was changed, a new diagnosis made, or whether a visit to the hospital or medical center was saved. Questionnaire results could be collected and processed by diagnosis and sent to the consulting physician. By associating the diagnoses with the feedback evaluation, research to make telemedicine more useful or to better assess its limitations could be more easily done.

Telemedicine: Practicing in the Information Age,
edited by Steven F. Viegas and Kim Dunn.
Lippincott–Raven Publishers, Philadelphia © 1998.

40

Pulmonology and Critical Care Medicine

Michael Charles Boyars

Department of Internal Medicine, University of Texas Medical Branch at Galveston, Galveston, Texas 77555

Many pulmonary diseases are of a chronic and slowly progressive nature and are well suited for telemedicine (Table 40-1). Certain conditions are of an acute and rapidly changing nature and are not appropriate for telemedicine (Table 40-2). Any time the patient is acutely clinically unstable, he or she should be taken directly to an acute-care facility for treatment. Clinically unstable conditions include episodes of hemodynamic instability, status asthmaticus or significant bronchospasm, significant hemoptysis, profound dyspnea of uncertain cause, acute respiratory acidosis, or any process with a rapidly deteriorating mental status. This chapter describes how to best use telemedicine to evaluate and follow respiratory patients.

PULMONOLOGY AND TELEMEDICINE

In the practice of pulmonology by telemedicine, the medical personnel on the patient end act as surrogates. The telemedicine room should have a desk directly in front of a large television screen. The controls for moving the camera should be on the desk in easy reach. The patient and the presenter should be in the viewing area at their location. There should be an x-ray viewbox with the recent chest x-rays (CXRs) in place. The old CXRs or computed tomography (CT) scans should be available for viewing if needed. A stethoscope with capabilities to transmit breath sounds is also necessary. The stethoscope should be placed at the apex on one side of the chest posteriorly and sequentially moved across the chest, pausing to hear one breath cycle. The examiner works his or her way to the bases and then repeats the process anteriorly.

DATA NEEDS

There are certain data that are helpful to review for every patient (Table 40-3). These data include a brief description of the present medical problem, recent and old CXRs, recent and old pulmonary function tests, and spirometry, as well as any recent and old arterial blood gas or oxygen saturation values.

TABLE 40-1. *Conditions suitable for telemedicine*

Chronic obstructive pulmonary disease
Asthma
Lung and mediastinal masses
Pulmonary infections
Interstitial lung disease
Pleural effusions
Obstructive sleep apnea

TABLE 40-2. *Conditions that are not suitable for telemedicine**

Status asthmaticus
Significant hemoptysis
Acute respiratory acidosis
Acute pneumothorax
Acute pulmonary thromboembolism
Any patient with hemodynamic instability
Any patient with acutely altered mental state
Any patient with the acute onset of significant dyspnea

*Except emergency settings.

TABLE 40-3. *Data needed before a telemedicine encounter*

System and complaint-directed history and physical examination
Recent and old chest x-rays and computed tomography scans
Recent and old pulmonary function tests, spirometry, and peak flows
Recent and old arterial blood gas and oxygen saturation values
Cigarette smoking and occupational history
Purified protein derivative status
Recent and old complete blood counts, if infection is considered
Sputum smear and culture results for routine bacteria, acid-fast bacillus, and fungus, if infection is considered possible

Chronic Obstructive Pulmonary Disease

Chronic obstructive pulmonary disease (COPD) remains a major health problem in U.S. society despite a more than 40% decrease in the number of cigarette smokers since the 1940s. COPD includes chronic bronchitis, emphysema, and asthma. The presenter should give the chief complaint first. It is important to know if this is an acute or chronic problem. Is the chief complaint dyspnea, chest pain, hemoptysis, fatigue, cyanosis, peripheral edema, or sleep disturbance? Tobacco use and occupational history are important to document risk factors for COPD. Family history for asthma or COPD should also be presented, as well as the patient's usual state of health, exercise capacity, and current medications. Be sure to state the last time the patient was on inhaled or systemic steroids, as well as the number and circumstances of previous hospitalizations, emergency room visits, and intubations in the past 2 to 3 years. If possible, the patient's baseline peak flow measurements and those during the illness are very helpful.

Other areas in the medical history to address are the presence and characteristics of cough and sputum, cyanosis, chest pain, dyspnea with quantitation, fever, chills, night sweats, hemoptysis, change in sleep patterns, and change in frequency of bronchodilator use. The physical examination should pay close attention to the rate and character of the respirations, as well as the presence of pursed lip breathing and central or peripheral cyanosis. The character of the breath sounds, particularly the length and intensity of the expiratory phase, should be noted, as well as evidence of extreme airway obstruction such as intercostal retraction, use of accessory muscles of respiration, and paradoxical respiratory movements.

Lung or Mediastinal Masses

Lung or mediastinal masses are a common reason for referral to a pulmonologist. The major differential diagnosis is between neoplastic and infectious etiologies. Accordingly, the history should pay particular attention to the presence of appetite or weight loss, fever, chills, night sweats, cough, sputum production, hemoptysis, cigarette smoking history, and past and present purified protein derivative (PPD) status, as well as history of prior treatment or prophylaxis for tuberculosis (TB) and occupational and travel history. Previous CXRs for comparison are invaluable for determining if the present findings represent a new process or an old, clinically inactive one. A CT scan of the thorax, if performed, should be available for review.

Pulmonary Infectious Diseases

Pulmonary infectious diseases are another common problem. Points in the medical history to be stressed are time and mode of onset of symptoms. Presence of predisposing factors, such as diabetes mellitus, silicosis, previous and present PPD status, acquired immunodeficiency syndrome (AIDS), cancer, or systemic chemotherapy, are important. The patient's previous area of residence, whether within this country or outside, is important to determine risk for TB and certain fungal infections. Any medication the patient has been recently taking, specifically antibiotics, should be noted. On physical examination, specific attention should be given to the fever pattern and presence of skin lesions or cutaneous abscesses, as well the physical examination of the chest. Naturally, the results of smears and cultures of sputum and blood should be available if obtained.

Infections in AIDS patients deserve special consideration. Important points in the history are recent CD4 counts and present medication, including any prophylaxis for *Pneumocystis carinii* pneumonia, TB, or atypical TB. The CXR is critically important to determine if the disease is unilateral or bilateral. Other factors should also be reviewed.

Interstitial Lung Disease

Interstitial lung disease is another common condition seen by the pulmonologist. Specific points in the history that deserve attention are mode and timing of onset, complete occupational history, history of previous radiation therapy to the chest, complete medication history going back 10 years, questioning about signs and symptoms of lupus, rheumatoid arthritis, and scleroderma, and family history of interstitial lung disease. In the physical examination, particular attention should be paid to the rate and pattern of breathing; character of the breath sounds; cutaneous signs of scleroderma; lupus or rheumatoid arthritis; and the presence of erythema nodosum, iritis, or lacrimal gland enlargement suggestive of sarcoidosis. Useful laboratory studies include recent and old CXRs as well as high-resolution CT scans of the thorax and recent and old pulmonary function tests.

Pleural Effusions

Pleural effusions are most commonly caused by infectious or malignant conditions. Therefore, the history should make mention of recent CXR and mammogram reports, because lung and breast carcinoma are the most common causes of malignant effusions. Previous and present PPD status, as well as previous treatment or prophylaxis for TB, is important. The patient should be asked for symptoms of fever, chills, night sweats, cough, sputum, hemoptysis, weight loss, and pleurisy. Congestive heart failure and chronic renal insufficiency can present with pleural effusion, and evidence for this can be sought in the history. The presence of poorly treated diabetes or hypertension or previous myocardial infarction are clues to the presence of previous cardiac or renal disease. Recent and old CXRs, as well as a recent complete blood count and results of thoracentesis and pleural biopsy, if performed, should be reported.

Obstructive Sleep Apnea

Obstructive sleep apnea is a common problem that is frequently underrecognized. If obstructive sleep apnea is considered, a history of daytime hypersomnolence, change in personality or increased irritability, morning headaches, observed severe snoring, and apneic episodes should be sought. On physical examination, evidence of a short, thick neck; enlarged tonsils; central obesity; and signs of right-sided heart failure should be noted.

Telemedicine: Practicing in the Information Age,
edited by Steven F. Viegas and Kim Dunn.
Lippincott–Raven Publishers, Philadelphia © 1998.

41

Infectious Diseases

David P. Paar and Norbert J. Roberts, Jr.

Department of Internal Medicine, University of Texas Medical Branch at Galveston, Galveston, Texas 77555; and Division of Infectious Diseases, University of Texas Medical Branch at Galveston, Galveston, Texas 77555

The model of telemedicine for the care of human immunodeficiency virus (HIV)-positive inmates is unique because the HIV care provider must remain intimately involved with the care given to HIV-infected individuals. The need for intimate involvement by the care provider is supported by published data that demonstrate improvements in quality of life and life span, as well as decreased cost of medical care, when people with HIV are cared for by HIV specialists (1). Because of the pivotal role that the subspecialist plays, it is anticipated that the patient will be intermittently transported to the subspecialist site for personal interactions, which establishes and maintains the patient-physician relationship and facilitates communication that may not otherwise occur over video. Taken as a whole, this model represents a dynamic interaction between the primary care providers at the remote site, the subspecialists, and the patient. Therefore, it is referred to as *HIV cooperative care*. In addition, video equipment is used for a variety of purposes. For example, patients can be seen by a physician assistant or other provider at the remote site, and the HIV-management plan can be discussed with the subspecialist via video; thus, the video equipment is used for teleconferencing rather than to directly examine the patient. At other times, it is necessary for the subspecialist to see a patient via video with the remote provider present and to use the video equipment for direct patient interaction with the subspecialist. Finally, the video equipment can be used to educate the remote presenters.

The following outline begins with the identification of an HIV-infected patient at a remote site and indicates how that patient entered into HIV cooperative care. Patients who are receiving ongoing HIV care enter into the system where appropriate.

For new patients, the referral system is laboratory based or at the request of the primary care provider. All patients who test positive for HIV enter the algorithm for evaluation and care in HIV cooperative care. At the remote site, providers interview the patient and obtain initial laboratory, radiology, and other diagnostic studies that are necessary for the assessment of an HIV-positive patient (2).

Certain interventions, such as initiation of prophylactic therapies or vaccination, occur automatically at the unit level based on the results of laboratory values. Once the initial data collection and preliminary interventions have been undertaken, the patient travels to the subspecialist for an initial evaluation. The preliminary information collected at the remote site is available to the subspecialist via a shared database.

HIV patients with acute problems can be triaged via telemedicine to determine if care can be provided at the remote site, at the emergency department, or a local emergency department.

ROLE OF THE REMOTE PRESENTER AND DATA ORGANIZATION

The remote presenter generally is a physician assistant with training in HIV care. The following outline shows how data should be organized during the process of care.

I. Data before the patient is seen: Once a patient is identified as HIV positive, the following data is collected over the ensuing 3 to 4 weeks. Three to 4 weeks are necessary because of the need to repeat certain baseline values, including CD4 and lymphocyte determinations and viral load (2). Also, certain interventions automatically occur based on the results of preliminary laboratory data.
   A. Historical data: demographic data, risk factors, Centers for Disease Control and Prevention (CDC) Category A/B/C staging criteria, initial history, and physical examination with extensive review of systems. Initial laboratory data and decision tree support are shown in Table 41-1.
   B. Radiologic data: Obtain chest x-ray (CXR). CXRs with significant findings including infiltrates, mass lesions, or effusions should be discussed with AIDS Care and Clinical Research Program (ACCRP) staff. There should be a weekly CXR teleconference to review newly diagnosed HIV-positive patients with abnormal CXRs. Before the CXR teleconference, the physician assistant performs a pulmonary review of systems, examines the patient, and has the following data ready to present to the ACCRP provider: history of cough, shortness of breath, sputum production, fever, chills, night sweats, and weight loss; purified protein derivative results; lung physical examination findings; and CXR. A plan for evaluation and management is developed at this point.

II. Data as patient seen: After all of the previous data is collected, the patient is seen. ACCRP personnel review and clarify key historical data and perform a physical examination. Because the CD4 count and viral load are available, the patient can be staged according to 1993 CDC Staging Criteria for HIV Infection (3), and the risk for progression of HIV-associated disease and death can be projected based on viral load (4). The patient is educated regarding the course of HIV disease and the potential benefits and side effects of antiretroviral therapy. Eligibility for ongoing clinical trials (if available) are assessed and discussed. Finally, a plan for therapy is developed. The patient may opt for no therapy, therapy on a clinical trial, or standard antiretroviral therapy.

TABLE 41-1. *Initial laboratory data and data-based interventions*

Laboratory test	Intervention
HIV positive	Pneumococcal vaccine Yearly influenza vaccine
Lymphocyte subset analysis Repeat 2 to 3 weeks later; if second value differs from first by more than 50%, obtain a third analysis	PCP prophylaxis if CD4 <200 cells/ml. Trimethoprim/sulfamethoxazole (Bactrim) 1 po MF Dapsone 100 mg po qd Aerosol pentamidine 300 mg po q mo MAC prophylaxis if CD4 <75 cells/ml. Azithromycin 1 g po q M Clarithromycin 500 mg po bid Rifabutin 150 mg po bid Refer to ophthalmology for retinal examination if CD4 <100 cells/ml.
Toxoplasma antibody	Toxoplasma prophylaxis if positive and CD4 <200 cells/ml. Bactrim provides both PCP and toxoplasmic prophylaxis. If patient is using dapsone for PCP prophylaxis, add pyrimethamine 25 mg q wk.
Viral load Repeat analysis 2 weeks later; if second value differs from first by more than 1 log, obtain a third analysis	Need for antiretroviral therapy should be determined by consultant.
Hepatitis serology (HCV Ab, HBsAg, HBcAb)	Initiate HBV vaccine series if HBcAb and HBsAg are negative.
Syphilis screen	If RPR is positive, treat with benzathine penicillin 2.4 million units IM q wk × 3.
Urinalysis	If positive for protein, repeat UA. If repeat UA is positive for protein, collect 24-hr urine for protein quantitation. If 24-hr urinary protein is >1.5 g, refer to nephrology for evaluation.
Serum chemistries, CBC with differential, CMV antibody	Abnormalities and need for interventions can be discussed with consultants.
PPD (a positive PPD is 0.5 mm in a positive individual)	If negative, perform a yearly PPD. If positive, initiate prophylaxis with INH, 300 mg po qd or 900 mg po twice weekly.
Pap smear	If shows dysplasia, the patient should be referred to gynecology. If dysplasia is absent, repeat Pap every 12 mos.

HIV, human immunodeficiency virus; PCP, *Pneumocystis carinii* pneumonia; MAC, *Mycobacterium avium* complex; HCV Ab, hepatitis C virus antibody; HBsAg, hepatitis B surface antigen; HBcAb, hepatitis B core antibody; HBV, hepatitis B virus; UA, urinalysis; CBC, complete blood cell count; CMV, cytomegalovirus; PPD, purified protein derivative; INH, isoniazid; Pap, Papanicolaou's smear; MF, medium frequency.

III. Data after patient is seen: For patients started on antiretroviral therapy, the following should occur:
   A. An evaluation at 4 weeks by the remote site personnel. This includes a review of therapy, specific side effects, problem-oriented examination, therapy-specific laboratory evaluation (e.g., zidovudine [ZDV]-complete blood count; didanosine [DDI]-amylase, lipase), and viral load determination. When the laboratory data are complete, the case can be discussed via telemedicine with an ACCRP provider, and further evaluation and management are discussed at that time.
   B. A routine evaluation every 3 months at which time a review of therapy-specific side effects, problem-oriented examinations, therapy-specific laboratory evaluation (e.g., ZDV-complete blood count; DDI-amylase, lipase), and viral load determination. When the laboratory data are complete, the case can be discussed via telemedicine with an ACCRP provider, and further evaluation and management are discussed at that time. Two of these quarterly evaluations should be performed at the subspecialty telemedicine site. However, approximately 2 weeks before the subspecialty telemedicine site visit, the unit providers should obtain the required laboratory evaluation, so results can be ready when the patient is seen.

IV. Data organization: Data are organized in flow-sheet format in an electronic database that is shared between the remote site and the subspecialist.

V. Data to monitor quality of care and resource use for improvement of clinical care are medication compliance, hospitalizations, costs of care, and satisfaction.

REFERENCES

1. Kitahata MM, Koepsell TD, Deyo RA, Maxwell CL, et al. Physicians' experience with the acquired immunodeficiency syndrome as a factor in patients' survival. *N Engl J Med* 1996;334:701–706.
2. Kaplan JE, Masur H, Holmes KK, et al. USPHS/IDSA guidelines for the prevention of opportunistic infections in persons infected with human immunodeficiency virus: an overview. *Clin Infect Dis* 1995;21[Suppl 1]:S12–31.
3. Castro KG, Ward JW, Slutsker L, Buehler JW, et al. 1993 revised classification system for HIV infection and expanded surveillance case definition for AIDS among adolescents and adults. *MMWR Morb Mortal Wkly Rep* 1992;41:1–19.
4. Saag MS, Holodniy M, Kuritzkes DR, O'Brien WA, et al. HIV viral load markers in clinical practice. *Nature Med* 1996;2:625–629.

Telemedicine: Practicing in the Information Age,
edited by Steven F. Viegas and Kim Dunn.
Lippincott–Raven Publishers, Philadelphia © 1998.

42

Allergy, Asthma, and Immunology

J. Andrew Grant

Department of Internal Medicine, University of Texas Medical Branch at Galveston, Galveston, Texas 77555

The diseases traditionally related to allergy, asthma, and immunology are among the most common disorders affecting the population at all ages (1). Allergic rhinitis affects approximately 80 million Americans and is a major cause of absence from school and work. Symptoms of rhinitis can be seasonal in keeping with the major pollen seasons or perennial in persons allergic to indoor allergens such as house dust mites, domestic pets, molds, and cockroaches. Although often considered a minor problem by those who do not have it, Bousquet and colleagues evaluated the impact of allergic rhinitis using a standardized questionnaire, the SF36 (2). They showed that this condition caused significant reduction in the quality of life that improved with effective therapy. They also evaluated the impact of bronchial asthma on patients and found those with bronchial asthma were less bothered by lower respiratory illness than upper, but obviously the risk of asthma is far greater (3).

Asthma affects about 5% of the population and causes more than 5,000 deaths annually in the United States (4). The prevalence, incidence, economic impact, and mortality of asthma have risen dramatically since 1980. One report followed patients with asthma for 25 years (5). More than half of the patients still had symptoms of asthma, abnormal pulmonary function, and increased hyperreactivity. Only 10% of the patients had lost all evidence of the disease, thus supporting the chronicity of asthma. Asthma is of special concern in adolescents and young adults, and in these age groups, ethnic factors are dramatic. The mortality among blacks is threefold to fourfold higher than in whites (4).

Cutaneous disorders, such as urticaria, atopic and contact dermatitis, drug reactions, and others, are seen in consultation by specialists in both dermatology and allergy-immunology. Anaphylaxis can be caused by drugs, foods, stinging insects, and many other factors and evaluation for long-term management often requires participation by an allergist. Finally, in the field of immunology, the most common disorders of concern are immunodeficiencies that cause recurrent infections. The most prevalent congenital immunodeficiency is for immunoglobulin A antibodies (up to 1 in 300 patients) (6). The most frequent symptoms of these patients are recurrent sinopulmonary infections, but often this condition is asymptomatic. Common variable immunodeficiency, also called *acquired hypogammaglobulinemia*, also causes recurrent sinopulmonary infections, usually beginning in adolescents and young adults. Certainly, the most common acquired immunodeficiency is due to human immunodeficiency infection that has become perhaps the most important cause of chronic serious disease in the population, and patients are seen in collaboration with specialists in both infectious diseases and allergy-immunology.

The diseases mentioned in the preceding paragraphs are traditionally the bulk of patients seen by specialists in the field of allergy, asthma, and immunology. These patients are also appropriate for management via telemedicine. Within Texas, there are approximately 175 physicians certified by the American Board of Allergy and Immunology, but they are heavily concentrated in the major population centers. Telemedicine is appropriate for evaluation of patients in rural areas and correctional facilities.

For this chapter, I have selected the development of a telemedicine program in asthma within the Texas Department of Criminal Justice (TDCJ) managed care system. This program could also be readily applied to rural areas of Texas. A review of *MEDLINE* yielded no reports of prior endeavors using telemedicine to manage asthmatic patients. As outlined in the preceding paragraphs, asthma is a condition of increasing importance as to prevalence, morbidity, mortality, and costs to society. At the University of Texas Medical Branch (UTMB) at Galveston, asthma is now the most frequent condition for emergency department visits and hospitalization in the pediatric population. In adult patients, asthma is also of increasing significance.

ASTHMA MANAGEMENT

There has been worldwide interest in asthma to improve the quality of care. This resulted in a consensus report from the Heart, Lung and Blood Institute at the National Institutes of Health (NIH) in 1991 and revised in 1997 (7). The World Health Organization issued a similar report in 1995. Finally, the American Academy of Allergy, Asthma, and Immunology published extensive practice parameters for management of asthma (8).

One essential feature of new proposals for asthma management is based on a better understanding of the pathophysiology of the disease. Traditionally considered a disease of bronchospasm, it is now clear that chronic asthma involves an intense inflammatory reaction in the lungs. In patients who must use bronchodilators more than two or three times weekly, it is recommended that antiinflammatory therapy be used. The most effective drugs of this class are corticosteroids. Oral and systemic drugs are effective for management of acute relapses, but inhaled corticosteroids have established efficacy for long-term control. These drugs improve patient quality of life and reduce both the morbidity and mortality of asthma. Other effects include

TABLE 42-1. *Definitions of asthma severity in chronic management*

Steps	Symptoms	Nighttime symptoms	Lung function
Step 4: severe persistent	Continual symptoms Limited physical activity Frequent exacerbations	Frequent	FEV_1 or PEF <60% of predicted
Step 3: moderate persistent	Daily symptoms Daily use of bronchodilators Exacerbations affect activity Exacerbations two or more times weekly	Two or more times weekly	FEV_1 or PEF 60% to 80%
Step 2: mild persistent	Symptoms more than twice a week but not daily Exacerbations possibly affect activity	Three or more times a month	FEV_1 or PEF >80%
Step 1: mild intermittent	Symptoms no more than twice weekly Exacerbations brief	Less than three times a month	FEV_1 or PEF >80%

FEV_1, forced expiratory volume in 1 second; PEF, peak expiratory flow.
Adapted from ref. 7.

reduced drug use, especially the need for bronchodilators and systemic steroids. Facility use, including hospitalization, is reduced. Pulmonary function testing and also objective measures of bronchial hyperreactivity improve with the use of inhaled corticosteroids. Finally, it has been shown that this class of drug actually reduces the inflammatory response in lung biopsies (9).

The most recent documentation of reduced resource use through asthma management and the use of inhaled steriods was published by the Harvard managed care system (10). Reduced resource use has obvious implications for reduced costs in the UTMB/TDCJ managed care system and improved health of Texas inmates.

NATIONAL INSTITUTES OF HEALTH ASTHMA GUIDELINES

The NIH asthma guidelines (7) allow the level of care and changes in care to be based on staging of asthma severity (Table 42-1). Four levels of severity have been established: (a) mild intermittent, (b) mild persistent, (c) moderate persistent, and (d) severe persistent. The levels are defined based on several criteria: symptoms, interference in daily activity, exacerbations of asthma, drug use, and measurements of pulmonary function. Recommended care is based on the severity (adapted for TDCJ managed care in Table 42-2). As patients change in terms of clinical parameters, they may move into a more severe or milder step (see Table 42-1). The doses and frequency of drugs can be modified, and drugs can be added or subtracted.

TABLE 42-2. *Stepwise approach to managing chronic asthma*

Steps	Long-term control drugs	Quick-relief drugs	Education and management
Step 4: severe persistent	Beclomethasone MDI six + puffs tid and prednisone 60 mg daily for 7 days; consider salmeterol MDI two puffs bid (non KOP) or theophylline SR 300 mg qd or bid	Albuterol MDI two puffs q4–6h prn and consider ipratropium MDI two puffs qid	Same as Step 1 Follow-up in 1 wk or prn Respiratory therapy evaluation Schedule for urgent telemedicine consultation
Step 3: moderate persistent	Beclomethasone MDI six to 10 puffs bid and consider theophylline SR 300 mg qd or bid	Albuterol MDI two puffs q4–6h prn	Same as Step 1 Follow-up in 2 wks Respiratory therapy evaluation Schedule for urgent telemedicine consultation
Step 2: mild persistent	Beclomethasone MDI two to six puffs bid	Albuterol MDI two puffs q4–6h prn	Same as Step 1 Peak flow measurement Review management based on measures and symptoms Follow-up in 2–4 wks
Step 1: mild intermittent	No daily drugs needed	Albuterol MDI two puffs prn (use more than twice weekly indicates Step 2 or higher)	Basic facts of asthma Inhaler and spacer use Roles of drugs Follow-up in 1–3 mos

MDI, metered dose inhaler; KOP, keep on person; SR, sustained release.
Adapted from ref. 7.

PATIENTS SUITABLE FOR TELEMEDICINE CONSULTATION

The present rate of specialty referral to the outpatient clinic facility in Galveston, Texas, is small, perhaps 15 to 30 asthmatic patients per year; however, the inpatient admissions are much higher. With more than 100,000 covered lives in the UTMB-based managed care system, a conservative estimate of the number of asthmatic inmates is 5,000. Thus, the use of specialists right now is low. Clearly, this can contribute to higher morbidity and economic costs of managing patients with asthma. The value of specialty care to reduce morbidity and costs has been shown (11,12). A qualitative review of available data suggests many TDCJ patients have moderate to severe disease and thus are quite appropriate for specialty and telemedicine consultation. Patients with mild-persistent or intermittent asthma can usually be managed by primary caregivers. Patients who fall into moderate-persistent asthma should be referred for a routine telemedicine consultation. Patients with severe-persistent asthma should have an urgent consultation.

Patients presenting to unit clinics with acute increases in asthma symptoms offer unique problems in management. A proposed scheme is provided in Fig. 42-1, with recommendations for treatment at the unit or at a regional emergency room. When stable, the patients would be evaluated according to the four steps (see Table 42-1)

Inmate presents with complaint of worsening dyspnea, wheezing, chest tightness, cough, or any combination of these:

Initial assessment

- Determine degrees of symptoms, length of this exacerbation, and drugs currently used.
- Examine patient for degree of distress. Listen to chest for breath sounds and note symmetry and depth of respiration. Use of accessory muscles or suprasternal retractions suggests severe exacerbation.
- Measure pulse and respiratory rate.
- If equipment is available, measure peak expiratory flow (PEF) and oxygen saturation.
- Consider potential triggers for symptoms (e.g., acute viral infection, sinusitis, pneumonia, exposure to toxic environment, heart disease).

Initial treatment

- Inhaled albuterol metered dose inhaler (MDI) two to four puffs up to three treatments at 20-min intervals.

Repeat assessment in 20–60 mins

- Evaluation of symptoms, chest examination, vital signs, PEF, and oxygen saturation.

↓ **Good response (mild episode)**	↓ **Incomplete response (moderate episode)**	↓ **Poor response (severe episode)**
• No wheezing or dyspnea	• Persistent wheezing and dyspnea	• Marked wheezing and dyspnea
• PEF >80% predicted or personal best	• PEF 50–80% predicted or personal best	• PEF <50% predicted or personal best
Management	**Management**	**Management**
• Continue albuterol MDI two to four puffs q4h for 1–2 days, then prn	• Continue albuterol MDI two to four puffs every hour	• Continuous inhaled albuterol and ipratropium by nebulization for an hour
• If on inhaled steroids, double dose for 7–10 days	• Oxygen to achieve ≥90% saturation	• Oxygen to achieve ≥90% saturation
• Treat any underlying condition	• Prednisone 60 mg po	• 100 mg prednisone po
• Discharge from unit clinic with follow-up in 3–7 days or prn		
↓		
• On follow-up visit, stage asthma and treat accordingly	↓	↓

Continued

FIG. 42-1. Management of acute asthma exacerbations in Texas Department of Criminal Justice unit clinics.

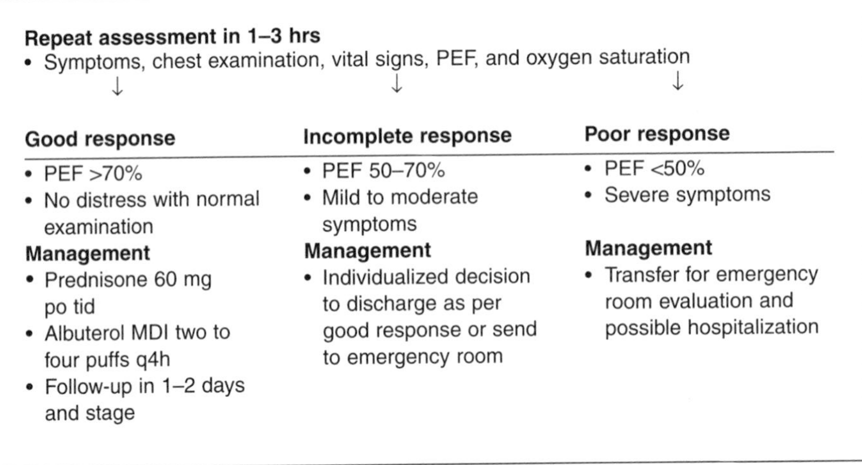

Repeat assessment in 1–3 hrs
• Symptoms, chest examination, vital signs, PEF, and oxygen saturation
Good response
• PEF >70%
• No distress with normal examination
Management
• Prednisone 60 mg po tid
• Albuterol MDI two to four puffs q4h
• Follow-up in 1–2 days and stage
Incomplete response
• PEF 50–70%
• Mild to moderate symptoms
Management
• Individualized decision to discharge as per good response or send to emergency room
Poor response
• PEF <50%
• Severe symptoms
Management
• Transfer for emergency room evaluation and possible hospitalization

FIG. 42-1. *Continued.*

and managed accordingly (see Table 42-2). Those in steps three and four would be considered for telemedicine.

TELEMEDICINE DATA AND EQUIPMENT

It is essential that data be collected from each patient before presentation via telemedicine. A proposed instrument for initial consultations is shown in Fig. 42-2. The questionnaire should be completed by unit personnel with the patient and then transmitted to UTMB Galveston for review by the allergy faculty before the actual presentation. A proposed follow-up questionnaire is provided in Fig. 42-3.

During the teleconference, this information should be presented by a nurse or physician's assistant. The allergy faculty will then elaborate on issues to obtain a complete history. The physical examination should be done by the nurse or physician's assistant. Having an electronic otorhinoscope is useful so that the allergy faculty can accurately examine the eyes, ears, nose, and throat. An electronic stethoscope for accurate examination of the heart and chest is also useful. Patients' skin can generally be examined, with most cameras providing sufficient resolution to diagnose common disorders. An essential laboratory instrumentation is measurement of peak expiratory flow (PEF). Optimally, it should be possible to measure forced vital capacity (FVC) and forced expiratory volume in 1 second (FEV_1). A routine part of laboratory evaluation is assessment of reversibility of reduced PEF or FEV_1 after administration of a bronchodilator. For follow-up of patients in unit clinics as well as telemedicine conferences, a key objective measure is frequent assessment of PEF. For emergency evaluation of patients, measuring oxygen saturation can be critical.

1. Have you been diagnosed with asthma by a physician?____________________
2. If so, when, and by whom?____________________
3. In the past year:
   a. Have you had episodes of coughing, wheezing, or shortness of breath?

      ____

   b. What things trigger your symptoms of coughing, wheezing, or shortness of breath?

Moldy places_____	Chemicals_____	Aspirin_____
House dust_____	Tobacco smoke_____	Other drugs_____
Cats_____	Strong odors_____	Foods_____
Outdoors_____	Perfumes_____	Cold weather_____
Exercise_____	Stress_____	Colds_____

      Other things (name)____________________

   c. Have you used any medications that help you breathe better?____________

      If yes, name the medications:____________________

      ____

   d. How often have you had asthma attacks? ____________________
   e. How many times have you been to a clinic or emergency room for asthma?

      ____

4. How many times have you been hospitalized for asthma in your life?

   ____

   When was the last time?____________________
5. Have you ever been on a ventilator?____________________

   When? ____________________
6. In the past month, have you had coughing, wheezing, or shortness of breath
   a. At night that awakened you?__________ How many nights? __________
   b. After running or other activity?____________________
   c. How far can you walk without getting short of breath?____________________
   d. What have your asthma symptoms been?
      i. Cough____________
      ii. Wheezing____________
      iii. Shortness of breath____________
      iv. Chest tightness____________
      v. Coughing up sputum____________
   e. What medications have you taken for asthma in the past month?

i. Asthma inhalers	Puffs used each time	How many times used daily?
__________	__________	__________
__________	__________	__________
__________	__________	__________

Continued

FIG. 42-2. Data to be obtained on patients before initial asthma telemedicine consultation.

ii. Tablets Dose Times taken daily

Tablets	Dose	Times taken daily
__________	__________	__________
__________	__________	__________
__________	__________	__________

f. What other medications have you taken in the past month?

Drug	Dose	Times taken daily
__________	__________	__________
__________	__________	__________
__________	__________	__________

7. What other illnesses or hospitalizations have you had?__________
8. Any family members have asthma?_____ Who?__________
9. Have you ever smoked?__________
   a. Cigarettes, cigars, pipe?__________
   b. At what age did you start smoking?__________
   c. How many packs of cigarettes a day?__________
   d. Have you stopped smoking?________ When did you stop?________
10. Do you ever have symptoms of runny nose, sneezing, congested nose, postnasal drip?__________
    a. What time of the year?__________
    b. What makes these symptoms worse?__________
11. How many times a year do you get attacks of sinus with yellow or green drainage from your nose?__________
12. Do you have heartburn?__________
13. Does food ever come up into your throat?__________

FIG. 42-2. *Continued.*

After the history and physical examination, the allergy faculty provide a verbal diagnosis and outline of treatment to the patient and presenter. A flow sheet of common diagnoses and treatments is provided in Fig. 42-4. Follow-up for patients with asthma in stage four usually is at 1 to 3 months and those in stage three are at 3 to 6 months and as required.

PRESENTER

Obviously, having the same presenter in each unit is advantageous. Having presenters instructed at length by allergy faculty and staff in general principles is essential. This can be done by videotapes to be prepared by the allergy staff for this purpose. Features of the educational program for the presenters include pathophysiology of asthma; triggers; complications; key historical features; typical examination, including use of electronic equipment; fundamentals of assessment; common

How many days in the past week have you had chest tightness, cough, shortness of breath, or wheezing (whistling in your chest)? 0___1___2___3___4___5___6___7___

How many nights in the past week have you had chest tightness, cough, shortness of breath, or wheezing (whistling in your chest)? 0___1___2___3___4___5___6___7___

Do you perform peak flow readings? Yes___No___

If yes, did you bring your peak flow chart? Yes___No___

How many days in the past week has asthma restricted your physical activity? 0___1___2___3___4___5___6___7___

Have you had any asthma attacks since your last visit? Yes___No___

Have you had any unscheduled visits to a the clinic, including to the emergency department, since your last visit? Yes___No___

How many puffs of your short-acting inhaled beta-agonist (quick-relief medicine) do you use per day? Average number of puffs per day__________________

How many of your short-acting inhaled beta-agonist inhalers did you go through over the past month? Number of inhalers in past month__________________

How well controlled is your asthma in your opinion?

Very well controlled__________

Somewhat controlled__________

Not well controlled__________

List the medications you have taken for asthma since your last teleconference.

Asthma inhalers	Puffs used each time	How many times used daily
____________	____________	____________
____________	____________	____________
____________	____________	____________

Tablets	Dose	Times taken daily
____________	____________	____________
____________	____________	____________
____________	____________	____________

What other medications have you taken in the past month?

Drug	Dose	Times taken daily
____________	____________	____________
____________	____________	____________
____________	____________	____________

FIG. 42-3. Data to be obtained on patients before follow-up asthma telemedicine consultation.

Medical diagnoses in the field of allergy

Bronchial asthma caused by allergies
Bronchial asthma not allergic
Asthma stage__________
Chronic obstructive pulmonary disease
Allergic rhinitis (hay fever)
Rhinitis not due to allergies
Sinusitis (acute or chronic)
Urticaria (hives)
Atopic dermatitis (eczema)
Angioedema
Anaphylaxis

Drug therapy

Long-term control medications for asthma

Beclomethasone (Vanceril/Beclovent) MDI__________________puffs bid or tid
Cromolyn (Intal) two puffs tid or__________________
Nedocromil (Tilade) two puffs tid or__________________
Salmeterol xinafoate (Serevent) two puffs qhs or bid
Theophylline (Theo-Dur) 300 mg bid or__________________
Zafirlukast (Accolate) 20 mg bid

Quick-relief medications for asthma

Albuterol (Proventil/Ventolin) MDI two puffs q4–6h prn
Prednisone________mg qd or bid for______days; then taper over________days
Ipratropium (Atrovent) two puffs q6h prn

Treatment of sinusitis

Antibiotics
Azithromycin (Zithromax Z pack) dose pack as directed
Cefuroxime (Ceftin) 250 mg bid for___________days
Amoxicillin/clavulanate (Augmentin) 875 mg bid for__________days
Trimethoprim/sulfamethoxazole (Bactrim DS) bid for__________days
Other______________________________
Oxymetazoline hydrochloride (Afrin) prn for 3–5 days

Treatment of allergic rhinitis (hay fever)

Antihistamines
Hydroxyzine (Atarax) 25 mg bid prn or______________
Other_______________________
Nasal steroids
Beclomethasone (Vancenase/Beconase)
two puffs/nostril bid or_________
Decongestants
Pseudoephedrine (Sudafed) 30 or 60 mg q6h prn
Antihistamine-decongestants

Continued

FIG. 42-4. Common diagnoses, drugs, and educational goals for asthma telemedicine consultation. MDI, metered dose inhaler.

Treatment of gastroesophageal reflux

H_2 blocker

Patient education

Basic facts of asthma

Use of MDI

Use of spacer

Measurement of peak expiratory flow

Role of medications

Plan for management of asthma attacks

Next scheduled asthma teleconference date________________________

FIG. 42-4. *Continued.*

therapeutic plans, including properties of common drugs; staging asthmatic severity; peak flow use; and metered dose inhaler use.

PATIENT EDUCATION

A major feature of the NIH guidelines for asthma management is patient education. Again, videos should be developed by the allergy staff for this purpose. Features of this educational program include the basic facts of asthma, role of medications (e.g., quick-relief drugs versus long-term control drugs), use of devices (e.g., metered dose inhaler, spacer), measurement of peak flow, and a plan for management of asthma attacks. The value of peak flow measurement and adjustment of care accordingly has been demonstrated (13).

FACTORS TO MONITOR IN OUTCOMES

The follow-up instrument in Fig. 42-3 assesses asthma symptom severity, PEF, frequency of asthma attacks, visits to clinic or emergency department, and drug use.

It is likely that TDCJ's organized program will duplicate the findings of the free-world studies that have found that asthma management improves patient quality of life and reduces cost of care.

REFERENCES

1. Evans R. Epidemiology and natural history of asthma, allergic rhinitis, and atopic dermatitis. In: Middleton E, Reed C, Ellis E, et al., eds. *Allergy: principles and practice*, 4th ed. St. Louis: Mosby, 1993:1109–1136.
2. Bousquet J, Bullinger M, Fayol C, et al. Assessment of quality of life in patients with perennial allergic rhinitis with the French version of the SF-36 Health Status Questionnaire. *J Allergy Clin Immunol* 1994;94:182–188.

3. Bousquet J, Knani J, Dhivert H, et al. Quality of life in asthma. I. Internal consistency and validity of the SF-36 questionnaire. *Am J Respir Crit Care Med* 1994;149:371–375.
4. Sly RM, O'Donnell R. Stabilization of asthma. *Ann Allergy Asthma Immunol* 1997;78:347–354.
5. Panhuysen CI, Vonk JM, Koeter GH, et al. Adult patients may outgrow their asthma: as 25-year follow-up. *Amer J Respir Crit Care Med* 1997;155:1267–1272.
6. Puck JM. Primary immunodeficincy diseases. *JAMA* 1997;278:1835–1841.
7. National Institutes of Health. Expert panel report 2: guidelines for the diagnosis and management of asthma. NIH publication No. 97-4051, April 1997.
8. Spector SL, Nicklas RA, eds. Practice parameters for the diagnosis and treatment of asthma. *J Allergy Clin Immunol* 1995;96:707–870.
9. Laitinen LA, Laitinen A, Heino M, Haahtela T. Eosinophilic airway inflammation during exacerbation of asthma and its treatment with inhaled corticosteroid. *Am Rev Respir Dis* 1991;143:423–427.
10. Donahue JG, Weiss ST, Livingston JM, et al. Inhaled steroids and the risk of hospitalization for asthma. *JAMA* 1997;277:887–891.
11. Vollmer WM, O'Hollaren M, Ettinger KM, et al. Specialty differences in the management of asthma. A cross-sectional assessment of allergists' patients and generalists' patients in a large HMO. *Arch Int Med* 1997;157:1201–1208.
12. Storms B, Olden L, Nathan R, Bodman S. Effect of allergy specialist care on the quality of life in patients with asthma. *Ann Allergy Asthma Immunol* 1995;75:491–494.
13. Ignacio-Garcia JM, Gonzalez-Santos P. Asthma self-management eduction program by home monitoring of peak expiratory flow. *Am J Respir Crit Care Med* 1995;151:353–359.

Telemedicine: Practicing in the Information Age,
edited by Steven F. Viegas and Kim Dunn.
Lippincott–Raven Publishers, Philadelphia © 1998.

43

Hematology/Oncology

Sue Prill and Jack B. Alperin

Department of Oncology, University of Texas Medical Branch at Galveston, Galveston, Texas 77555; and Departments of Internal Medicine, Human Biological Chemistry and Genetics, and Pathology, University of Texas Medical Branch at Galveston, Galveston, Texas 77555

Patient access to appropriate healthcare has been a continuing problem in the United States. It has been difficult providing primary care physicians to rural or underpopulated areas. Rural areas are even more underserved by subspecialists who typically choose to live and work in university centers or areas of larger populations. Telemedicine has long been anticipated as the answer, at least in part, to the physician shortage in underserved areas (1). Some patients are not well served by this technology, while others are ideal for this mechanism. Additionally, there are other uses for telemedicine (such as continuing education) that are being investigated. Specialists in hematology/oncology have begun to explore the usefulness of telemedicine for their patient population (2,3). This chapter discusses some of the issues involved in using this technology and its applications in the specialty of hematology/oncology.

AREAS WELL SERVED BY TELEMEDICINE

There are specific groups of patients or patients in certain geographic areas that can be served by telemedicine.

Rural Areas

Patients who live in rural areas often are examined by primary care physicians who identify medical problems or diagnoses that require input, recommendations, treatment, or any combination of these that are directed by medical specialists (4). The specialists, however, often practice in university settings or metropolitan areas, possibly requiring that patients from rural areas travel great distances to see the specialist.

Prison Population

Inmates in prisons pose a unique set of problems because transportation to a specialist can be a major undertaking. Telemedicine can be a method to bring prison inmates before physicians. Many states are investigating the use of telemedicine in this population (5). This application may prove extremely useful given the problems of transportation, security, and other issues unique to a prison population.

Outlying Clinics

Many hematology and oncology practices have begun to address patient access problems by establishing outreach clinics, or extensions of the primary office (and personnel) to those areas with too few patients to justify a full-time hematologist/oncologist. These clinics are manned on specific days of the week or specified days in the month, depending on the number of patients and the staffing requirements for each clinic area. Telemedicine links can be used by the specialist to provide both patient follow-up and support or to give the local physician recommendations and options for care.

HEMATOLOGY/ONCOLOGY PATIENT TYPES

There are three types of patient situations that occur in the practice of hematology/oncology: new patients, follow-up patients, and acute problems.

New Patients

A new patient is usually a patient who has been examined by another physician and has an abnormality that is unexplained or has a diagnosed blood dyscrasia or cancer. Telemedicine can provide the initial encounter between the patient, the specialist, and the primary physician. This allows the hematologist/oncologist to guide the primary care doctor in obtaining the necessary tests or information needed to complete the diagnosis and initiate treatment. Thus, when the patient finally attends the hematology/oncology clinic, data are available to further manage the patient's problems.

Follow-up Patients

Patients who have been previously treated or are under treatment must be followed regularly for recurrence of disease or to evaluate the effectiveness of treatment. Telemedicine allows the primary physician and the specialist to see and evaluate the patient and review blood counts and other laboratory data so that further management can be planned.

Acute Problems

Patients with acute problems present to their local physician with new, unexpected complaints or symptoms that may be related to their blood dyscrasia or cancer signaling recurrent disease. Telemedicine provides a link between the provider and the specialist to assist quickly in appropriate triage of the patient.

SPECIFIC PATIENTS BY SPECIALTY

The following list contains some examples of the hematology/oncology diagnoses or problems that can be evaluated, managed, or both via telemedicine. Some of these patients may be seen initially via telemedicine with subsequent visits to the hematology/oncology clinic; others may be seen first in the clinic or hospital setting where treatment or recommendations are initiated and then followed subsequently via telemedicine.

- Hematology
  - Anemia
  - Thrombocytopenia
  - Bleeding disorders
  - Leukemia
  - Lymphoma
  - Myelodysplasia
  - Polycythemia
  - Nonmalignant leukocyte disorders
- Oncology
  - Carcinoma
  - Lymphoma
  - Chemotherapy-related leukopenia and thrombocytopenia
  - Hospice care
- Acute problems
  - New symptoms
  - New tumor masses
  - New lymphadenopathy

Problems that are not well served by telemedicine because of the need for immediate evaluation are as follows:

- Chest pain
- Acute neurologic changes
- Sudden changes in blood count

APPROPRIATE PATIENT EVALUATION VIA TELEMEDICINE

The use of telemedicine for evaluation of patients is attractive and can assist in better use of physicians and medical facilities by providing care to underserved patient groups; however, caution must be used in the establishment of this technology. There are patients who are well served by telemedicine and can benefit from its availability, but one must be aware that not all patients can be evaluated this way.

Physician Problems

Telemedicine does not give the physician the benefit of complete physical examination, and the specialist must often rely on another physician or a physician-extender to provide results of the physical examination. These observations may not be completely accurate, or they may include subjective assessments that differ from those of the specialist.

Patient Problems

Some patients are not comfortable with the new technology. This may limit the ability to obtain accurate medical information from patients because some may feel disconnected from the physician seen via telemedicine.

Telemedicine versus Real Time

Despite enthusiasm for this technology, there are situations in which the use of telemedicine is not appropriate. Telemedicine appointments are complicated due to the interaction of at least two physicians' schedules and the patient, the availability of telemedicine facilities, and the limitations of the encounter. Any situation in which delay may put the patient's life at risk, such as progressively worsening dyspnea, bleeding, anemia, or chest pain, must be evaluated immediately by a physician. Patients scheduled for certain types of treatment (e.g., chemotherapy, evaluation of intravenous access) should be seen by the specialist or specialist extender.

EDUCATIONAL USES OF TELEMEDICINE

In addition to the use of telemedicine in the evaluation and management of patients, the system can be used for educational purposes.

Patient Encounter

The local physician can participate in the evaluation of the patient via telemedicine and often does a limited physical examination under the direction of the specialist. In this way, the local physician is directly involved in the care of a patient that he or she would ordinarily refer to the specialist for care (6).

Lectures

Telemedicine can be used to provide lectures for small groups of physicians or their extenders. Grand rounds at an area university center could be transmitted to physicians in remote areas. Designated specialists could provide lectures on topics of interest such as anemia or pain control.

EVALUATION OF PATIENT VISIT

Evaluation of the effectiveness of the encounter should be undertaken by the patient, the primary care provider, and the specialist (7). Questions regarding the accessibility, cost, technical problems, and overall efficacy using this technology should be asked. After completion of these evaluations, there must be a mechanism for feedback, so that problems can be identified and adaptations made in future encounters.

ADVANTAGES OF THE USE OF TELEMEDICINE

Overall, the use of telemedicine has many advantages and few drawbacks to its use. There are obviously situations in which its use is not appropriate because of some limitations, but clearly it can provide a link that is often lacking between the patient and the physician today. Telemedicine is a technology whose time has come and will certainly see more use as availability increases.

Personnel Resources

Telemedicine allows for the management of many complicated subspecialty problems in geographic areas not normally serviced, as in rural areas or prisons. This benefits the specialist (who can provide medical services to more patients over a large area without spending a lot of time traveling), the patient (who is not required to travel long distances to see a specialist), and the primary care physician (who has access to consultation with specialists and educational opportunities).

Cost-effectiveness

Costly travel by the patient, the specialist, or both is eliminated. In some instances, arrangements can be made for necessary workup before the telemedicine appointment. This provides an opportunity to see the patient with the necessary information immediately available, rather than having two or more office appointments.

Triage

Telemedicine can provide an opportunity to identify those patients who need to travel to the specialist's office for more direct physician-specialist-patient encounters and those who do not.

REFERENCES

1. Perednia DA, Allen A. Telemedicine technology and clinical applications. *JAMA* 1995;273:4834–4888.
2. Doolittle GC, Allen A, Wittman C, Carlson E, Whitten P. Oncology care for rural Kansas via telemedicine: the establishment of a teleoncology practice [Abstract]. *Proc of ASCO* 1996;15:326.
3. Fintor L. Telemedicine: scanning the future of cancer control. *JNCI* 1993;85:183–184.
4. Pushkin D. Opportunities and challenges to telemedicine in rural America. *J Med Syst* 1995;19:59–67.
5. Appleby C. A prison plugs in. *Hosp Health Netw* 1995;69:56–58.
6. Swett HA, Holaday L, Leffell D, et al. Telemedicine: delivering medical expertise across the state and around the world. *Conn Med* 1995;59:593–602.
7. Bashur R. Telemedicine effects: cost, quality and access. *J Med Syst* 1995;19:81–91.

Telemedicine: Practicing in the Information Age,
edited by Steven F. Viegas and Kim Dunn.
Lippincott–Raven Publishers, Philadelphia © 1998.

44

Pediatrics

Sally Sue Robinson and Deborah E. Seale

Department of Pediatrics, University of Texas Medical Branch at Galveston, Galveston, Texas 77555; and East Texas Area Health Education Center, University of Texas Medical Branch at Galveston, Galveston, Texas 77555

The Special Services Division of the Department of Pediatrics at the University of Texas Medical Branch (UTMB) at Galveston and the Department of Nursing at Lamar University (LU) in Beaumont, Texas, have partnered to serve special-needs children via a telemedicine clinic.* Separated by a distance of approximately 80 miles, UTMB and LU are linked using high-speed telephone lines and two-way video/two-way audio conferencing technology. The patient, accompanying family members, and the presenting team in Beaumont are able to converse and visually interact with the evaluating team in Galveston. Thirty-four evaluations were completed involving 20 patients between October 15, 1996, and April 15, 1997. This service has been enthusiastically embraced by the evaluating team, the presenting team, and patients and their families. The first 6 months of clinic operations are reviewed, delineating the process used and an evaluation of the process.

CLINIC OPERATIONS

This section provides an overview of the UTMB/LU clinic operations at the presenting (patient) site and the evaluating (specialist) site. First, the clinic schedule is outlined, followed by a description of the patient population and the factors used to select patients for the telemedicine clinic. Second, the personnel required to support both sites is delineated. Specifications for the facilities along with the equipment and materials used at each site for the telemedicine application are discussed last.

Clinic Schedule

The first UTMB/LU clinic was held on October 15, 1996. The telemedicine clinic is scheduled for a 2.5 hour session twice a month, resulting in a total of 5 hours of

*In November of 1997, a second clinic was opened in Nacogdoches, Texas, through a partnership with Stephen F. Austin State University.

clinic per month. The first and third Tuesday afternoons of the month are reserved as the regular clinic times to assure the availability of the room and equipment well in advance. Approximately 30 to 45 minutes are scheduled for each patient evaluation, allowing three to four patients to be seen per session.

Patients

The patients being served by the UTMB Special Services Division are largely economically disadvantaged, of minority ethnicity, and between the ages of 3 weeks and 20 years. Their medical problems are severe, multiple, and frequently lifelong. When these children return home, they require extensive community support systems and intricate health-management plans. The Special Services Division provides services to more than 500 special-needs children in 34 counties throughout Texas.

Patients from this population were chosen for the telemedicine clinic based on two factors: They were geographically closer to the presenting site and they did not require any intervention that was too technical to be performed locally. Usually these patients are known to the evaluating team and are being followed for determination of progress and modification or qualification of recommendations.

Personnel

Presenting Site

The minimum number of persons at the presenting site is two: one to present or demonstrate the evaluation and one to direct the camera and the remote control. In addition, it is helpful to have another individual who assists in making appointments, greeting the patient, obtaining consents and vital signs, and placing the patient in the examining room. All personnel, medical or technical, should be reminded of their responsibility of confidentiality.

With the pediatric special-needs patient, the presenter should have the basic personality of adaptability and ease with children. It would be preferable that this individual have background training in pediatrics and in child development, but this is not an essential ingredient, because the process itself teaches both the medical and developmental aspects of the evaluation of these children. An additional benefit could be obtained if the presenter is the person caring for the child, such as the school nurse, the local primary care physician, or the office nurse, as there would be increased communication and teaching at that time. For billing purposes, it would be preferable that the presenter be licensed as a pediatric nurse practitioner, primary care physician, or physician's assistant. Of course, the presenter should be gentle, respectful, and maintain confidentiality. During the telemedicine evaluation the presenter is responsible for the following:

1. Facilitating the remote examination
2. Describing his or her findings on physical diagnosis

3. Manipulating the patient to demonstrate his or her particular physical problems so that the team can evaluate from a distance with a satisfactory degree of comfort and accuracy
4. Performing, under direction, the developmental evaluations thought to be indicated

Evaluating Site

The evaluating healthcare team includes a pediatrician with experience in rehabilitation and developmental problems, an occupational therapist, a physical therapist, a speech therapist, a dietitian, and, when appropriate, a psychologist or social worker. The day before each clinic session, the schedule of appointments is listed and the team predetermines which therapists need to be present at what time.

Nonhealthcare providers involved in clinic operations at the evaluating site include the appointment scheduler, the camera operator, and an operations researcher. The scheduler, who is the same for the telemedicine clinic as for the traditional clinic, does not attend clinic regardless of the venue. The protocol for notification, reminders, directions, and maps is the same as for the traditional clinic with one exception: If the appointment being scheduled is the patient's first visit to the telemedicine clinic, a brief explanation of the equipment, process, and travel savings is provided by a pediatric nurse practitioner or physician and willingness to participate is determined.

The camera operator at the evaluating site assures that the presenting site can see the evaluator on the screen at all times. The camera operator may be a member of the healthcare team or someone specifically assigned that responsibility.

The operations researcher works with the presenting and evaluating team to identify ways to enhance service delivery and to conduct research on the effectiveness of this mode of delivery.

Facilities, Equipment, and Materials

Presenting Site

The room at the presenting site should be big enough to hold three to six adults plus the patient and also have enough space to demonstrate gait. A room 25 ft in length is recommended. If the room is too large (e.g., an auditorium) the feeling of intimacy is destroyed. We have found in the UTMB/LU program that if the walls are painted a light blue, we are better able to see skin color and physical features. Some storage capacity is required to secure medical records and house testing materials. Although a sink is optimal for maintaining sanitary conditions, using any of the variety of hand wipes available is acceptable. Handicapped parking and facility access is essential. An area separate from the examination room that is suitable for intake, patient family waiting, and exit interviews is needed.

The only essential equipment in the room is a gurney and a floor mat. Due to the fragile nature of many special-needs patients, having a basic emergency code box available for stabilization while waiting for assistance if something unexpected happens is advised. A phone and facsimile are needed to transfer patient information and communicate with technical and clinical staff privately. The auxiliary camera facilitates capturing views of the patient from all angles and heights.*

In addition to the patient record and consent and exit interview forms, therapists in the UTMB/LU program have developed an evaluation kit composed of materials needed for the evaluations to be conducted by the presenter.

The following is a list of specifications for the presenting site:

Facilities
- Seating for three to six adults
- 15×25-ft room
- Light blue walls
- Storage capacity
- Sink or sanitary wipes
- 36-in. doorways
- Handicapped parking
- Waiting area

Equipment
- Gurney
- Floor mat
- Emergency code box
- Tabletop workspace
- Phone and facsimile
- Auxiliary camera

Materials
- Patient record
- Consent forms
- Exit interview forms

Testing and developmental tools
- Composite of: Revised Gesell Developmental Schedule and the Denver II
- Goniometers
- Cavicide (Metrex Research Corporation, Parker, CO)
- Vest with buttons and zippers
- Medium ball
- Pediatric stairs

Evaluating Site

The requirements at the evaluating site are minimal. The room should be large enough to seat six to eight adults, be relatively quiet, and have adequate air conditioning to handle the people and the television. Tabletop workspace, such as a conference table, is desired. A phone and facsimile are used by the evaluating team to receive and return phone calls from their home departments in an emergency, as well as to send or receive patient information from the presenting site.

---

*Specifications for the conferencing equipment and transmission facilities used at both sites are provided in Chapter 12.

The phone is also necessary as a backup for communications should there be problems with transmission or video equipment during the clinic. For this reason, the phone and fax machine should not be on the same transmission line as the video system.

The following is a list of specifications for the evaluating site:

Facilities
- Seating for three to six adults
- Tabletop workspace
- Private, quiet

Equipment
- Phone and facsimile
- Materials
- Patient record

Handling of Patient Records

The presenter has a copy of the last clinic visit that gives her or him demographic information, diagnosis, recent problems, and suggested solutions. The presenting location keeps that copy and adds the information from the clinic visit, which includes vital signs, updated demographics, local patient resources, and recommendations. No one has access to this information except the presenting team and the parent or guardian. The main medical record is kept at UTMB, which is a typed clinic note plus the written summary of the therapist's evaluation. This information is kept in the main medical record department and in a "shadow" file in the secretary's office. No one has access to the information except the evaluating team and the parent or guardian. UTMB/LU plans to tape the visits, on parental request, to document progress and to assist the parent with training of school personnel and local caregivers.

EVALUATION

During the first 6 months of the UTMB/LU program, ten of the thirteen sessions scheduled were completed (Table 44-1). Operating with limited core staff, three clinic sessions were canceled to allow for vacations, holidays, and spring break. There was no downtime due to technical failure. All sessions were held for the scheduled 2.5 hours, resulting in 25 hours of clinic operation.

Of the 36 appointments scheduled, 34 (94%) evaluations were completed involving 20 patients. The average length of the evaluations was 40 minutes.

The show rate remains extremely high as long as the family receives the appointment and understands the directions to the new clinic location. The ease of going to an appointment locally has increased the show rate. The typical show rate for a similar clinic session in Galveston is 75%.

No one invited to participate in telemedicine has declined. Half of the patients have returned for more than one visit, and 71% (24) of all visits involved return patients. No one who was asked to return for another visit refused.

TABLE 44-1. *Clinical statistics*

	Number	Percentage
Clinic sessions		
Sessions scheduled	13	100
Sessions completed	10	77
Hours in operation	25	100
Appointments		
Scheduled	36	100
Kept (i.e., show rate)	34	94
Average length in minutes	40	NA
Patients		
Total patients seen	20	100
One encounter only	10	50
More than one visit	10	50
Two visits	8	40
Three visits	0	0
Four visits	2	10

NA, not applicable.

All of the patients were seen as follow-up visits for existing, ongoing conditions. A list of diagnoses for the patients seen in the first 6 months is as follows:

Spina bifida
Spastic diplegia (cerebral palsy)
Status post (S/P) encephalopathy
S/P traumatic brain injury, attention deficit with hyperactivity
S/P premature birth, bronchopulmonary dysplasia
S/P traumatic brain injury
Anoxic encephalopathy
Congenital heart disease, failure to thrive, developmental delay
S/P gunshot wound to the head
Gastroschisis
Mental retardation (MR), porencephaly
Seizure disorder/MR
Attention deficit with hyperactivity
Bilateral femoral hypoplasia
Anoxic brain injury

The patients were all known to the evaluating team and were being followed for determination of progress and modification or qualification of recommendations.

Family, Caregiver, and Community Involvement

Because the distance is reduced, it is easier for both extended family members and local caregivers who help support the patient and family to attend the appointments. Being present during the patient evaluation helps answer questions and teaches the extended family about the special-needs child. In addition, community social and healthcare service providers, such as home health aides, physical therapists, and school nurses, have attended because it is a feasible distance. These providers have been able to discuss their concerns and obtain clarification about recommendations and treatment plans. The interaction between the evaluating team and the local caregivers has been invaluable in establishing a better treatment plan for the child.

Reactivity, Acceptance, and Satisfaction

There does not seem to be much need to explain the technology to the patient, his or her family, or to the other personnel that attend the appointment. The television is such a part of everyday life that it is not strange to have it talking and interacting with you. The children talk back and wave to the television as if the therapist were in the room. There does not seem to be a measurable difference with the interaction of the children and the therapists using the interactive television. Occasionally, younger children are too distracted by the television to perform the developmental tasks for evaluation, and occasionally the parents are shy of being on television.

Each parent or caregiver was asked to evaluate the experience based on comfort level, information obtained, time saved, and days off work saved. The response has been overwhelmingly positive. The single biggest item of satisfaction is the time saved for the families and caregivers. There have been no negative comments.

Effectiveness

The UTMB/LU evaluating team has found that occasionally some areas are difficult to evaluate, such as muscle tone. By observing the presenter's demonstration and listening to his or her interpretation of the experience, however, evaluators are able to determine adequately a decrease or increase in tone. There is also the difficulty of assessing the degree of contracture without the laying on of hands. Again, this limitation has been overcome with a degree of satisfaction and accuracy that is comfortable to the therapists by training the presenter to conduct the assessment and report his or her findings. Despite the limitations, the therapists' responses to telemedicine have been enthusiastic.

The evaluating team has been able to effectively evaluate progress, determine the need for a face-to-face clinic visit, give feedback from a psychological evaluation to a family, assist in following a behavioral feeder and giving the family reassurance, determine that new equipment for the patient is necessary, determine that new school placement may be needed, give information to the local healthcare team, and determine significant social or family problems.

Efficiency

For the evaluating team, it is more efficient to have the patient come to the traditional clinic setting where the team can rotate in and out of examination rooms seeing multiple patients in a short period. However, the benefits of family, caregiver, and community involvement are lost. This involvement could be maintained if the team traveled to the patient, but the time, distance, and low volume of patients at any one locale makes this solution prohibitive. If the pediatrician were to travel to see patients alone, the benefit of the input from the rest of the team would be lost. Unlike any other venue of service, the involvement of the entire healthcare team is coupled with the involvement of the family, caregivers, and community support network with telemedicine. With the team grouped together for the entire visit, the information shared between team members has increased communication and assisted in forming a consensus on the treatment plan. Similarly, interactions with the child, family, and community caregivers attending the clinic with the patient also influence the treatment plan. This interaction has been a very positive experience for the team and has stimulated a summation conference at the end of the traditional clinic, in which each team member typically evaluates separately. In addition, the interaction has been a positive experience for the patient, as the messages given are uniform, and the treatment plan is a consensual plan not only with the team but also with the local healthcare team and caregivers.

Obviously, the downside of this benefit to care is the relative inefficiency of all team members being present while the other is doing the evaluation. Table 44-2 provides the frequency of involvement in telemedicine visits by each of the team members. Some of the inefficiencies can be eliminated by planning before the conference which team members need to be present for the evaluation. For example, if there are no oral-motor problems, the speech therapist need not be present.

The inefficiencies of having multiple team members present are exacerbated when the patient is late or a "no show," the billable units are wasted for the entire team at both sites. Assisting the patient and his or her family with easy instructions, maps, telephone numbers, handicapped parking, and occasionally Medicaid transportation has facilitated UTMB/LU's high show rate and minimized the impact.

Because scheduling appointments is more complicated for telemedicine than a traditional clinic, inefficiencies arise here as well. As with any appointment, the scheduler must arrange for the availability of the patients and their families as well as the evaluating team. In addition, the presenting team must be available. Next, the rooms and equipment at both sites must be scheduled and adequate bandwidth on the transmission line must be reserved. For optimal evaluations, a minimum of 768 Kbps

TABLE 44-2. *Participation at the evaluating site*

Healthcare personnel	Number	Percentage of participation
Pediatrician	34	100.00
Nurse practitioner	32	94.00
Occupational therapist	34	100.00
Physical therapist	34	100.00
Speech therapist	30	88.00
Dietitian	34	100.00
Social worker	4	12.00
Psychologist	1	0.03

transmission speed is needed for the video system. However, the UTMB/LU system has functioned at 384 Kbps. The logistics of these arrangements can become complicated and require coordination at both sites. Setting a regular clinic schedule well in advance has simplified scheduling the rooms, video equipment, and bandwidth. Electronic mail has made scheduling between the healthcare teams at each site easier.

Role Shifts

As the UTMB/LU clinic matured, there were some slight shifts in the roles of the team members. The presenter is a pediatric nurse practitioner who has assumed a larger role in making appropriate referrals locally. After the evaluation, the presenter may assist in referrals to local primary care providers or social service agencies, then monitor patient follow-through. UTMB/LU has found that this has become a very important part of the visit. Once a new problem has been delineated during the evaluation, the presenter, who is much more familiar with the local resources, can facilitate the appropriate referrals and follow-up locally. The evaluating healthcare team could never provide this kind of patient advocacy from a distance.

Also, the information specialist who serves as the camera operator at the presenting site has become much more involved in patient evaluations. In addition to providing technical support, the information specialist has learned a great deal about multiple medical conditions and has felt a part of the medical team.

Finally, the evaluating team has worked together as an interdisciplinary team for years. In this format, they have become more like a transdisciplinary team. If a team that functioned as a multidisciplinary team were to begin this process anew, they would rapidly progress to an interdisciplinary approach.

Technology

Early in the process, it was observed that the UTMB/LU program needed two cameras to accurately assess the patients, particularly with gait and watching manipulation of objects by the child. So an auxiliary camera was added at the presenting site to supplement the camera attached to the videoconferencing equipment. The use of two cameras at the presenting site is a good example of the learning that is necessary for maximal equipment use when assessing the patient.

Although the single videoconferencing camera is sufficient at the evaluating site, we at UTMB/LU found support for camera operation was needed. Because the evaluators become too involved in the interaction to watch their position on the screen, we have found that it is helpful to have an individual who is not evaluating the patient directing and focusing the camera on the evaluator. Currently, a nurse practitioner has responsibility for operating the camera at the evaluating site. Perhaps once the evaluating team is trained in how to effectively use the camera to aid in patient evaluation for each discipline, the role of camera operator can be rotated among team members.

Although many peripherals are available to assist the subspecialist in his or her evaluations, the evaluation of children with special needs has not required special pieces of equipment such as otoscopes, ophthalmoscopes, or endoscopes. There are document cameras available that could view a radiograph or evaluate skin conditions closely. At this point, we have not used them. Written information to assist the patient or the presenter is faxed from site to site. Prescriptions are called in to the local pharmacy.

CONCLUSION

In summary, the first 6 months of UTMB/LU clinic operations showed many positive results. The patients and their families were unanimous in their enthusiasm for the reduction in distance traveled and the amount of time saved. Preliminary impressions indicate that the reduction in physical demands and stress placed on these fragile children and their accompanying guardian by the decreased travel has led to more effective patient evaluations. The attention spans and physical abilities of most of these children decline with the fatigue that often accompanies extended travel. Guardian attention and interaction can also be affected by the stress and fatigue associated with managing the needs of these children en route and during the "wait time" frequently associated with appointments at the traditional clinic. The higher no-show rate in the traditional clinic indicates that these barriers sometimes lead to the patient receiving limited or no follow-up care. In addition, participation by the local healthcare and social support agencies during the evaluation has led to more effective management of the patient's care locally. Similarly, having the evaluating team together in the room throughout the evaluation has led to a more coordinated treatment plan.

In the future, health outcome studies need to be conducted to measure short- and long-term recovery patterns of patients being cared for in the traditional clinic setting versus telemedicine. Also, at present, there are no specific practice guidelines for telemedicine consultation that differ from accepted rules of conduct and ethics. When reimbursement is established, there will undoubtedly be rules of referral and other established criteria.

Telemedicine: Practicing in the Information Age, edited by Steven F. Viegas and Kim Dunn.
Lippincott–Raven Publishers, Philadelphia © 1998.

45

Teleophthalmology

Bernard F. Godley, Helen K. Li, and Rosa A. Tang

Department of Ophthalmology and Visual Sciences, University of Texas Medical Branch at Galveston, Galveston, Texas 77555

Telemedicine can no longer be considered a technology in search of an application. With more than 30 years of evolution, telemedicine's role as a physician extender has been explored in military, space, prison, and rural medicine settings. There has been renewed interest in its applications in part due to advances in communications and computer technology and because of the potential to improve the efficiency of healthcare delivery, particularly in underserved populations. Telemedicine offers the promise of improved access to subspecialty consultation, and its feasibility in ear, nose, and throat; dermatology; and ophthalmology has been reported (1–3). The use of telemedicine for diagnosis and management of retinal diseases has previously been limited by technical difficulties in photographing the fundus and the acquisition, digitization, and recovery of high-resolution images diagnostically comparable to color photographs and patient and provider acceptance of the modality (3). Although real-time videoconferencing is preferable in some areas of telemedicine, such as acute care, the evaluation of high-quality still images, which have been acquired, transmitted, stored, and later reviewed, may leverage the specialist's time most effectively (4).

The University of Texas Medical Branch (UTMB) at Galveston provides tertiary healthcare for the Texas Department of Criminal Justice (TDCJ) prison system. One pilot study of retinal disease frequency and severity indicated that inmates with complications of trauma and diabetic retinopathy were among the most common reasons for referral to the UTMB retina subspecialty clinics for evaluation and treatment (5). The cost and difficulty of transporting shackled prisoners between the prison units and the UTMB/TDCJ tertiary care facility is unknown. A routine follow-up visit to the retina clinic can involve a multiday trip for an inmate with temporary stays in other prison units. In North Carolina's prison system, for example, the cost of transporting shackled prisoners to a tertiary care center averages $1,000 per day for a 1-day visit (1). In addition to cost, access is an issue as inmates often refuse to travel to UTMB, or appointments are missed due to complex travel and security considerations.

Whether teleophthalmology can improve the access and efficiency of retinal consultations in a large prison system remains to be seen. Initial studies on teleophthalmology consultation in civilian populations for retinal diseases have yielded promising results, although the medical peripherals presented some limitations. One study reported that although the fundus examination had good patient acceptance, 8% of patients complained of the bright lights needed for the photographic technique (2). Operation of the fundus camera was difficult to master, and the narrow field of view made interpretation of the fundus images difficult.

New technologies have the potential to supplant many of these problems. A new generation of nonmydriatic fundus cameras can provide high-resolution, wide-angle digital still images of the fundus, are technically easy to use, need lower light intensities, and do not require pupillary dilation. A study is under way using this nonmydriatic peripheral situated in a remote prison unit with an integrated service data network connection to UTMB to investigate the role of teleophthalmology in diagnosing diabetic retinopathy.

This chapter proposes clinical and informational guidelines for teleophthalmology consultation for retinal disorders with store and forward technology. This paradigm has been developed specifically for the correctional institution setting; however, the protocols are also applicable to the civilian setting with minimal modification. The protocols are designed to focus the remote health provider, the patient presenter, and the retina consultant on the pertinent clinical information required for an effective consultation.

PATIENT REFERRAL

Patients should be considered for retinal consultation using store-and-forward technology if they have a subacute or chronic retinal disease that does not require immediate or emergency evaluation. Symptoms and signs that herald a serious retina problem needing immediate evaluation include sudden loss of vision, pain, photopsias and floaters, visual field defect, and loss of red reflex. The ideal patients for teleophthalmology consultation are diabetic patients who have had an initial face-to-face evaluation at the retina clinic, who have been diagnosed with a stable level of nonproliferative diabetic retinopathy, and for whom subsequent follow-up has been arranged for several months to a year. A telemedicine consultation has the potential to substitute for one or more follow-up visits. Other appropriate referrals can include newly diagnosed diabetics or stable diabetics in whom a significant visual change has occurred. Although there is evidence to support the diagnostic value of telemedicine in the diagnosis of diabetic retinopathy, further studies are needed to substantiate its value in diagnosing other retina diseases and in the long-term management of diabetic retinopathy.

ROLE OF THE PATIENT PRESENTER

In the setting of a store and forward system, the presenter's role is to capture and transmit high-quality fundus images along with pertinent clinical information for storage and review by the consultant. The presenter should read a statement to the

Teleophthalmology Consultation Form
Retina Service

Patient name____

Visual acuity________OD______OS______

TDCJ #____

UH #____

Date____________________

Age_____Sex_____Race____Red reflex______OD______OS______

Chief complaint:____

____

____

____

Past medical history:

Diabetes	No_____Yes_____If yes, how long?________
Hypertension	No_____Yes_____
Elevated cholesterol	No_____Yes_____
Chronic renal failure	No_____Yes_____
Coronary artery disease	No_____Yes_____

Other diseases:______________________ Medications:______________________

Ocular history:______________________ Prior eye surgery or laser:____________

(Please fax the last two ophthalmology clinic notes, if present)

Consultant's report and recommendations:______________________________

____

____

____

Signature____

Follow-up: UTMB retina clinic____________Duration______________________

Teleophthalmology______________________________________

Diagnostic certainty (1–10)________________Image quality (1–5)______________

FIG. 45-1. An example of a teleophthalmology consultation form. TDCJ, Texas Department of Criminal Justice; UH, University of Houston; UTMB, University of Texas Medical Branch.

patient describing the teleophthalmology consultation and ask the patient to sign a consent form. The increasing availability of nonmydriatic cameras should make the technical aspects of photography much easier than was possible with previously available cameras. The new technology also obviates the need to perform pupillary dilation, which reduces the time of the consultation, improves patient comfort, and decreases the likelihood of iatrogenic complications.

CLINICAL DATA COLLECTION

Clinical data (Fig. 45-1) should be collected and sent digitally or by fax to be available to the consultant when the images are reviewed. Demographic information, chief complaint, past medical history, medications, and past ocular history, including prior surgery or laser treatments, are required, as well as visual acuity in both eyes and an assessment of media clarity. In addition, copies of the prior two consultations (if available) should be forwarded.

PROVIDER FEEDBACK

The signed consultant's report is sent to the remote care provider and to the patient's medical record. The consultant's report includes a diagnosis and recommendations for treatment and follow-up. Depending on the clinical findings, the con-

Teleophthalmology Evaluation Form

Retina Service

Patient name________________________

Date of consultation________________________

UHC #________________________

TDC #________________________

Age____________ Sex____________ Race____________

Provider satisfaction: Answer 1 (lowest) to 10 (highest) for the first three questions:

1. Was the consultation report returned in a timely fashion?_____
2. Did the consultation meet your expectations?_____
3. Did the consultation change or guide the patient's management?_____
4. Did the consultation replace a trip to the UTMB retina clinic? Yes_____ No_____

Patient satisfaction: (answer yes or no)

1. Was the examination comfortable?_____
2. Do you think that the concerns about your eye were adequately addressed?_____

FIG. 45-2. An example of a teleophthalmology evaluation form. UHC, University Hospital Clinic; TDC, Texas Department of Corrections; UTMB, University of Texas Medical Branch.

sultant may recommend that the patient be evaluated urgently or routinely in person at UTMB or that subsequent follow-up be done using teleophthalmology.

EVALUATION OF TELEOPHTHALMOLOGY CONSULTATION

The consultant's report includes an evaluation of photographic quality (see Fig. 45-1) and diagnostic certainty. Data on provider satisfaction with the teleophthalmology consultation process and the patient satisfaction rating is recorded (Fig. 45-2). A logbook of patient examinations should be kept at the examination site.

REFERENCES

1. Norton SA, Burdick AE, Phillips CM, Berman B. Teledermatology and underserved populations. *Arch Dermatol* 1997;133:197–200.
2. Crump WJ, Levy BJ, Billica RD. A field trial of the NASA telemedicine instrument pack in a family practice. *Aviat Space Environ Med* 1996;167:1080–1085.
3. Loshin DS, Caputo MP. Application of telemedicine in the diagnosis of posterior fundus ocular disease. *Invest Ophthalmol Vis Sci* 1995;36:S429.
4. Kvedar JC, Edwards RA, Menn ER, et al. The substitution of digital images for dermatologic physical examination. *Arch Dermatol* 1997;133:161–167.
5. Kapoor S, Khorrami A, Syblik D, Freeman D, Godley BF. Spectrum of retinal diseases in a prison population. *Invest Ophthalmol Vis Sci* 1998;39:S846.

Telemedicine: Practicing in the Information Age,
edited by Steven F. Viegas and Kim Dunn.
Lippincott–Raven Publishers, Philadelphia © 1998.

46

Establishment of Telemedicine as an Integral Component in the Evaluation and Care of Neurosurgical Patients in the Texas Department of Criminal Justice Hospital

Jeff W. Chen

Department of Surgery, University of Texas Medical Branch at Galveston, Galveston, Texas 77555

The neurosurgery service at the University of Texas Medical Branch (UTMB) at Galveston became involved in the telemedicine program for the evaluation and care of patients in the Texas Department of Criminal Justice (TDCJ) system in February 1996. Protocols were developed for the referral of patients to the Neurosurgery Telemedicine Clinic. All patients who could normally be seen by the traditional clinics were candidates for telemedicine evaluations. These patients included new consultations, clinic and hospital follow-ups, and postoperative follow-ups. Emergency neurosurgical problems were excluded from telemedicine evaluations. Teleconferencing was used to train the presenters at the distant site in the neurologic examination. This allowed for the consistent communication of neurologic findings to the neurosurgeons in Galveston. The establishment of telemedicine as an integral component of the neurosurgery service's care and treatment of TDCJ patients is described in this chapter.

BACKGROUND

The telemedicine system was established in the TDCJ by UTMB to facilitate the healthcare of prison inmates in 1993. The neurosurgical services became involved with the use of telemedicine in the evaluation of neurosurgical patients in February 1996.

Surveys of neurosurgical practices in the United States have found that, in most general neurosurgery practices, 70% to 80% of cases deal with the spine and peripheral nerves, while the remaining 20% to 30% deal with cranial problems (1). The TDCJ neurosurgical cases fit a similar profile (2). The majority of the TDCJ neurosurgical clinic patients have neck, back, or peripheral nerve problems. Hence, the long bus rides across Texas to UTMB in Galveston are not appreciated and often exacerbate the pain. Telemedicine evaluations allow the rapid and efficient triaging of neurosurgical patients. This has the potential to increase compliancy and decrease the "no-show" rate.

Neurosurgical evaluations have traditionally carried a certain mystique of complexity. This mystique may lead to a certain reluctance on the part of distant presenters to evaluate patients by telemedicine because of a difficulty in communicating findings. To obviate such perceptions about neurosurgical patients, UTMB established guidelines for which patients to include and exclude for telemedicine evaluations. Distance learning using telemedicine was performed to train the distant presenters in the neurologic examination. An abbreviated neurologic examination was established for the purpose of telemedicine evaluations.

METHODS

Equipment

The telemedicine setups and the peripherals available at the distant prison sites have been described previously in Chapters 12–14 (2). The neurosurgery service used the existing systems without modifications.

Selection of Patients for Telemedicine

Table 46-1 outlines UTMB's inclusion and exclusion criteria for neurosurgery evaluations via telemedicine. Neurosurgical emergencies with a rapid change in neurologic or mental status were evaluated in nearby emergency rooms for stabilization and treatment. Some were eventually transferred to UTMB. All new consultations, hospital, clinic, and postoperative follow-ups were candidates for telemedicine. There were some limitations on which patients could be seen by telemedicine, depending on the location of the patient's unit relative to a telemedicine site.

TABLE 46-1. *Inclusion and exclusion criteria for neurosurgery telemedicine patients*

- Telemedicine clinic evaluations
  - Stable neurologic examination
  - Back and leg pain
  - Neck and arm pain
  - Carpal tunnel, ulnar nerve compression
  - Postoperative checks
- Emergency room evaluations
  - Acute trauma (cranial or spinal)
  - New neurologic deficits or mental status changes
  - Newly diagnosed brain or spine tumor
  - Aneurysmal subarachnoid hemorrhage
  - Intracranial hemorrhage

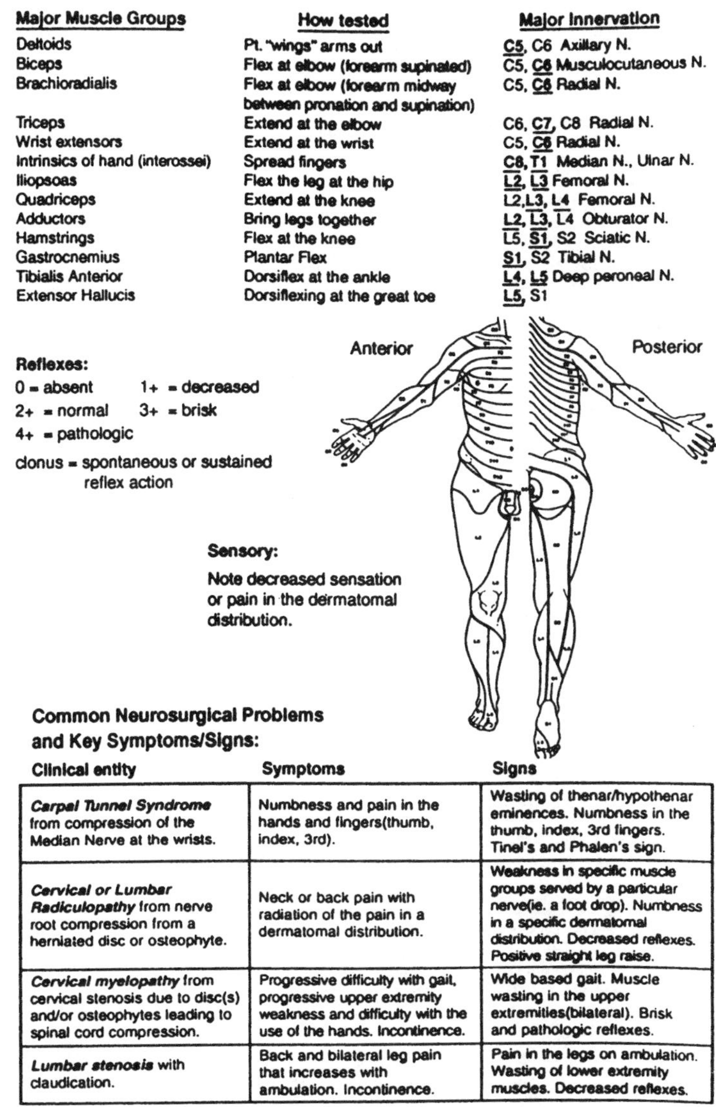

Major Muscle Groups	How tested	Major Innervation
Deltoids	Pt. "wings" arms out	C5, C6 Axillary N.
Biceps	Flex at elbow (forearm supinated)	C5, C6 Musculocutaneous N.
Brachioradialis	Flex at elbow (forearm midway between pronation and supination)	C5, C6 Radial N.
Triceps	Extend at the elbow	C6, C7, C8 Radial N.
Wrist extensors	Extend at the wrist	C5, C6 Radial N.
Intrinsics of hand (interossei)	Spread fingers	C8, T1 Median N., Ulnar N.
Iliopsoas	Flex the leg at the hip	L2, L3 Femoral N.
Quadriceps	Extend at the knee	L2, L3, L4 Femoral N.
Adductors	Bring legs together	L2, L3, L4 Obturator N.
Hamstrings	Flex at the knee	L5, S1, S2 Sciatic N.
Gastrocnemius	Plantar Flex	S1, S2 Tibial N.
Tibialis Anterior	Dorsiflex at the ankle	L4, L5 Deep peroneal N.
Extensor Hallucis	Dorsiflexing at the great toe	L5, S1

Reflexes:

0 = absent 1+ = decreased

2+ = normal 3+ = brisk

4+ = pathologic

clonus = spontaneous or sustained reflex action

Sensory:

Note decreased sensation or pain in the dermatomal distribution.

Common Neurosurgical Problems and Key Symptoms/Signs:

Clinical entity	Symptoms	Signs
Carpal Tunnel Syndrome from compression of the Median Nerve at the wrists.	Numbness and pain in the hands and fingers(thumb, index, 3rd).	Wasting of thenar/hypothenar eminences. Numbness in the thumb, index, 3rd fingers. Tinel's and Phalen's sign.
Cervical or Lumbar Radiculopathy from nerve root compression from a herniated disc or osteophyte.	Neck or back pain with radiation of the pain in a dermatomal distribution.	Weakness in specific muscle groups served by a particular nerve(ie. a foot drop). Numbness in a specific dermatomal distribution. Decreased reflexes. Positive straight leg raise.
Cervical myelopathy from cervical stenosis due to disc(s) and/or osteophytes leading to spinal cord compression.	Progressive difficulty with gait, progressive upper extremity weakness and difficulty with the use of the hands. Incontinence.	Wide based gait. Muscle wasting in the upper extremities(bilateral). Brisk and pathologic reflexes.
Lumbar stenosis with claudication.	Back and bilateral leg pain that increases with ambulation. Incontinence.	Pain in the legs on ambulation. Wasting of lower extremity muscles. Decreased reflexes.

FIG. 46-1. The University of Texas Medical Branch (UTMB) at Galveston guide to neurosurgical evaluation. This is general information on the neurologic examination that has been imprinted on two sides of a 4×6-in. card. The UTMB guide was distributed to the presenters at the distant sites to allow easy reference. The guide facilitates communication between the distant presenters and the neurosurgeons at UTMB. HX, history; HTN, hypertension; DM, diabetes mellitus; TB, tuberculosis; IVDA, intravenous drug abuse; HIV+, human immunodeficiency virus positive.

THE UNIVERSITY OF TEXAS
MEDICAL BRANCH at GALVESTON

NEUROSURGERY TELEMEDICINE EXAMINATION

Pertinent HX: Chief Complaint

CHARACTERIZATION OF SYMPTOMS
—PAIN(Localization, Radiation, Duration, Exacerbating/Relieving Factors)
—WEAKNESS(Localization, Exacerbating/Relieving Factors)
MEDICAL PROBLEMS(ie. HTN, DM, TB, Sickle Cell, IVDA, HIV+)
MEDICATIONS
PRIOR SURGERIES (Especially for the Same Complaint)

Mental Status Examination:

-GENERAL ALERTNESS
-ORIENTED TO PERSON, PLACE, TIME
-APPROPRIATE RESPONSES
-FOLLOWS COMMANDS

Glasgow Coma Score (GCS=E+V+M [3-15])

Eyes (E)		Verbal (V)		Motor (M)	
-Spontaneously open	4	-Oriented	5	Obeys commands	6
-Opens to voice	3	-Confused speech	4	Localizes to pain	5
-Opens to pain	2	-Inappropriate speech	3	Withdraws to pain	4
-No opening of eyes	1	-Incompr. Sounds	2	Flexes to pain	3
		-No Sounds	1	Extends to pain	2
				No movement	1

Physical Examination:

Pupils: Size, Reactivity, Asymmetry, Irregularity
Cranial Nerves:
I: Smell: test ability to smell coffee grounds/mints
II: Vision: test visual acuity with chart; visual fields
III: Pupillary reactivity; signs of ptosis; look up/down/medial
IV: Look down and medial
VI: Look lateral
V: Motor: clench teeth; Sensory: over forehead, maxilla, jaw
VII: Motor: symmetry in raising eyebrows, closing eyes
VIII: Auditory: Ability to hear bilaterally
IX-X: Palatal sensation; gag reflex
XI: Shoulder shrug
XII: Tongue movement-note deviation to one side
Extraocular Movements: conjugate, smooth, any nystagmus?

Motor Exam:

—Visual inspection for signs of muscle wasting, asymmetry, fasciculations
—Grading of muscle strength:
5=normal strength 4=nearly normal but there is giveaway(may grade further as 4- or 4+)
3=anti-gravity strength only (unable to give any resistance)
2=movement with gravity eliminated 1=flicker of movement 0=no movement

Pupil Gauge (mm)

2 3 4 5 6 7 8 9

FIG. 46-1. *Continued*

Training of Distant Presenters

A brief introduction to the neurologic examination with particular emphasis on the testing of different muscle groups and reflexes was distributed to physician's assistants and nurses who were the examiners at the distant sites. This served as a template for the information database on each neurosurgical patient. An example of the UTMB guide to the neurosurgical evaluation is presented in Fig. 46-1. Using the telemedicine system, teleconferencing with the examiners was done. This allowed interactions between the distant presenters and the UTMB neurosurgeon that improved their comfort in communicating their findings from the neurosurgical examination.

RESULTS

From February 1996 to February 1997, 81 neurosurgical evaluations were conducted in the TDCJ using telemedicine. The distribution of problems evaluated is depicted in Table 46-2. The clinical problems encountered are grouped according to whether they are referable to the neck (cervical spine), back (lumbar spine), peripheral nerve (carpal tunnel or ulnar neuropathy), or to a brain tumor. Clinical problems under the miscellaneous category included patients evaluated for minor head injury, possible ventriculoperitoneal shunt problems, or skull defects. The distribution of cases seen parallels that seen in a general neurosurgery practice (1). Table 46-3 demonstrates the distribution of the clinical encounters. A significant number of the visits (31%) were for postoperative wound checks and routine postoperative assessment of the patient's neurologic function. As in free-world practice, postoperative patients were routinely seen 7–10 days after surgery for suture or staple removal and a wound check, and subsequently at 6 weeks postoperatively.

Careful tutoring of the examiners at the far end allowed the detection of neurologic signs that had significance in the patient treatment algorithm. Examples include pathologic reflexes, wasting of muscle groups, Tinel's sign, and Phalen's sign. The far-end cameras allowed the evaluation of postoperative wounds.

TABLE 46-2. *Distribution of clinical problems*

Clinical problem	Number of patients (percentage of total)
Cervical spine	28 (34.6)
Lumbar spine	21 (25.9)
Brain tumor	14 (17.3)
Peripheral nerve	10 (12.3)
Miscellaneous	8 (9.9)
Total	81 (100)

TABLE 46-3. *Types of clinical encounters*

Type of clinical encounter	Number of patients (percentage of total)
Initial visit	16 (20)
Clinic follow-up	40 (49)
Postoperative follow-up (within 90 days of surgery)	25 (31)
Total	81 (100)

All of the distant telemedicine units were equipped with the ability to obtain routine spine x-rays. These "hard-copy" images can be viewed by the neurosurgeon at UTMB by having the distant presenter place the x-rays on the viewbox or the document camera.

CONCLUSION

Careful tutoring of examiners at the distant sites has allowed the neurosurgical evaluation of patients via telemedicine at UTMB. This is a useful adjunct to the "hands-on" clinic visit. The patients are more likely to be compliant when they do not need to travel such long distances.

REFERENCES

1. Pevehouse BC, Gary Siegel Organization, Inc., eds. *1995 Comprehensive neurosurgical practice survey.* Park Ridge, IL: The American Association of Neurological Surgeons and Congress of Neurological Surgeons, 1996.
2. Chen JW. Tele-neurosurgery. *Telemed Today* 1997;Jan/Feb:16.

Telemedicine: Practicing in the Information Age,
edited by Steven F. Viegas and Kim Dunn.
Lippincott–Raven Publishers, Philadelphia © 1998.

47

Orthopedics

Stanley D. Allen and Emmie H. Ko

Department of Orthopaedics and Rehabilitation, University of Texas Medical Branch at Galveston, Galveston, Texas 77555; and Department of Orthopaedic Surgery, University of Texas Medical Branch at Galveston, Galveston, Texas 77555

WHO CAN BE SEEN WITH TELEMEDICINE?

Consultations requiring orthopedic care can be divided into three categories: (a) new patients, (b) established patients, and (c) emergency consultations. Established patients consist of those undergoing conservative management and those requiring postoperative follow-up. The multitude of patients' chief complaints are varied and can range from a simple, mildly sprained ankle to a complex, previously operated lumbar spine. The telemedicine program at the University of Texas Medical Branch (UTMB) at Galveston and the Texas Department of Criminal Justice (TDCJ) is used for orthopedic conditions involving the spine, hip, knee, shoulder, elbow, hand, foot, and ankle. Many disorders seen have distinct visual characteristic appearance and can be diagnosed with simple diagnostic tests. This is especially true for much of the hand disorders seen.

New Patients

New patients in the UTMB/TDCJ telemedicine program undergo an interactive consultant-patient consultation starting with a routine orthopedic history and physical examination facilitated by the primary care physician (PCP) at the remote site. Inmates are screened to eliminate unnecessary travel to Galveston and those not requiring specialty management by the orthopedist. Examples of patients who are screened and have an elective surgical problem but do not wish to have surgery include patients with bunions, claw or hammer-toe deformities, ganglion cysts, mild malunions, and osteoarthritis of the hip or knee.

New patients who have a disorder that deserves a trial of conservative management of nonsteroidal antiinflammatory medication, physical therapy, or both, which is available nearby to their home site, become established patients. The remainder of patients fall into the category of needing special procedures, further investigation, inpatient intervention, or surgery. Commonly encountered situations requiring transport to Hospital Galveston (HG) include disorders not amenable to diagnosis via telemedicine and disorders requiring casting; joint aspiration; steroid injections; and radiographic studies such as magnetic resonance imaging, computed tomography, and myelograms. Disorders that are not easily diagnosed via telemedicine frequently involve the knee, either because the remote presenter is unfamiliar with aspects of a knee examination or the result of such examinations consists of a subjective feel of laxity (e.g., Lachman test for anterior cruciate ligament insufficiency).

For many patients, an evaluation over telemedicine pinpoints a specific diagnosis and identifies whether the patient desires surgery and the scheduling of surgery. When the patient is then transported to HG, one simply confirms the diagnosis, answers further questions regarding the surgery, and obtains informed consent.

The ability to feel confident about decisions made strictly based on a telemedicine evaluation is dependent on several factors: (a) the experience of the consultant, (b) the experience of the remote presenter, and (c) the quality of the equipment.

Established Patients

The follow-up of uncomplicated surgical procedures is one of the most effective and cost saving uses of telemedicine. Surgical incisions can be inspected, and joint range of motion can be easily demonstrated via telemedicine. Suture or skin staples can then be instructed to be removed by the presenter at the remote site. Additionally, if radiographs and casting are available at the remote site, the monitoring of fracture healing can be done effectively. The decision when to remove or replace casts and when to begin weightbearing or range of motion exercises can be made without the patient traveling. Similarly, monitoring interval progress, or the lack of interval progress, in patients undergoing physical therapy can be done entirely via telemedicine. At any time that the patient is not exhibiting interval progress, therapy can be changed, surgery can be planned, or arrangements to have the patient evaluated at HG can be made.

Emergency Patients

Evaluation of emergencies is an area in which telemedicine can have a significant impact. Having a specialist available would be of benefit to the primary practitioner in any situation. The ability to see the patient and his or her injury would give the specialist more information on which to make his or her recommendation.

Telemedicine can be used as a triage tool. The decision about where and in what time frame the patient should receive treatment would be an ideal use of this technology. For limb-threatening injuries (e.g., knee dislocation), immediate transport to the nearest emergency room would be required. For less severe but nevertheless emergent cases (e.g., minimally displaced hip fracture), immediate transport to Galveston via ambulance would be indicated. For less severe injuries (e.g., minimally displaced closed wrist or finger fracture), splinting and referral to Galveston the next day or next clinic should be safe and cost effective. These decisions would be better made by an orthopedic surgeon than a nurse who has minimal experience in bone or joint injuries and is usually available at night on the unit.

Through telemedicine, the consultant can assist the healthcare provider who may not be comfortable with orthopedic injuries. If necessary, he or she could direct the PCP on appropriate initial management by knowing what to look for (e.g., compartment syndrome) or what type of immobilization should be used (e.g., splint, traction).

REMOTE SITE

Different tools than other fields of medicine are used for the evaluation and treatment of orthopedic patients. Although orthopedists do not need stethoscopes or otoscopes that can transmit signal, there are items that are unique to the specialty.

Radiographs

Other physicians use radiographs for diagnosis and to follow treatment, but no specialist is as dependent on viewing the actual radiographs as orthopedists. The remote site must have the facilities to view radiographs and ideally the capacity to produce new studies in a timely manner. The technology available today allows the interpretation of most films, and the availability of this degree of technology is essential for an orthopedic telemedicine consultation.

Ambulation

UTMB orthopedists did not realize how important watching a patient walk was until they could not view this at the remote site. It is important that during design and development of the remote site there is an adequate walkway area and that the cameras are positioned so that the consultant can view at least several steps.

Casting

If one wants to use video medicine to follow patients postoperatively or to follow the healing of fractures, there should be the means to remove and apply splints and casts. The provider at the remote site must be trained in the removal and especially the application of casts if he or she is going to be required to do this.

Dressing Changes and Suture Removal

Likewise, if postoperative care is to be provided through video, there must be the capability of changing dressings and removing sutures.

REMOTE PRESENTER

The success of orthopedic telemedicine can be significantly altered by whether the presenter or PCP at the remote site is well trained. This is especially true in the field of orthopedics. The PCP must know how to perform an examination of the extremities and a basic neurologic examination, be versed in many of the terms used by orthopedists (e.g., *varus*, *valgus*, *proximal*, *distal*), and sometimes perform special examinations (e.g., anterior drawer, Lachman test). In many cases, the consultant is dependent on the opinions of the remote presenter, and the subspecialist must have confidence in his or her physical examination skills. The ideal individual as remote presenter would be a physician assistant who is interested in and has been trained in the evaluation of bone and joint problems.

PRESENTATION

How the patient is presented in telemedicine depends on the consultant's preference. Many of our nonorthopedic colleagues at UTMB want the remote presenter to obtain the basic history of the illness along with medication, allergies, and so on and show the consultant the pertinent physical findings. The consultant may ask for further information or a specific examination. We have opted to obtain the information from the patient and direct the physical examination as indicated. As the remote presenters become more comfortable and proficient in orthopedic evaluation, having the remote presenter obtain the basic history will enhance clinic efficiency.

Telemedicine: Practicing in the Information Age,
edited by Steven F. Viegas and Kim Dunn.
Lippincott–Raven Publishers, Philadelphia © 1998.

48

General Surgery Telemedicine

Thomas A. Broughan and Sally Abston

Department of Surgery, University of Oklahoma Health Science Center, Tulsa, Oklahoma 74129; and Department of Surgery, University of Texas Medical Branch at Galveston, Galveston, Texas 77555

For the Division of General Surgery at the University of Texas Medical Branch (UTMB) at Galveston, telemedicine is used solely in the care of the ever-growing Texas prison population, which encompasses some 134,000 inmates currently. Telemedicine allows the general surgeon to visit multiple prison unit infirmaries at the press of a button. It is appreciated that the constraints of having a jailed patient population stifle some of the potential that telemedicine could offer. In its present form, telemedicine for the general surgeon is most often applied for diagnosis and postoperative follow-up during a weekly clinic. Some triage of surgical acuity is conducted at this time as well. Finally, a small amount of treatment is undertaken, predicated by the level of training of the staff at the other end of the monitor.

USES OF TELEMEDICINE

Diagnosis

Telemedicine has proved useful at UTMB for diagnosing superficial conditions that can be readily seen on a monitor. These conditions include various subcutaneous masses and soft tissue infections. It is important that the examining camera be mobile and flexible to observe patients in a variety of body positions. Recessed anatomic areas and darker skin tones can challenge the resolution of the camera lighting apparatus. General surgical conditions are more visual than auditory (also available via telemedicine). However, the second valuable sense in general surgery, palpation, is not yet available through telemedicine.

Triage

Triage is another potentially valuable use for telemedicine in general surgery. Currently in the Texas Department of Criminal Justice (TDCJ), a single general surgery clinic is held weekly. Patients whose acuity of illness allows are deferred to the weekly clinic, while others are brought hundreds of miles to the UTMB emergency room for evaluation. If the telemedicine facilities were available at all hours, on-call personnel could determine which patients could be treated locally, deferred to a scheduled clinic, or brought to the emergency room. One would need to judge if the resources required to provide 24-hour telemedicine coverage would be worthwhile in terms of patient care and cost.

Postoperative Follow-up

Postoperative follow-up has emerged as one of the most significant telemedicine uses for general surgery. The surgeon-patient relationship has already been established. The operation and immediate postoperative care have been conducted in the home hospital. Protocols can be developed for history and physical examination on the postoperative patient via telemedicine that obviate a long-distance return trip to the surgeon. In fact, follow-up can be more frequent. Patients participating in clinical trials can have ongoing laboratory work and examinations. Minor complaints and wound problems can be satisfactorily addressed long distance, and patients with more significant problems can be triaged to the outpatient facility or the emergency room.

STAFF TRAINING

Much of what can be accomplished in telemedicine depends on the level of training and the eagerness of the healthcare person to participate with whom the telemedicine surgeon is interacting. The remote healthcare provider has the better opportunity to obtain a brief history and vital signs. Before the onscreen telemedicine visit, protocols can be developed to ensure collection of data. The telemedicine staff should be enthusiastic about working with the camera and lighting until the telemedicine surgeon can adequately see the pathology. The remote healthcare provider should be able to perform basic physical examinations such as a hernia or abdominal examination. The staff member becomes the surgeon's hands in the telemedicine encounter and can be a nurse or a physician's or surgeon's assistant. One might also envision the general surgeon interacting with a family medicine physician or internal medicine specialist as a consultant.

The issue of performing procedures at the far end of the telemedicine circuit is likely to be more complicated. The person performing the procedure must be qualified, and credentialing and the issuance of privileges must be properly undertaken. It would be difficult for the surgeon to be responsible long distance for the conduct of a telemedicine procedure. This was not an issue originally foreseen by the American College of Surgeons' proscription on itinerant surgery, but the surgeon's responsibility for procedures conducted at a distance from his or her home hospital will likely require resolution.

The treatment arm of telemedicine for surgery may have great growth potential but is now currently limited by the level of training of the person with the patient. Because nurses and physician's assistants are used, UTMB surgeons have been able to obtain suture and skin staple removal, incision and drainage of superficial abscesses, ordering of blood work and x-rays, and dispensation of medications (e.g., antibiotics) for superficial soft tissue or wound infections via telemedicine. Eventually, digitization of imaging and transmission of endoscopy and laparoscopy will allow the telemedicine general surgeon to be more actively involved in a patient's care. Virtual surgery is in the development phases in the military, but its civilian application may be more limited due to ethical and legal reasons.

CONCLUSION

The telemedicine experience in general surgery for the TDCJ has only scratched the surface of the potential for this modality. Its further development will depend on organization, need, cost, technology, resolution of licensure and credentialing issues, and perhaps further refinement of the principles of itinerant surgery. Telemedicine is of particular use for preoperative screening of superficial, straight-forward surgical conditions and postoperative follow-up of many conditions. Acute surgical conditions could be increasingly triaged through telemedicine if the staffing and expense of 24-hour availability are reasonable. Telemedicine challenges the surgeon to practice without the sense of touch, and it is interesting to explore the importance of touch in a variety of clinical situations. The role of telemedicine in general surgery is very much under investigation, and this report can only be considered preliminary.

Telemedicine: Practicing in the Information Age,
edited by Steven F. Viegas and Kim Dunn.
Lippincott–Raven Publishers, Philadelphia © 1998.

49

Plastic Surgery and Telemedicine

John S. Mancoll and Linda G. Phillips

Department of General Surgery, University of Texas Medical Branch at Galveston, Galveston, Texas 77555

Telemedicine is an evolving technology designed to assist physicians and patient caregivers in delivering healthcare to patients at a remote site. In its most simplistic form, telemedicine is a way of providing patient information between healthcare providers who are physically separated from the patient. The transfer of information could include a thorough history and physical, laboratory results, x-ray results, and even photographic images as today's technology is evolving.

Plastic surgery is a "specialized field of surgery concerned with the repair of deformities and the correction of functional deficits" (1). Surgeons for centuries have documented patient problems with detailed drawings outlining their surgical procedures and transferring this information amongst their colleagues. In more modern times, the telephone has been the centerpiece of communication between primary care providers and their consultants. Plastic surgeons are frequently asked to help manage difficult patient problems over the telephone. Based on the description of the problem, plastic surgeons are asked to suggest intermediate care and assess the urgency in which the patient should be seen by the specialist. The obvious limitations of an "audio only" form of telecommunication system is that it relies heavily on the subjective assessment of the referring physician. Often, the referring physician is uneasy or unfamiliar with the problem that he or she is confronting, and therefore accurate transfer of information about the patient's problem is difficult. Many patients who are referred to a plastic surgeon have long-standing, non–life-threatening medical problems and immediate consultation is not usually necessary.

In more recent years, this audio-only form of communication has been supplemented with photographs and whatever additional information can be sent by fax. Today, it is possible to fully evaluate the plastic surgery patient via telemedicine with information that includes detailed history and physical, x-rays, laboratory studies, and anatomic-specific photographs (both still life and real-time video). The obvious advantage of this modern technology is more accurate assessment of the patient problem and perhaps the ability to manage these problems from a remote site. Thus, not every patient now needs to be referred to a tertiary care center or to the plastic surgeon's office for treatment of his or her problem. This potential shift to managing patients in this manner should not be difficult for most plastic surgeons, because they have been providing patient care by a less formal but similar means for years.

SYSTEM REQUIREMENTS

The plastic surgery patient usually has problems that can be seen on the surface. This characteristic makes remote physical examinations easy to perform. The successful evaluation of patients via telemedicine requires the system to enable the consulting physician to see accurate colors on the video monitor. Therefore, anything that would cause shadowing or distortion of the colors of the skin would give a false impression to the examiner. Although medical peripheries exist for performing dermatologic examinations, these tend to only enable the physician to do close-up evaluation. Although this form of examination is highly detailed, it tends to be awkward and unnatural. But medical peripherals are being developed that will offer a more global view of skin lesions. In many cases, plastic surgeons remove moles or other types of lesions from the skin regardless of their color. Either the location of the lesion is a problem for the patient or the other characteristics warrant removal. This technology can enable the surgeon to understand the location and size of the lesion and still make surgical plans.

The medical peripherals needed for the physical examination of plastic surgical patients are not unique to plastic surgery. The presently available otoscope can be used for examining the oral and nasal cavities. To evaluate the septum or other more posterior nasal or pharyngeal structures, flexible endoscopy equipment can be used. Ophthalmologic examinations with the telemedicine ophthalmoscope, slit lamp, or both can be used for evaluation of the orbital contents.

In patients being referred because a bony injury has been suspected, digital x-rays or standard radiographic studies can be done. These images can then be forwarded to the consulting surgeon. If standard radiographs are done, these images can be scanned, and the scanned images forwarded. If digital radiograph technology exists at the institution, the digital image can be forwarded. Therefore, accurate preoperative assessment and operative planning of fractures can be done based on this information. All subsequent postoperative visits, including both physical examination and radiographic studies, can also be managed in this way.

The most important component for successful telemedicine evaluation of plastic surgery is the adequate training of the presenter at the remote site. It may be unnecessary for a physician to present the patient if a physician's assistant or qualified nurse can be adequately trained. To help facilitate this evaluation, it is recommended that a set of problem-driven protocols be used to help in the assessment and history-taking process. This information can be forwarded to the consulting physician before either the live video examination or as part of the stored and forwarded consultation. The training of the remote site person can be via on-site training, through videotaped sessions, or in the live session, having the consulting physician demonstrate which examination maneuver he or she would like performed. Although telemedicine evaluation processes may initially be cumbersome and time consuming, as this technology is further used, the expedition of telemedicine will improve as the experience of the presenter increases.

USES AND LIMITATIONS OF TELEMEDICINE FOR PLASTIC SURGERY

In general, all plastic surgery patients are candidates for telemedicine; however, because plastic surgery is such a broad field, some areas are more conducive than others. Plastic surgeons, by definition, operate on all areas of the body. The discipline of plastic surgery incorporates multiple, recognized, subspecialty areas. These include aesthetic surgery and craniofacial, pediatric, maxillofacial trauma, microsurgery, urogenital, burn, hand, and wound care. Certain areas of plastic surgery warrant specialized comments.

Aesthetic Surgery

Aesthetic surgery is one of the few areas in plastic surgery in which telemedicine may have a limited role. Although adequate patient examination may be possible with today's technology, the distance between the patient and the surgeon may not be tolerated. Many patients seeking aesthetic surgery are very uncomfortable about disrobing for examination. Patients who are unhappy with how their breasts, hips, or thighs look may be reticent about displaying their imperfections to "strangers" or the camera. It is important for the plastic surgeon to make the patient feel as comfortable as possible and establish a rapport during the initial interview. This is necessary to help alleviate some of the anxieties associated with seeing a plastic surgeon. It remains to be seen if the level of patient comfort necessary to establish a good relationship between the surgeon and the plastic surgical aesthetic patient is possible through telemedicine.

The relationship established between the plastic surgeon and the aesthetic patient is critical to a successful outcome. The plastic surgeon spends much time counseling the patients regarding their concerns both before and after surgery. The confidence and trust that is inherent in this relationship may not be possible to achieve at a distance. These patients have high expectations with regard to what surgery can achieve, and a significant amount of one-on-one interaction must transpire between the surgeon and the patient before surgery. The single most important cause of patient dissatisfaction after aesthetic surgery is patients' unrealistic expectations of what surgery can accomplish.

Hand Surgery

Hand surgery is one field in plastic surgery in which telemedicine can play a significant role. Patients with hand injuries or elective hand complaints can be seen and have their problem documented with both physical examination and x-ray findings, and this information can be sent via the electronic format to the referring physician. For this form of examination to be successful, however, it is imperative that a well-trained presenter be present. Much of the diagnosis in hand surgery is based on physical examination and proper maneuvering of the wrist, hand, or digits. Proper history taking can be enhanced by the use of protocol questions, which can be supplied by the consulting physician to the referring physician. Once the initial electronic communication has been obtained, the consulting physician can determine if additional in-person physical examination is necessary before recommending treatment or if additional diagnostic studies are needed. Additionally, postoperative follow-up visits can all be done over the telemedicine system, and this can include store-and-forward formats, live video formats, or both. Postoperative wound checks and subsequent hand rehabilitation progress can easily be monitored via telemedicine.

Pediatric Plastic Surgery

Pediatric plastic surgery is a field that is very broad. Congenital anomalies of all sorts, including craniofacial, extremity, and truncal anomalies, are generally dealt with by plastic surgeons with interest in this region. In many cases, parents bring their children to see a plastic surgeon regarding congenital anomalies within days or weeks after birth. Most patients are not surgical candidates at this age. Their immaturity and size make anesthesia extremely risky for elective surgery. Therefore, telemedicine is useful as an initial way for families to touch base with a plastic surgeon and receive reassurance that their child's problem can be corrected. Additionally, some congenital anomalies, such as arterial/venous malformations, are managed initially by observation only. Because many congenital anomalies may regress over time, yearly checkups can be performed with this system.

In many cases, it is only necessary to check the color and consistency of the skin to determine if lesions are regressing or if they need more urgent management. Simple store and forward information can be done in this population of patients, and this information can be stored for yearly comparison. In our clinic, for patients who must travel great distances, we monitor with periodic photographs sent by either a family doctor or the patient's parents. We review the photographs, and, when the time is appropriate for surgery, we have the patient come to the clinic. Telemedicine can provide the same information and can enhance the periodic checks by including the ability to have real-time video examinations.

Maxillofacial Trauma

Maxillofacial trauma includes injuries to facial structures, including skin and underlying bone. It is conceivable that emergency physicians in remote areas with immediate concerns could call in a plastic surgical consult by sending live video, store-and-forward documentation (including physical findings and x-rays), or both to their consulting physician. With the patient in the emergency room, the consulting physician could review the documentation and suggest treatment alternatives. Additionally, the consulting physician could prompt the on-site physician if additional diagnostic studies would be helpful before the patient leaves the emergency room.

With the advent of medical peripheries, ophthalmic examinations, nasal endoscopy, and intraoral examinations can be obtained with remarkable accuracy via telemedicine. Because very few severe maxillofacial injuries need to be addressed in the emergent setting, these patients can even be scheduled for surgery after having an examination from the remote site. Additionally, the information that is sent to the plastic surgeon can be disseminated to other consulting services (e.g., neurosurgery, ophthalmology, orthopedics). Therefore, telemedicine affords the unique ability to consult multiple specialties and provide the same information without the risk of accidentally deleting important information. Additionally, the use of telemedicine should save time and promote accurate delivery of care. Postoperatively, these patients can be followed. Telemedicine may also help to identify potential problems, such as enophthalmos or lagophthalmos, which are late findings after maxillofacial injury.

Telemedicine enables plastic surgeons to follow along with the patient's primary care provider on the progression of the patient's recovery. If problems develop, they can be detected at an earlier time, hopefully providing a better overall outcome.

Burn Care

Treatment of burn patients can be divided into acute care and reconstructive care. In the acute-care setting, plastic surgery's involvement is determined by the arrangements within the community. Most acute burn care is provided for by general surgeons with plastic surgical consultation in more sensitive areas such as the face and hands. Accurate assessment of burn depth can be determined from photographs in conjunction with the emerging technology, such as laser Doppler and surface oxygen tension. This information is possible to transmit in electronic format to the consulting physician coupled with photographic documentation (i.e., store and forward or live video) and helps the plastic surgeon in providing a treatment plan.

Burn Reconstruction

In the reconstructive phase, burn patients are followed mainly for their scar healing. Many patients require frequent visits to determine if scar patterns in particular areas are causing functional deformities and thus require surgical intervention. Assessment of the healing wound includes analyzing its color and firmness and looking at the range of motion of the tissues around it. Virtually all of this can be determined from simple photographs. The consistency of the scar is something that can be taught to the on-site care provider, and this information can be passed on to the consulting surgeon.

Telemedicine offers an exciting potential to follow a large number of postburn patients in their rehabilitative phase. It is here that the plastic surgeon must be intimately involved. Some scars are treatable by physical therapy only. Once all the benefits of physical therapy have been exhausted, and the patient is still having problems, surgical releases are warranted. Digital images coupled with functional measurements (i.e., goniometer) can enable plastic surgeons to manage these patients from outlying rehabilitation centers or even the patient's home.

Microsurgery

The subspecialty of microsurgery is an aspect of plastic surgery that transfers various types of flaps around the body as needed for reconstruction. Surgeons reconnect the arterial and venous blood supplies usually with the aid of an operating microscope. Postoperative monitoring of the flap is critical. If either an arterial or venous occlusion occurs, immediate operative reexploration is indicated. The earlier occlusion can be identified, the greater the chances that the flap can be salvaged. The ability to accurately assess the flap is important in detecting problems. The color of the flap, capillary refill, and turgor are subjective parameters that are monitored to alert plastic surgeons of a problem.

Presently, various systems are available for monitoring the attempt to make monitoring a more objective assessment. These systems use clinical data, including temperature, oxygen tension, or laser Doppler readings of blood flow. Although each of these systems provides numeric or analog outputs, their interpretation still requires expertise.

Telemedicine would be a real advantage to the microsurgeon. If a question about the status of a flap was to arise, a bedside examination could be performed with the telemedicine system. If one of the monitoring systems were in place, the information coming from the monitoring system could be sent on-line to the surgeon at home, and the trends in the data, coupled with the on-hand clinical evaluation, could make the decision to explore more timely.

CONCLUSION

All patients that would normally be referred to a plastic surgeon are potential patients who could be seen in the telemedicine setting. The only possible exception are patients who request aesthetic surgery. Additionally, patients being referred for breast or gynecologic reconstruction may have a difficult time being examined via telemedicine. The main limitation for aesthetic surgery patients is the significant degree of trust and understanding that must be obtained between the surgeon and the patient before undergoing surgery. Although patient satisfaction using the telemedicine system has been achieved, aesthetic surgery is a personal relationship in which the less-than-human interaction, which is inherent in the telemedicine system, is a potential detriment. All of the patients with cutaneous problems can be evaluated via telemedicine, and consultation referral plans can adequately be determined based on history and physical, photographs, x-rays, and laboratory studies. The majority of the time, the store and forward format is adequate for achieving these goals. Some patients, such as those undergoing hand rehabilitation or extremity rehabilitation after reconstruction, may be better served by real-time video sessions. All postoperative follow-ups could be successfully treated by telemedicine. Wound assessment, timing of when to remove sutures, timing to start physical therapy or occupational therapy, when to return to work, and all of the information necessary to make these decisions can easily be obtained by telemedicine.

It is clear that in the future the plastic surgeon will rely heavily on telemedicine in his or her daily practice. The ability to care for patients who have difficulty traveling to the plastic surgeon's office and are being referred from remote sites will be enhanced the most. Which of the populations of patients who call on the skills of plastic surgeons will benefit the most is still unclear. As plastic surgeons' experience with telemedicine increases, this question should be easily answered.

REFERENCE

1. McCarthy J. Introduction to plastic surgery. In: *Plastic surgery*. Philadelphia: WB Saunders, 1990.

Telemedicine: Practicing in the Information Age,
edited by Steven F. Viegas and Kim Dunn.
Lippincott–Raven Publishers, Philadelphia © 1998.

50

Thoracic Surgery

Scott K. Alpard and Joseph B. Zwischenberger

Department of Surgery, University of Texas
Medical Branch at Galveston, Galveston, Texas 77555

Patients referred by their primary care provider to a thoracic surgery telemedicine clinic should be pressessed and referred based on a problem-oriented approach. Screening should take place before the telemedicine referral, as not every thoracic surgical condition can be properly evaluated via telemedicine. Telemedicine can offer the great advantage of access to thoracic surgeons to areas that would not otherwise have access to those subspecialists' assessment and care. This chapter focuses on thoracic conditions most likely to be and capable of being referred for consultation via telemedicine and provides an algorithmic approach to suspecting, diagnosing, and treating various thoracic conditions.

ESOPHAGEAL DISORDERS

Dysfunction of the esophagogastric junction results in physiologic diminution of pressure in the lower esophageal sphincter (LES), with resultant gastroesophageal reflux (GER) (Fig. 50-1). The most common symptoms of GER are chest pain, heartburn, regurgitation, and dysphagia. All neuromuscular disorders of the esophagus can cause symptoms of dysphagia, spasm, or both.

The most common neuromuscular disorder is achalasia. Achalasia is the diminished to absent peristalsis of the esophageal body with incomplete relaxation of the LES.

Initial Studies

Barium swallow and esophagoscopy are the key initial studies in esophageal disorders. Barium swallow provides information on anatomic detail and esophageal motility. A sliding hernia has an elevated esophagogastric junction, whereas the less common paraesophageal hernia has a normally located esophagogastric junction with herniation of the stomach into the thorax. Achalasia causes dilation and tortuosity of the esophagus, smooth luminal narrowing at the esophagogastric junction, and decreased to absent peristaltic waves. When esophageal cancer is present, a barium swallow demonstrates the level of stricture and irregular narrowing of the esophagus with proximal dilation.

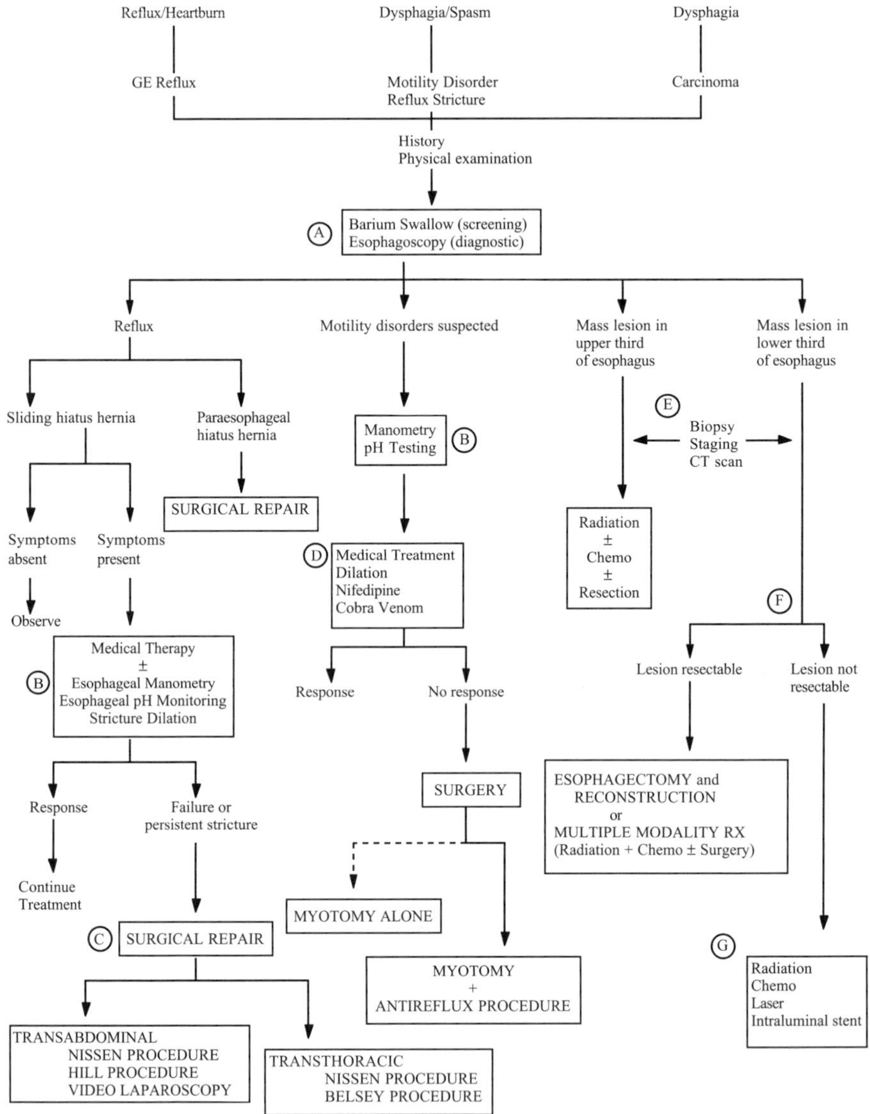

FIG. 50-1. Algorithm for esophageal disorders. GE, gastroesophageal; CT, computed tomography; chemo, chemotherapy; RX, treatment.

Esophagoscopy allows direct visualization, including the extent of a hiatal hernia, the presence or absence of any stricture, location and degree of esophagitis, and the presence of a mass. Biopsies can be taken to determine the degree of esophagitis and to rule out esophageal carcinoma. Esophagoscopy can also confirm the extent of mucosal involvement of esophageal carcinoma.

Manometric Studies

Manometric studies of the esophagus show a deviation from normal (i.e., 20 mm Hg) pressure in the LES. It is also important to assess the uncoordinated changes in pressures as a food bolus nears the esophageal sphincter and passes into the stomach. Symptoms can be reproduced by instilling 0.1 N hydrochloric acid into the esophagus at 5 ml per minute. The amount of gastroesophageal reflux can be determined by measuring esophageal pH for 24 hours. The presence of reflux, the number of episodes, and the amount of time to return to normal pH provide important diagnostic information.

Medical Therapy

Medical therapy is the preferred treatment strategy for most patients with severe, erosive esophagitis. The goals of management for GER are relief of symptoms, healing of esophagitis, prevention of complications, and maintenance of remission. Changes in lifestyle may control GER in up to 20% of patients. The pathophysiology of GER is addressed by promotility therapy; however, cisapride only offers control in 50% to 60% of cases, while metoclopramide and bethanechol are limited by side effects. In patients with relapsing, nonerosive GERD (mild-to-moderate gastroesophageal reflux disease), initial therapy with histamine H_2-receptor antagonists is suggested. Acid suppression using histamine receptor antagonists controls GER in 50% to 60% of patients. Proton pump inhibitors (e.g., omeprazole and lansoprazole) provide the most effective control of GER (80% to 100%) and should be used by patients with severe reflux esophagitis or complications, such as peptic stricture or Barrett's esophagus. However, proton pump inhibitors can only be used for limited periods because of the risks of bacterial overgrowth and gastric carcinoid tumors.

Medical treatment of achalasia is recommended as the initial, and sometimes the only necessary, treatment. Dilation of the esophagus, using Hurst or Maloney dilators, only provides a transient effect, whereas pneumatic dilation has been shown by Wehrman et al. (see Bibliography) to be effective in approximately 75% of patients. Relief of dysphagia is readily accomplished in most patients using polyethylene or mercury-filled dilators or balloon dilators. Balloons provide advantages over rigid dilators, including a decreased risk of stricture recurrence, a need for fewer treatment sessions to achieve end-diameter dilation, and less procedural discomfort. Low-compliance balloons have been shown to obtain initial symptomatic success in 87.5% of patients. Pneumatic dilation with low-compliance balloons has been reported as a safe and effective treatment of achalasia. However, when esophageal acid exposure was measured after dilation, clinically relevant GER occurred in only 5% of patients.

Drug therapy, using nifedipine, has some effect in decreasing the symptoms of achalasia (e.g., decreasing LES tone, allowing esophageal emptying by gravity). Antacids and H_2 blockers are most effective when reflux and esophagitis are present. Anticholinergic drugs have been used to decrease sphincter spasm, with mild success. Botulism toxin injections into the sphincter have shown relief of symptoms in select patients.

Surgical Repair

Surgical repair is indicated when medical therapy fails, severe symptoms persist, stenosis remains unresolved, or reflux esophagitis does not clear. Surgical repair attempts to improve esophagogastric junction competence and increase LES pressure. The choice of operation depends on the need for concomitant repair of other intraabdominal disease, experience of the surgeon, and the ability to restore the esophagogastric junction below the hemidiaphragm to provide increased LES pressure. Two procedures are accomplished transabdominally: the Nissen and the Hill.

The Nissen procedure uses the fundus of the stomach to wrap (360 degrees) the distal esophagus. Crural repair is carried out concomitantly. The uncut Collis-Nissen procedure provides acceptable short-term control of GERD. The laparoscopic Nissen procedure has also been reported as safe, effective treatment for refractory GERD.

The Hill procedure is a posterior gastropexy, in which the anterior wall of the stomach near the lesser curvature and posterior wall is attached to the median arcuate ligament and followed by crural repair. It results in accentuation of the esophagogastric angle, tightening of the cardiac sling musculature, increased sphincter support, and hiatal narrowing.

The transthoracic approach allows a cut Collis (to elongate the esophagus) and a Nissen (360-degree wrap) or the Belsey Mark IV procedure. For the Belsey Mark IV procedure, the esophagogastric junction is freed and the fundus of the stomach is used to partially wrap the distal esophagus to create a valve effect, as opposed to the sphincter effect of the (360-degree) Nissen. The hernia is then reduced, and the crura are reapproximated.

ESOPHAGEAL CARCINOMA

Symptoms of esophageal carcinoma include weight loss and dysphagia, progressing to obstruction. Esophageal carcinoma accounts for 2% of all reported cancers. The most common cell type is squamous cell carcinoma in the upper and middle esophagus. Adenocarcinoma occurs with increasing frequency closer to the esophagogastric junction.

Treatment Strategy

Once the diagnosis of carcinoma has been confirmed, the level and extent of the lesion should be established. The presence or absence of metastasis is the most important factor in determining treatment strategy for carcinoma of the esophagus. To determine the extent of the disease, a computed tomography (CT) scan of the thorax and upper abdomen, including the liver, is used. Palpable scalene nodes should also be biopsied. The best available method for locoregional staging of esophageal carcinoma is endoscopic ultrasound (EUS). EUS is accurate in staging mediastinal lymph nodes (80% sensitivity, 87.5% specificity, and 86.5% accuracy). Conventional 7.5-MHz ultrasound systems have been shown by Natsugoe et al. (see Bibliography) to be ineffective. A newer, 20-MHz linear-radial switchable probe is a useful method for staging superficial esophageal cancer. EUS is limited by tumor stenosis, the ability to distinguish between malignant and benign lymph nodes, and the ability to distinguish between mucosal and submucosal cancer. To fully evaluate those patients with esophageal carcinoma, the EUS transducer must pass through the entire tumor to the cardia to scan the celiac axis.

Treatment Goals

The goals of treatment are (a) relief of dysphagia, (b) resection of the tumor, and (c) pathologic staging of the disease. When resectable, esophagogastrectomy is the most common method of resection. For the Ivor-Lewis procedure the esophagus is mobilized by a thoracic or thoracoabdominal approach. The alimentary tract is reconstructed by bringing the stomach into the thorax to replace the native distal esophagus. An alternative approach is total esophagectomy and reconstruction by right thoracotomy with celiotomy with or without distal cervical dissection by stomach or colon interposition. Another method is transhiatal esophagectomy and cervical esophagogastrostomy. Radiation therapy has been used as adjuvant therapy before and after esophagectomy. Combined chemotherapy and radiation therapy have been used before resection and reconstruction, but no clear advantage has been shown by any multiple modality therapy.

Palliative Therapy

Patients not candidates for resection, reconstruction, or both undergo palliative therapy. Radiation therapy, used with moderate success, has been coupled with dilation of the esophagus. Chemotherapy is another palliative option and can be used in combination with radiation therapy. The neodymium:yttrium-aluminum-garnet laser has been used when an obstructive component is present. The recent advances in esophageal and tracheobronchial stents provide another option to palliate an obstructive component.

THORACIC OUTLET SYNDROME

Thoracic outlet syndrome (TOS) is caused by compression at the thoracic inlet because of impingement or compression of the subclavian artery, subclavian vein, or brachial plexus secondary to abnormalities of the first rib, musculi scalenus anticus, clavicle, or cervical rib (Fig. 50-2). The differential diagnosis includes reflex sympathetic dystrophy, referred pain from carpal tunnel syndrome, ulnar nerve entrapment syndrome, and cervical disc or nerve dysfunction from spinal cord pathology, including degeneration or tumor. Apical thoracic diseases, including superior sulcus tumor or suppurative lesions, can also cause symptoms of TOS. The diagnosis of TOS is particularly difficult because no specific test is diagnostic and the patient's psychiatric background appears contributory. Disability support and pain medications serve as potential for secondary gain.

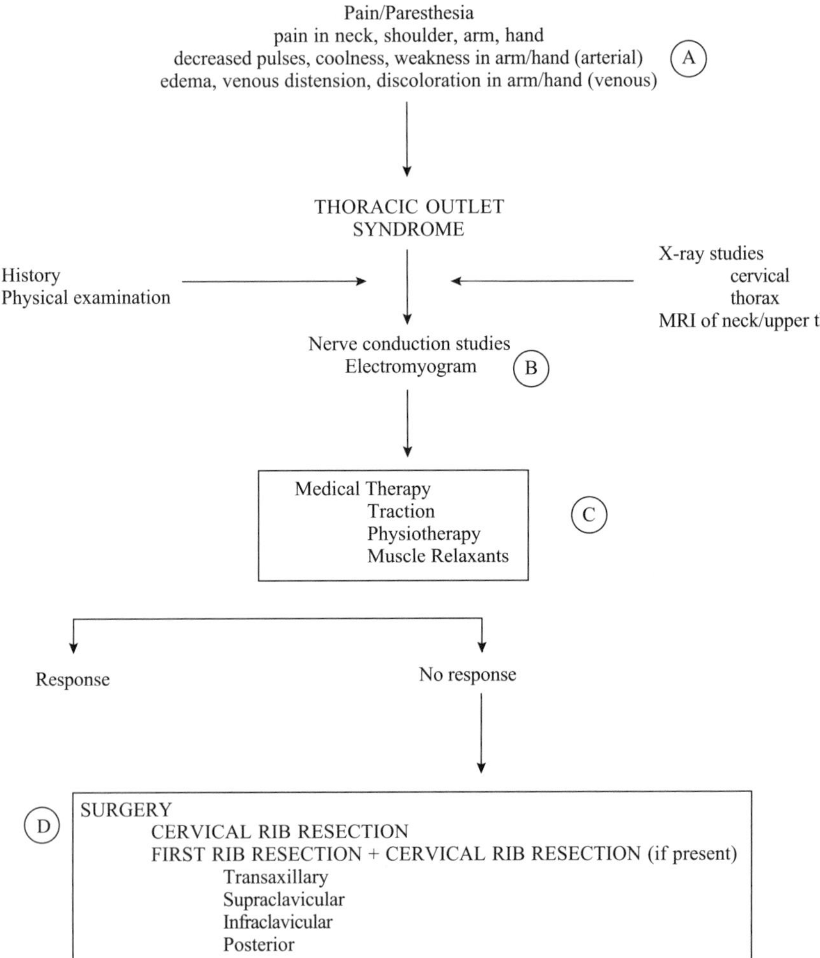

FIG. 50-2. Algorithm for thoracic outlet syndrome. MRI, magnetic resonance imaging.

Symptoms

Pain and paresthesias are common symptoms, usually occurring over the ulnar nerve distribution. Pain involves the neck, shoulder, arms, and hand. Subclavian arterial compression produces pain, color, and temperature changes, as well as ischemia manifested by loss of pulse, claudication, thrombosis, or weakness and fatigability of the arm and hand. Subclavian vein compression causes edema, venous distention, upper extremity discoloration, and, if thrombosed, the Paget-Schroetter syndrome (axillary vein thrombosis). To demonstrate these symptoms, a number of maneuvers are used. Adson's maneuver (full inspiration with neck extension, while turning the head to the contralateral side), the costoclavicular test (drawing shoulders down and back), and the hyperabduction test (arm abducted to 180 degrees) all produce diminution of the radial pulse. Nerve compression can produce symptoms similar to subclavian artery compression—pain, color and temperature changes, and ischemic manifestations—or it can result in symptoms similar to Raynaud's phenomenon or disease.

Diagnosis

Physical examination is paramount in making the diagnosis of TOS. The diagnosis is supported by nerve conduction studies, electromyograms, and the exclusion of other diagnoses. Nerve conduction studies are performed by stimulating the ulnar nerve in the supraclavicular fossa, in the upper arm, and below the elbow and wrist. Action potentials in the hypothenar or first dorsal interosseous muscles are recorded. Ulnar nerve compression is suggested by a reduction from the normal value of 72 m per second across the thoracic outlet. Magnetic resonance imaging (MRI) with T1-weighted imaging allows evaluation for mass lesions compressing the nerve rods.

Medical Therapy

TOS is often a diagnosis of exclusion. Once the diagnosis is presumed, medical therapy should be initiated, starting with muscle relaxants and physiotherapy. Most patients respond to cervical traction and physiotherapy, including heat, massage, neck exercises, musculi scalenus anticus strengthening, and postural changes.

Surgical Therapy

First rib resection can be accomplished through a supraclavicular, infraclavicular, transaxillary (most common), or posterior (least common) approach. During rib resection, it is important to avoid undue traction on the brachial plexus or damage to the subclavian artery or vein. The patient must be counseled regarding continued physiotherapy and the possibility of less than 100% recovery. When a cervical rib is present, cervical rib resection is combined with first rib resection, which provides the best outcome. Division of the musculi scalenus anticus alone has had poor patient response.

MASSIVE HEMOPTYSIS

Massive hemoptysis, the expectoration of blood or bloody sputum, is the loss of more than 600 ml of blood within 24 to 48 hours (Fig. 50-3). Massive hemoptysis is most likely associated with pulmonary infarction or tuberculosis. The history should focus on previous infections, especially tuberculosis; exposures to any known pulmonary disease; evidence of bleeding disorders or systemic illnesses; and any previous acute infections. The severity of the hemoptysis is not correlated with any specific diagnosis, although bronchitis and pneumonia rarely result in massive hemoptysis.

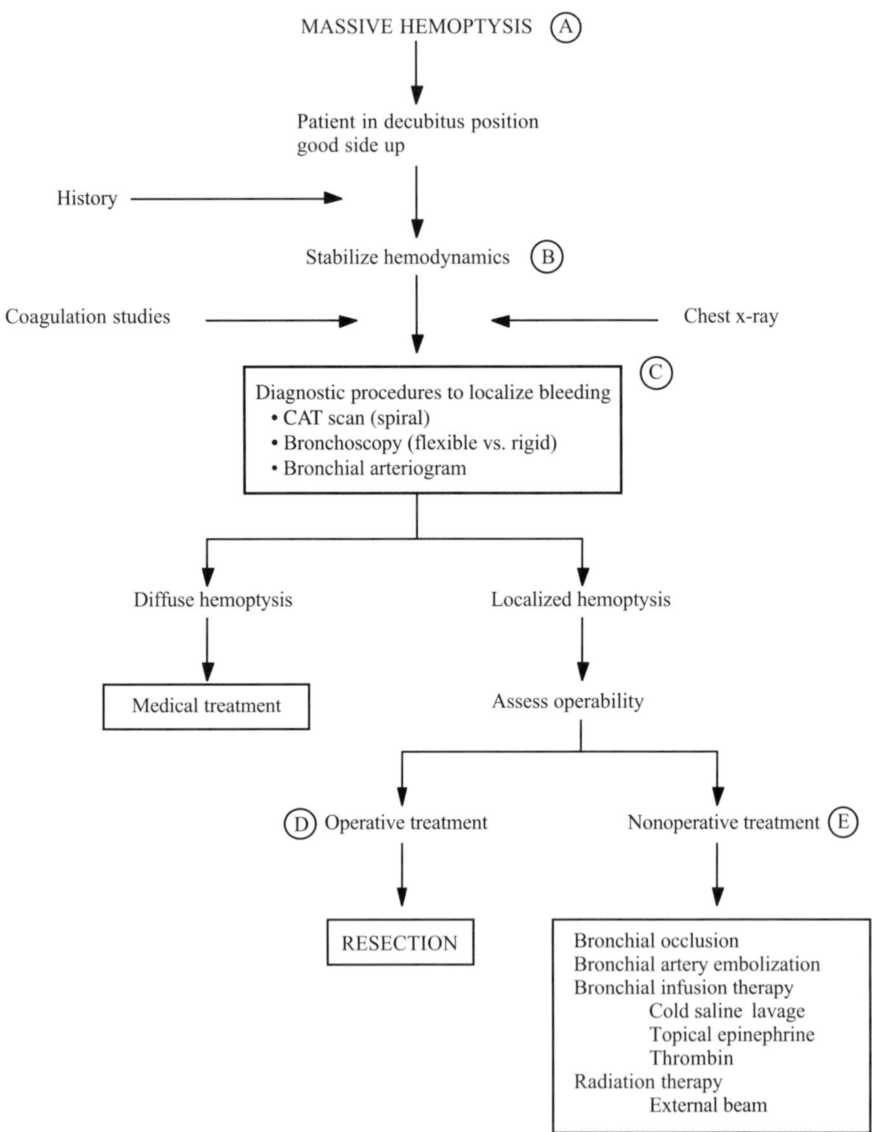

FIG. 50-3. Algorithm for massive hemoptysis. CAT, computerized axial tomography.

Treatment Priorities

As massive hemoptysis is life threatening, the first priorities in treatment are to maintain the airway, optimize oxygenation, and stabilize hemodynamics. If the bleeding site is known, the patient should be placed with the bleeding lung in the dependent position to prevent aspiration. Once the patient is stabilized, diagnostic and therapeutic interventions should be rapidly initiated.

Bronchoscopy

Rigid bronchoscopy is preferred when massive hemoptysis is present to provide an airway and aspirate voluminous quantities of bloody secretions. A flexible bronchoscope can be used through the rigid bronchoscope to identify specific bleeding points. Bronchoscopy can identify a localized lesion or diffuse bleeding in the tracheobronchial tree. If diffuse bleeding is found, cultures and bronchial biopsies may help determine the origin of the diffuse disease.

Surgical Treatment

Surgery is the most definitive form of therapy, because it removes the source of bleeding. Resection is carried out only after identifying the specific lobe or segment from which bleeding is occurring. A double-lumen tube is used to control the airway, ensuring ventilation to the good lung and preventing intraoperative filling of the dependent lung during resection.

Controlling Bleeding

If inoperable, occluding the involved bronchus with a balloon occluder temporarily prevents flooding of the good lung and can also transiently stop the bleeding. Other techniques used to control ongoing bleeding include bronchial artery embolization, cold saline lavage of the involved lobe or segment, epinephrine-soaked pledgets (1:10,000), and instillation of 10 ml of 1,000 U/ml topical thrombin through a flexible bronchoscope. If malignant disease is responsible, external beam and brachytherapy are available for use. Laser eradication can be used for localized endobronchial lesions.

SOLITARY PULMONARY NODULE

Solitary pulmonary nodule is an isolated, round intrapulmonary lesion less than 4 cm in diameter, usually discovered incidentally on a chest film of an asymptomatic patient (Fig. 50-4). Many malignant and benign processes can manifest as a solitary pulmonary nodule on chest x-ray. Approximately 10% of the solitary pulmonary nodules in the general population and 40% in the clinical setting are malignant. The likelihood of a malignant tumor correlates with the age of the patient, size of the nodule, history of a prior malignant lesion, and a history of smoking. Approximately 5% of small-cell lung cancer (SCLC) patients present with an asymptomatic peripheral tumor (solitary pulmonary nodule) on routine chest x-ray.

Recurrent bacterial pneumonia is two or more episodes of nontuberculosis pneumonias at least 1 month apart. Symptoms include persistent cough, sputum production, fever, and abnormal breath sounds.

If the lesion has been present with no changes documented for more than 1 year, the patient should be followed with serial chest films every 6 months for a period of 2 years. After 2 years, annual chest films are appropriate. Any new lesion, change

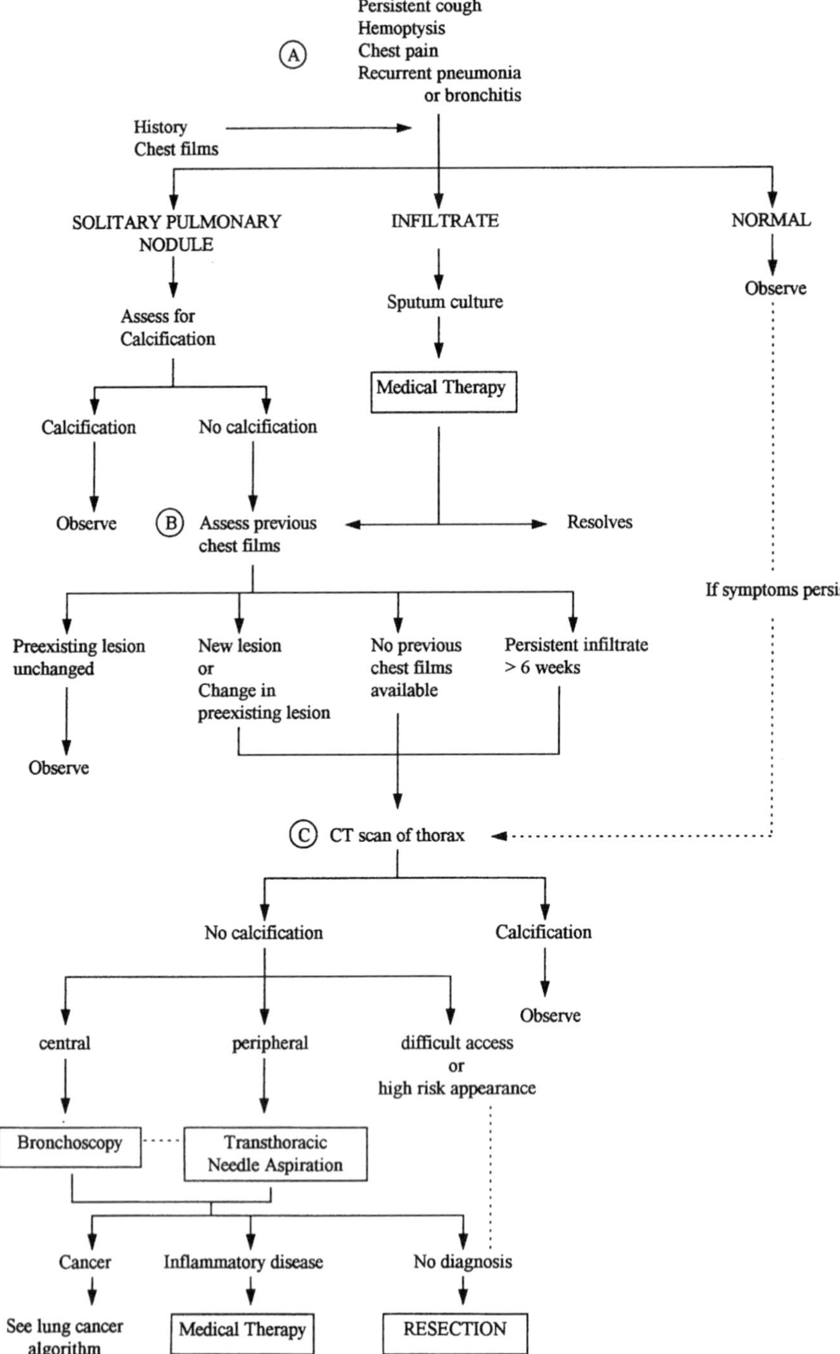

FIG. 50-4. Algorithm for solitary pulmonary nodule. CT, computed tomography.

in previous lesion, or persistent infiltrate greater than 6 weeks must be evaluated farther.

CT scan of the thorax confirms the solitary nature of the lesion and describes the relationship to adjacent structures. CT also allows evaluation of the mediastinum, for extension or lymphadenopathy. Bronchoscopy, under fluoroscopic control, with washings, brushings, and biopsies establishes a diagnosis in one-third of patients with malignant disease.

Bronchoscopy and transthoracic fine-needle aspiration are nonoperative diagnostic approaches. Transthoracic fine-needle aspiration, under fluoroscopic or CT guidance, is preferred to bronchoscopy when the lesion is peripheral or if the diagnosis is not made or inaccessible by bronchoscopy. When a diagnosis is not obtained, open thoracotomy is necessary. Thoracoscopy offers minimal invasion for diagnosing the solitary nodule if the lesion is relatively peripheral and accessible. Thoracoscopy is nearly 100% sensitive and 100% specific with minimal mortality and decreased morbidity.

PRIMARY CHEST WALL TUMOR

Primary chest wall tumors are uncommon, usually originating from osseocartilaginous or adjacent soft tissues, especially muscle (Fig. 50-5). They can present as a palpable mass with or without pain or as an abnormality on chest x-ray. Location, size, and tumor extension all influence treatment.

Diagnosis

Histologic diagnosis and cell type is imperative. If the chest wall tumor is less than or equal to 3 cm, excisional biopsy with 2-cm margins of normal tissue may be therapeutic as well as diagnostic. If the chest wall tumor is greater than 3 cm, biopsy is required (core needle or, more commonly, incisional). Open biopsy is the method of choice, and it is important to collect tissue from nonnecrotic areas. Light microscopy alone is insufficient for diagnosis. Electron microscopy, special stains, immunohistochemical techniques, flow cytometry, and monoclonal antibody studies may also be necessary.

If the lesion is malignant, the presence of metastatic disease must be evaluated. Fibrosarcomas and chondrosarcomas metastasize to the lungs, while plasmacytomas may be the initial manifestation of multiple myeloma.

Metastatic Disease

If metastatic disease is identified, local radiation therapy for pain relief, and systemic chemotherapy are used. Chemotherapy should be used for plasmacytoma; however, resection is required if no response occurs. Chemotherapy has also been used to treat Ewing's sarcoma and fibrosarcoma.

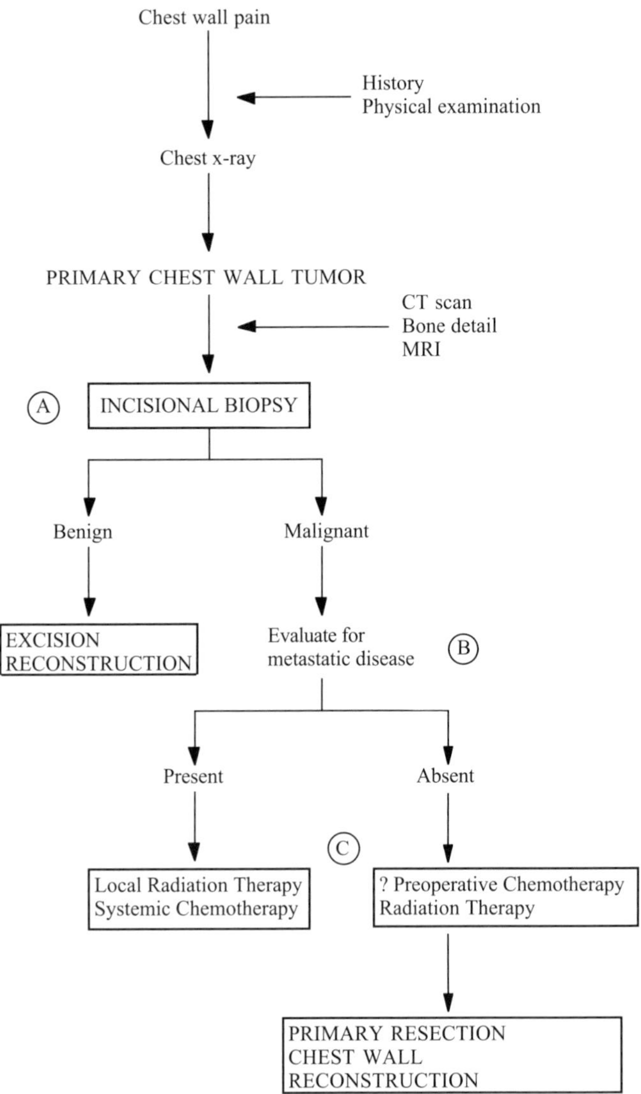

FIG. 50-5. Algorithm for primary chest wall tumor. CT, computed tomography; MRI, magnetic resonance imaging.

Surgical Therapy

When tumors show little to no response to medical therapy, or benign lesions are present, resection with reconstruction is required. The best methods of reconstruction include using myocutaneous flaps with microvascular anastomosis, omental flaps, and supplemental split thickness skin grafts. Structural integrity is maintained with ribs, fascia lata, Prolene mesh, or Gore-Tex patches.

LUNG ABSCESS

Lung abscesses are most commonly caused by the aspiration of a foreign body into the tracheobronchial tree, often preceded by an altered state of consciousness induced by alcohol or anesthesia (Fig. 50-6). Lung abscesses are characterized by fever, chills, cough, expectoration of foul-smelling sputum, hemoptysis, and signs of toxicity.

Primary Therapy

Primary therapy should include antibiotics, percussion, and postural drainage. Broad spectrum antibiotics are initiated until cultures are available to guide further therapy. Antibiotics have been shown by Wiedemann and Rice (see Bibliography) to be effective in 90% of cases. Before antibiotics, mortality ranged from 35% to 70% but has since dropped to 3.5%.

Repeat Bronchoscopy

When initial bronchoscopy and postural drainage fail to accomplish successful drainage, a repeat bronchoscopy should be done. Therapeutic response can be prolonged, and antibiotic therapy should be continued for 6 to 8 weeks, provided symptoms of sepsis and constitutional symptoms are resolving.

Surgical Therapy

If the patient fails treatment or progresses on a septic course, direct drainage is necessary. Approximately 10% of patients require external drainage or surgical therapy. Percutaneous drainage, especially with interventional radiologic techniques, may be successful. The other option is definitive resection of the involved lung parenchyma by wedge resection or lobectomy. With modern antibiotics, the use of a double-lumen endotracheal tube, improved anesthesia techniques, and thorough preoperative preparation (fluid and blood), the mortality rate for resection has fallen to less than 10%.

LUNG CANCER

Lung cancer is the most common cause of cancer death in the United States (Fig. 50-7). The major cell types are squamous cell, adenocarcinoma, large cell, and small cell. The common symptoms associated with lung cancer include cough, sputum production, hemoptysis, wheezing, and dyspnea. In primary lung cancer, the physical examination may be completely normal. One-half of patients present with metastases, commonly going to the brain, bone, liver, and adrenals. The chest x-ray is the most common study leading to a diagnosis. The presentation can be in different forms such as a solitary nodule, linear atelectasis, lobar atelectasis, distal abscess formation, hilar adenopathy, pleural effusion, or elevation of the diaphragm.

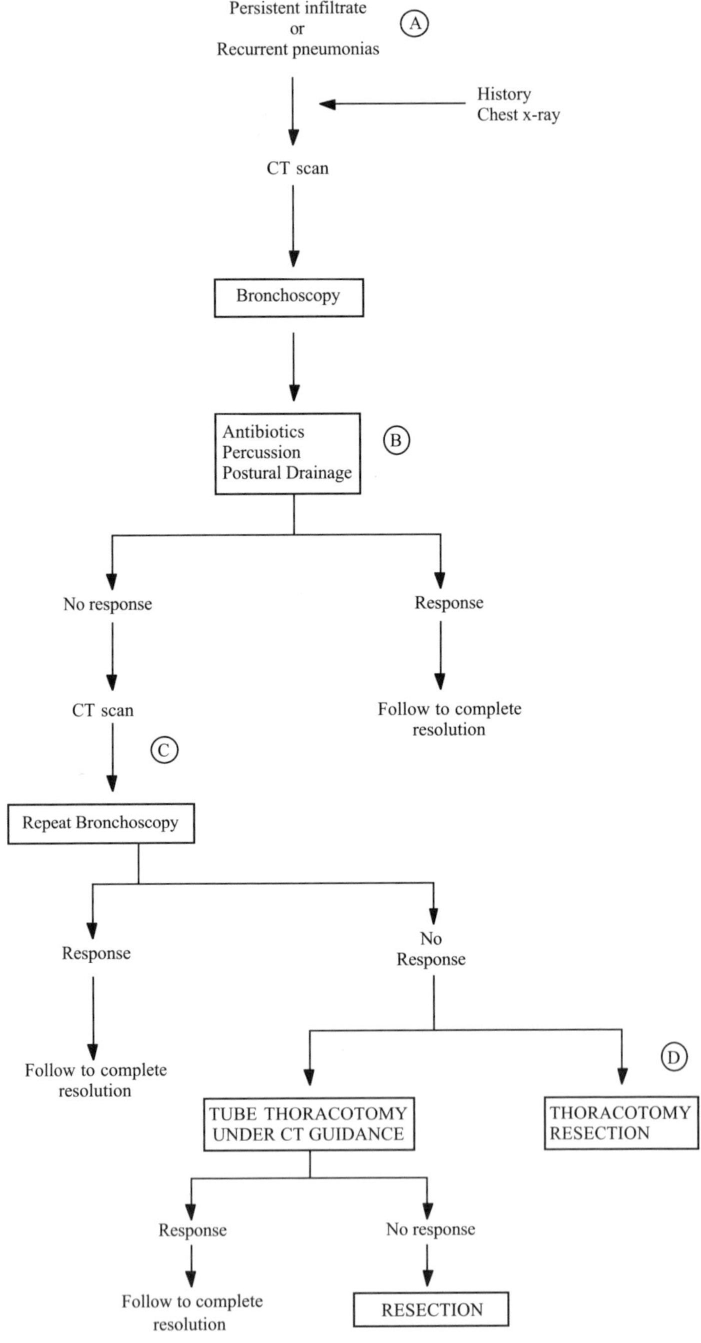

FIG. 50-6. Algorithm for lung abscess. CT, computed tomography.

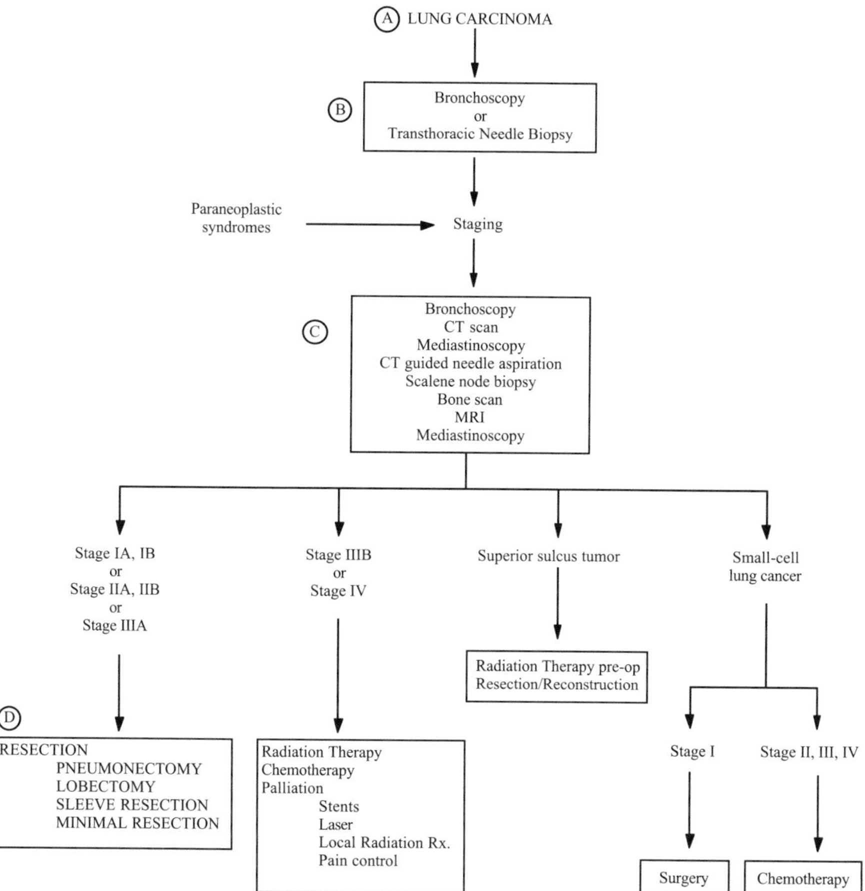

FIG. 50-7. Algorithm for lung cancer. CT, computed tomography; MRI, magnetic resonance imaging; pre-op, preoperative; Rx, therapy.

Diagnosis

Bronchoscopy, performed with washings, brushings, and biopsies, is the method of choice for diagnosing and staging central lesions and assessing operability. The anatomy dictates whether pneumonectomy is necessary, lobectomy is feasible, or if the tumor extends into the trachea. Sputum cytology, either before or after bronchoscopy, increases the diagnostic yield. The diagnostic success rate for peripheral lesions can be improved with fluoroscopic guidance.

Transthoracic needle biopsy is appropriate to establish a diagnosis when bronchoscopy or sputum cytology fails to and may be the only procedure needed if the patient is not a candidate for resection. Staging is mandatory to assess the potential for resectability.

Cancer Staging

Accurate staging of lung cancer requires tissue confirmation of mediastinal nodes through sampling or complete node dissection. CT scanning is the most sensitive and accurate method for noninvasive evaluation of the mediastinum, with spiral CT used for evaluation of select mediastinal invasion. CT of the thorax and upper abdomen provides the location and extent of the tumor and the presence or absence of mediastinal lymphadenopathy. Transthoracic needle biopsy, by CT guidance, is used increasingly to sample enlarged mediastinal nodes. However, only a positive aspirate is helpful to define staging. Liver and adrenal metastases are identified and confirmed by needle aspiration. When the chest wall is involved, a CT scan is of limited benefit. Although used by some, MRI has no advantage over CT except when there is involvement of the bony thorax.

Video-assisted thoracoscopy (VAT) allows for evaluation and biopsy within the pleural space and at the pulmonary hilum. Routine VAT staging in patients with lung cancer is advocated by some as safe, reduces the need for exploratory thoracotomy, and can identify patients with localized lung cancer at high risk for postoperative recurrence.

Mediastinoscopy or mediastinotomy is indicated when enlarged mediastinal nodes are found on CT scan, because CT cannot reliably differentiate the benign reactive nodes from malignant. Surgical staging with mediastinoscopy has a role in accurately determining stage I or II disease. When enlarged nodes are present, their exact location must be identified at time of biopsy. Mediastinotomy provides access to lymph node–bearing groups not available to mediastinoscopy at the aortopulmonary window. Any palpable, identified, enlarged lymph node should be biopsied. Scalene nodes have an especially high positive yield.

A bone scan is warranted when bone pain or elevated levels of alkaline phosphatase are present, but it is very sensitive and susceptible to false-positives. Therefore, biopsy confirmation of metastases is needed before the disqualification of a patient from resection. A negative bone scan can rule out metastatic disease. A positive bone scan requires confirmation by standard x-rays, MRI, and needle biopsy.

Therapy

In non–small-cell lung cancer (NSCLC), complete resection with lobectomy is the preferred treatment. When unable to tolerate lobectomy, segmental or wedge resections and external radiotherapy are appropriate. VAT is useful in wedge resection for those patients with poor pulmonary reserve. In patients with stage II NSCLC, combined modality therapy offers improved outcome. In patients with stage IIIA NSCLC, cisplatin-based neoadjuvant chemotherapy before surgical resection has shown some improved survival in phase II and phase III trials. However, morbidity is increased.

Chemotherapy is the mainstay treatment for patients with all stages of SCLC in three- or four-drug regimens, to produce a response in 75% to 90% of patients. Complete resection, mediastinal lymph node sampling, and postoperative chemotherapy are indicated in the patient with stage I SCLC. Patients with limited stage SCLC are treated with a combination of chemotherapy and chest radiation. Patients with extensive stage SCLC and performance status can be treated with combination chemotherapy.

MALIGNANT PLEURAL EFFUSION

Pleural effusion can occur with known malignancies or can be the presentation of an undiagnosed malignancy (Fig. 50-8). The site and amount can be identified with standard lateral and posteroanterior x-rays of the chest.

Initial Therapy

The initial thoracentesis should remove all pleural fluid to allow cytologic evaluation of the pleural fluid. Most malignant effusions are exudative, and one-third are bloody. In those patients with malignant pleural effusions, cytology is positive for neoplastic cells in 60% of initial pleural fluid specimens. The remainder of patients (40%) require repeat thoracentesis, pleural biopsy, thoracoscopy, or other procedures to detect the presence of cancer.

If the effusion is controlled, the primary malignancy should be treated with either radiation therapy or chemotherapy.

Diagnosis

If, after thoracentesis and pleural biopsy, the diagnosis is not established, bronchoscopy, mediastinoscopy, or thoracoscopy should be used to identify the etiology of the pleural effusion. VATS thoracoscopy has a high degree of accuracy in diagnosing pleural-based malignancies or tuberculosis when cytology and pleural biopsies have failed. When adequate visualization is achieved, a pathologic diagnosis of benign disease can also be made with approximately 100% specificity. VATS lung biopsy is a safe alternative to open lung biopsy by thoracotomy for the accurate diagnosis of diffuse interstitial or infectious lung disease.

Further Therapy

If the effusion is not controlled after thoracentesis on greater than two occasions, a thoracostomy tube should be placed to remove any fluid still present. The placement of the tube combined with suction can result in pleural symphysis. If so, no further treatment is required. In more than 50% of patients, however, the effusion persists, and further treatment is necessary. Pleurodesis with a sclerosing agent administered through a chest tube is the most widely used therapy. Many different materials have been placed in the pleural space to achieve pleural symphysis, including doxycycline, bleomycin, radioactive gold, quinacrine, nitrogen mustard, and talc. Talc has been generally accepted as the most effective sclerosant for chemical pleurodesis and, as a result, should be considered the procedure of choice in the treatment of symptomatic malignant pleural effusions. A slurry of 5 g of United States Pharmacopeia talc and 20 ml of 1% lidocaine (Xylocaine) in 100 cc saline is instilled through the thoracostomy tube while the patient is turned 360 degrees. Repeat thoracentesis is appropriate for the

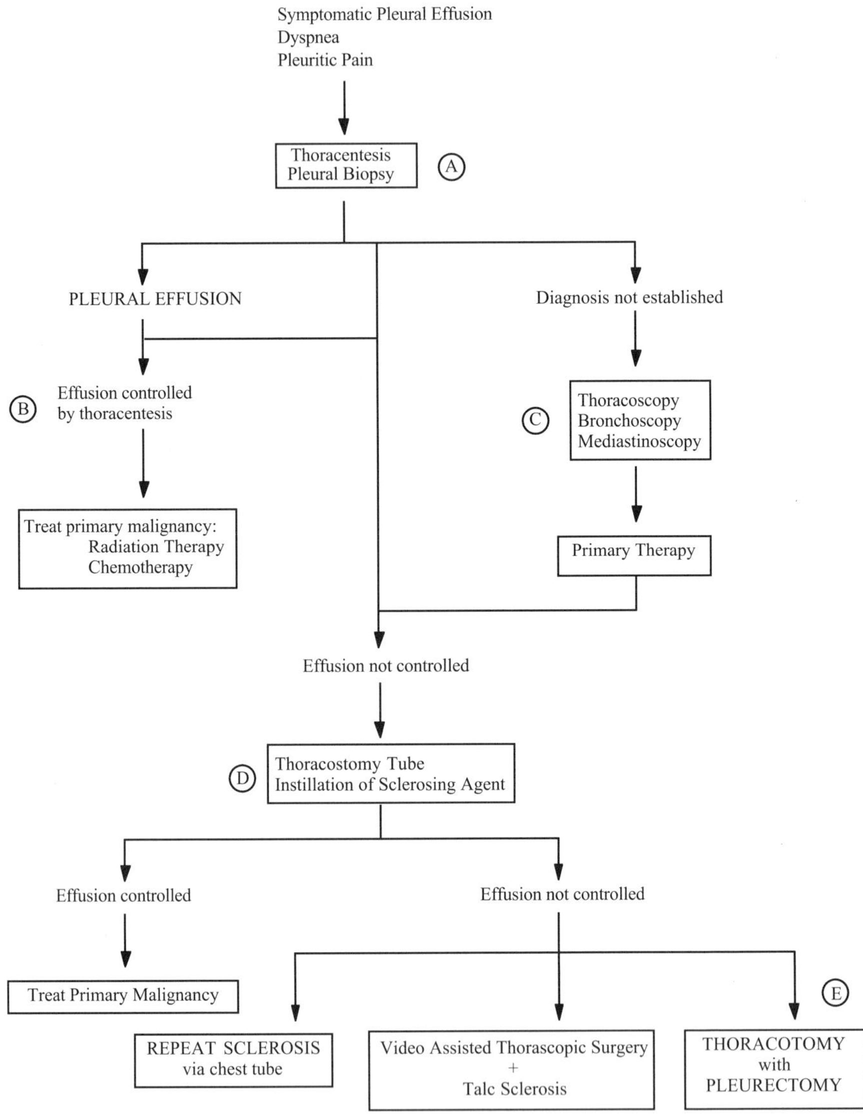

FIG. 50-8. Algorithm for malignant pleural effusion.

patient with limited survival and a slowly recurrent effusion. Pleuroperitoneal shunting remains an option for those patients whose lung is trapped by tumor.

Pleurectomy is an option when the patient is in good general condition, has an anticipated life span of longer than 6 months, and in whom the effusion is the primary problem. VATS affords excellent visualization of the entire pleural surface, biopsy to confirm the diagnosis, and allows effective talc insufflation to be performed for sclerotherapy of malignant effusions.

BIBLIOGRAPHY

Esophageal Disorders and Carcinoma

DeVault KR. Current management of gastroesophageal reflux disease. *Gastroenterologist* 1996;4:24–32.

Marks RD, Shukla M. Diagnosis and management of peptic esophageal strictures. *Gastroenterologist* 1996;4:223–237.

Natsugoe S, Yoshinaka H, Morinaga T, et al. Ultrasonographic detection of lymph-node metastases in superficial carcinoma of the esophagus. *Endoscopy* 1996;28:674–679.

Naunheim KS, Landreneau RJ, Andrus CH, Ferson PF, Zachary PE, Keenan RJ. Laparoscopic fundoplication: a natural extension for the thoracic surgeon. *Ann Thorac Surg* 1996;61:1062–1065.

Pera M, Deschamps C, Taillefer R, Duranceau A. Uncut Collis-Nissen gastroplasty: early functional results. *Ann Thorac Surg* 1995;60:915–920.

Wehrmann T, Jacobi V, Jung M, Lembcke B, Caspary WF. Pneumatic dilation in achalasia with a low-compliance balloon: results of a 5-year prospective evaluation. *Gastrointest Endosc* 1995;42:31–36.

Thoracic Outlet Syndrome

MacKinnon SE, Novak CB. Evaluation of the patient with thoracic outlet syndrome. *Semin Thorac Cardiovasc Surg* 1996;8:190–200.

Novak CB, Collins ED, MacKinnon SE. 1995. Outcome following conservative management of thoracic outlet syndrome. *J Hand Surg [Am]* 1995;20:542–548.

Urschel HC Jr. The transaxillary approach for treatment of thoracic outlet syndrome. *Semin Thorac Cardiovasc Surg* 1996;8:214–220.

Urschel HC Jr, Razzuk MA. Upper plexus thoracic outlet syndrome: optimal therapy. *Ann Thorac Surg* 1997;63:935–939.

Massive Hemoptysis

Cahill BC, Ingbar DH. Massive hemoptysis. Assessment and management. *Clin Chest Med* 1994;15:147–167.

Kato R, Sawafuji M, Kawamura M, Kikuchi K, Kobayashi K. Massive hemoptysis successfully treated by modified bronchoscopic balloon tamponade technique. *Chest* 1996;109:842–843.

Ramakantan R, Bandekar VG, Gandhi MS, Aulakh BG, Deshmukh HL. Massive hemoptysis due to pulmonary tuberculosis: control with bronchial artery embolization. *Radiology* 1996;200:691–694.

Solitary Pulmonary Nodule

Mack MJ, Hazelrigg SR, Landreneau RJ, Acuff TE. Thoracoscopy for the diagnosis of the indeterminate solitary pulmonary nodule. *Ann Thorac Surg* 1993;56:825–830.

Midthun DE, Swensen SJ, Jett JR. Approach to the solitary pulmonary nodule. *Mayo Clin Proc* 1993;68:378–385.

Primary Chest Wall Tumor

Ayabe H, Tagawa Y, Hara S, et al. Resection and reconstruction of full thickness chest wall. *Jap J Thorac Surg* 1996;49:21–25.

Kao CC, Rand RP, Stridde BC, Marchioro TL. Techniques in the composite reconstruction of extensive thoracoabdominal tumor resections. *J Am Coll Surg* 1995;180:146–149.

Schwarz RE, Burt M. Radiation-associated malignant tumors of the chest wall. *Ann Surg Oncol* 1996;3: 387–392.

Lung Abscess

Wiedemann HP, Rice TW. Lung abscesses and empyema. *Semin Thorac Cardiovasc Surg* 1995;7: 119–128.

Lung Cancer

Darling CE. Staging of the patient with small cell lung cancer. *Chest Surg Clin North Am* 1997;7:81–94.
Edelman MJ, Gandara DR, Roach M III, Benfield JR. Multimodality therapy in stage III non–small cell lung cancer. *Ann Thorac Surg* 1996;61:1564–1572.
Govindan R, Ihde DC. Practical issues in the management of the patients with small cell lung cancer. *Chest Surg Clin North Am* 1997;7:167–181.
Shepard FA. The role of chemotherapy in the treatment of small cell lung cancer. *Chest Surg Clin North Am* 1997;7:113–133.
Urschel JD. Surgical treatment of peripheral small cell lung cancer. *Chest Surg Clin North Am* 1997;7: 95–103.

Malignant Pleural Effusion

Fenton KN, Richardson JD. Diagnosis and management of malignant pleural effusions. *Am J Surg* 1995; 170:69–74.
Waller DA, Morritt GN, Forty J. Video-assisted thoracoscopic pleurectomy in the management of malignant pleural effusion. *Chest* 1995;107:1454–1456.
Yim AP, Chan AT, Lee TW, Wan IY, Ho JK. Thoracoscopic talc insufflation versus talc slurry for symptomatic malignant pleural effusion. *Ann Thorac Surg* 1996;62:1655–1658.
Yim AP, Chung SS, Lee TW, Lam CK, Ho JK. Thoracoscopic management of malignant pleural effusion. *Chest* 1996;109:1234–1238.

Telemedicine: Practicing in the Information Age,
edited by Steven F. Viegas and Kim Dunn.
Lippincott–Raven Publishers, Philadelphia © 1998.

51

Epilogue

Steven F. Viegas and Kim Dunn

Departments of Orthopaedics and Rehabilitation, Anatomy and Neurosciences, and Preventive Medicine and Community Health, University of Texas Medical Branch at Galveston, Galveston, Texas 77555; and Department of Internal Medicine, Texas Department of Criminal Justice, University of Texas Medical Branch at Galveston, Galveston, Texas 77555

Over the time since the writing of this book began, the technology and network options available for use in the University of Texas Medical Branch (UTMB) at Galveston and Texas Department of Criminal Justice (TDCJ) telemedicine program have changed significantly. It appears that these changes will continue at an even faster rate; however, several things appear to be unchanged. These are that telemedical technology and some type or combination of network capabilities will be increasingly integrated into routine healthcare delivery.

An observation on the change in technology is that desktop technology has continually improved in its resolution and speed of transmission capabilities, making it more comparable to full-size room units. Both in the experience of developing the UTMB/TDCJ telemedicine program and in the lessons learned in the expansion of the telephone and the cellular networks, the importance of ease of access and availability to communicate have proven to be of critical importance for the expansion of a program. We believe that this translates into a future expansion that will include many more telemedicine access sites or workstations that go where the healthcare provider is located.

In light of the expectation that technology and networks will change dramatically, one may understandably ask, "Why purchase or lease technology now?" First, our belief is that telemedicine technology will be integrated into your healthcare delivery system and it should not be a stand-alone program or separate from routine healthcare delivery patterns. If it makes sense to integrate telemedicine technology into one's healthcare delivery program, it should be done in such a way as to facilitate and allow the particular healthcare providers who are using the technology to practice sound medical assessment and treatment of the patient population. If you think about how much the way medicine is practiced has changed in the past 1, 5, or even 10 years, you will realize that the answer is actually very little. If this is true, a telemedicine program you build with today's technology, if it addresses the needs of the healthcare provider today, will most likely address the needs tomorrow, because those needs do not change that quickly.

Another reason for entering into the practice of telemedicine now is that the sooner one becomes involved in the practice of telemedicine, the faster one becomes experienced with the application and approach of delivering healthcare through a telemedicine network. Some practitioners ask for or prefer to have a protocol in place to outline the patients who are optimal for telemedicine and the treatment guidelines that should be used and followed to diagnose and treat those patients. On the other hand, this is not the usual request or case in an actual practice situation, and therefore some prefer to "just do it." Whether the healthcare provider has the "just do it" approach or wishes to have a clearly outlined protocol or set of guidelines for his or her entry into telemedicine, it is of critical importance to have, as your vanguard, champions of telemedicine. "Champions" are individuals who are willing to work constructively through the typical foibles of new programs and technologies to improve the efficiency, quality, and organization of the program. At UTMB, the program has been blessed with a long list of such champions, many of whom are listed as authors in this book and many more who have been just as instrumental in the success of the telemedicine and distance education programs who are not listed.

As telemedicine becomes a part of the healthcare provider's mindset, it begins to be included in the list of possible solutions for various problems and possible opportunities for tomorrow. Telemedicine will be an integral part of the future of medicine, and it is already affecting a reengineering of healthcare.

Subject Index